T0093937

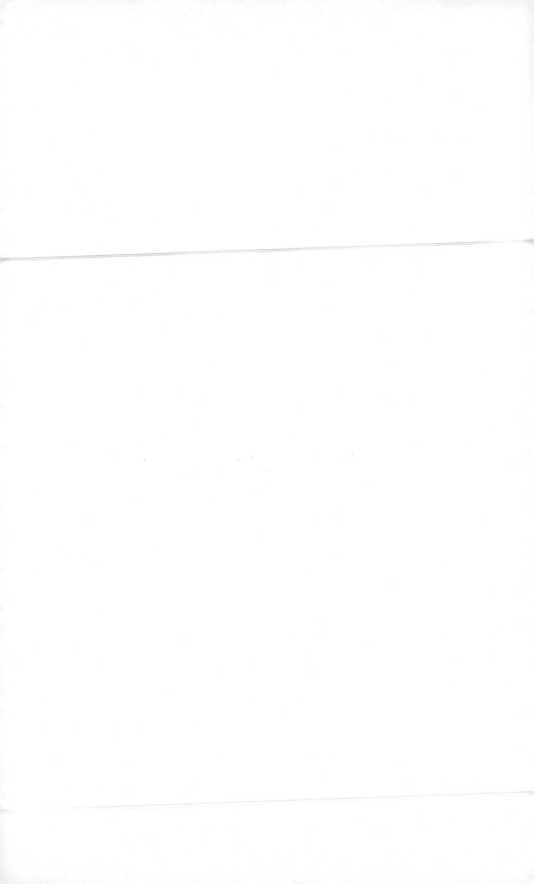

Exertional Heat Illness

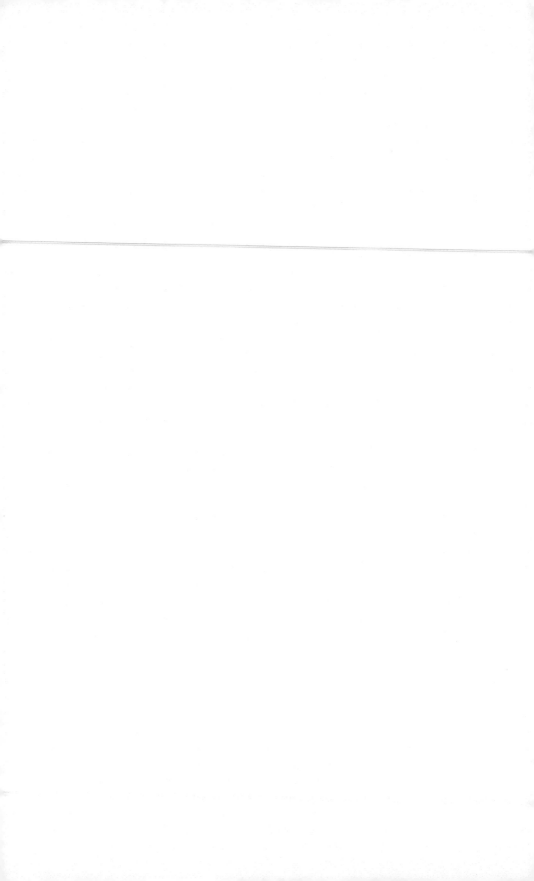

William M. Adams • John F. Jardine
Editors

Exertional Heat Illness

A Clinical and Evidence-Based Guide

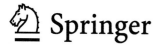
Springer

Editors
William M. Adams
Department of Kinesiology
University of North Carolina at Greensboro
Greensboro, NC
USA

John F. Jardine
Korey Stringer Institute
University of Connecticut
Storrs, CT
USA

ISBN 978-3-030-27804-5   ISBN 978-3-030-27805-2   (eBook)
https://doi.org/10.1007/978-3-030-27805-2

This Springer imprint is published by the registered company Springer Nature Switzerland AG
The registered company address is: Gewerbestrasse 11, 6330 Cham, Switzerland

Preface

The idea for this book arose from collaborative work and many conversations that we have had with friends and colleagues who share an interest on the topic of exertional heat illness. Having a resource such as this available for clinicians and scientists is essential for disseminating the knowledge necessary to enhance the health and safety of the physically active—first, to provide them with a current and comprehensive overview of the prevention, recognition, treatment, and care of the various medical conditions that fall within the realm of exertional heat illness, and second, to provide a setting-specific (i.e., athletics, military, occupational, and road race medicine) discussion on exertional heat illness for the consideration of the medical providers working in these settings.

As medicine has evolved, and as it will continue to evolve, we have and will continue to garner new knowledge on how to reduce the risk of mortality and morbidity from a variety of pathologies afflicting the world's population. Exertional heat illness is unique in that it can appear in generally healthy and physically active individuals. The most severe form, exertional heat stroke, is life-threatening and requires immediate triage and care to optimize survival. What is fascinating about the topic of exertional heat illness, particularly exertional heat stroke, are the vast historical accounts of this condition, some dating back to the Roman Empire, that in some instances have shaped the course of history. As clinicians and scientists have begun to pursue the various facets of exertional heat illness, we have gained a deeper understanding of the etiology and pathophysiology involved, the complexities of which continue to steer the path for future research.

While we as clinicians and scientists have a better understanding of how to reduce risk, but more importantly, to ensure survival from exertional heat stroke, we are continually plagued with news from mass media surrounding young, seemingly healthy and fit individuals (i.e., athletes, laborers, and soldiers) dying from this survivable condition. The recent deaths of athletes Jordan McNair from the University of Maryland; Braeden Bradforth from Garden City Community College, Garden City, Kansas; Zach Polsenberg from Riverdale High School in Fort Myers, Florida; and other notable and highly profiled cases such as Korey Stringer and Max Gilpin are just a few among many young individuals who have succumbed to a medical condition that would have been 100% survivable had the appropriate policies and procedures been in place at the time of their collapse.

We believe this book provides clinicians and scientists at all levels of training and experience a practical, yet thorough, review of exertional heat illness that can be used as a resource to guide them in their practice/research. We also hope that this text can act as a conduit for medical providers from various fields of medicine (athletic training, emergency medical services, emergency room physicians, sports medicine and primary care physicians, etc.) who may encounter exertional heat illness to work closely together to guarantee that current evidence-based practices for the appropriate management and care of exertional heat illness are consistent and seamless throughout healthcare.

Greensboro, NC, USA   William M. Adams, PhD, LAT, ATC
Storrs, CT, USA   John F. Jardine, MD

Acknowledgments

William M. Adams would like to acknowledge the following individuals:

- First, and foremost, to all of the authors who contributed to the writing of this book. It is through their expertise on exertional heat illness as clinicians and scientists that this book was possible.
- Dr. John Jardine, a great friend and colleague, for his efforts and insights as coeditor for this book. His roles as an emergency department physician and medical director of the Falmouth Road Race—the latter being where he has helped treat >350 patients with exertional heat stroke—are a true testament to his dedication in ensuring that the health and safety of these athletes is prioritized.
- Dr. Douglas Casa for his mentorship and the many opportunities he provided to assist in making a positive and lifelong impact for the health and safety of athletes, soldiers, and laborers. His passion on topics related to exertional heat illness and preventing sudden death in sports and physical activity is contagious and has been an inspiration for me as I continue my career as a researcher in this field. Having Dr. Casa as a friend and colleague is truly an honor.
- Ms. Katherine Kreilkamp for her tireless efforts in making this book the product that it is. It was a pleasure working with her, and I hope to have the chance again in the future.
- Springer for seeing the value of this book as a clinical and evidence-based guide on this topic, which is an ever-present concern for physically active populations.

John F. Jardine would like to acknowledge the following individuals:

- Dr. William Adams for including me in this project. I felt that a clinical guide based on the science and evidence of prominent researchers would be most helpful to fellow clinicians to better understand this group of illnesses. Dr. Adams is a bright scientist and researcher in this field. This has been his brainchild, and I am honored to work with this talented colleague and friend.
- Dr. Douglas Casa and his staff at Korey Stringer Institute (KSI) for their dedication to the health and safety of athletes, laborers, and military personnel, with

contagious passion for the science, and for their collaborations and friendship. Understanding the science of heat illness, its treatment, and prevention has provided a special enthusiasm in my emergency medicine career.

- Board of Directors and staff at the Falmouth Road Race, for providing the platform upon which to build my career. Their support for me and our research at KSI has been incredible. Their dedication to their athletes' safety has transcended their race and become a standard against which to measure other events.

Contents

Editors

William M. Adams, PhD, LAT, ATC Department of Kinesiology, University of North Carolina at Greensboro, Greensboro, NC, USA

John F. Jardine, MD Korey Stringer Institute, Department of Kinesiology, University of Connecticut, Storrs, CT, USA

Contributors

Lawrence E. Armstrong, PhD Hydration & Nutrition, LLC, Newport News, VA, USA

Department of Kinesiology (Professor Emeritus), University of Connecticut, Storrs, CT, USA

Luke N. Belval, MS, ATC, CSCS Korey Stringer Institute, Department of Kinesiology, University of Connecticut, Storrs, CT, USA

Jacob S. Bowie, BS Human Performance Laboratory, Department of Kinesiology, University of Connecticut, Storrs, CT, USA

Department of Kinesiology, University of Connecticut, Storrs, CT, USA

Douglas J. Casa, PhD, ATC Korey Stringer Institute, Department of Kinesiology, University of Connecticut, Storrs, CT, USA

Aidan P. Fiol, BS Human Performance Laboratory, Department of Kinesiology, University of Connecticut, Storrs, CT, USA

Department of Kinesiology, University of Connecticut, Storrs, CT, USA

Andreas D. Flouris, PhD FAME Laboratory, Department of Exercise Science, University of Thessaly, Karies, Trikala, Greece

Gabrielle E. W. Giersch, MSc Korey Stringer Institute, Department of Kinesiology, University of Connecticut, Storrs, CT, USA

Andrew Grundstein, PhD Department of Geography, University of Georgia, Athens, GA, USA

Yuri Hosokawa, PhD, ATC Faculty of Sport Sciences, Waseda University, Tokorozawa, Saitama, Japan

Robert A. Huggins, PhD, ATC Human Performance Laboratory, Department of Kinesiology, University of Connecticut, Storrs, CT, USA

Department of Kinesiology, University of Connecticut, Storrs, CT, USA

Korey Stringer Institute, Department of Kinesiology, University of Connecticut, Storrs, CT, USA

Glen P. Kenny, PhD Human and Environmental Physiology Research Unit, School of Human Kinetics, University of Ottawa, Ottawa, ON, Canada

Elaine C. Lee, PhD Human Performance Laboratory, Department of Kinesiology, University of Connecticut, Storrs, CT, USA

Department of Kinesiology, University of Connecticut, Storrs, CT, USA

Rebecca M. Lopez, PhD, ATC, CSCS Athletic Training Post-Professional Program, Department of Orthopaedics & Sports Medicine, University of South Florida, Tampa, FL, USA

Kevin C. Miller, PhD, AT, ATC School of Rehabilitation and Medical Sciences, Central Michigan University, Mount Pleasant, MI, USA

Margaret C. Morrissey, MS Korey Stringer Institute, Department of Kinesiology, University of Connecticut, Storrs, CT, USA

Sean R. Notley, PhD Human and Environmental Physiology Research Unit, School of Human Kinetics, University of Ottawa, Ottawa, ON, Canada

Nathaniel S. Nye, MD, Maj, USAF, MC Sports Medicine Clinic, 559th Medical Group, Joint Base San Antonio-Lackland, TX, USA

Francis G. O'Connor, COL (ret.), MC, USA, MD, MPH Military and Emergency Medicine, Consortium for Health and Military Performance, Uniformed Services University of the Health Sciences, Bethesda, MD, USA

Julien D. Périard, PhD, MA, BEd, BSc Research Institute for Sport and Exercise, University of Canberra, Bruce, ACT, Australia

J. Luke Pryor, PhD, ATC, CSCS Exercise and Nutrition Sciences, University at Buffalo, Buffalo, NY, USA

Riana R. Pryor, PhD, ATC Exercise and Nutrition Sciences, University at Buffalo, Buffalo, NY, USA

William O. Roberts, MD, MS Sports Medicine Program, Department of Family Medicine and Community Health, University of Minnesota, Minneapolis, MN, USA

Rebecca L. Stearns, PhD, ATC Korey Stringer Institute, Department of Kinesiology, University of Connecticut, Storrs, CT, USA

Chapter 1
Overview of Exertional Heat Illness

William M. Adams and John F. Jardine

Exertional heat illness (EHI) has been documented for centuries, dating back more than 2000 years during the time of the Roman Empire and the military conquests that transpired [1]. Throughout history, EHI has continued to be chronicled in military [2–13], occupational [14–21], and athletic [22–26] settings, particularly in situations where individuals are performing strenuous exercise in hot environments. EHI describes a collective of specific medical conditions that are related to the effects of exertion-related heat illness that varies in severity and includes conditions such as heat exhaustion, heat syncope, and heat stroke, the latter being a medical emergency capable of causing death if not properly treated.

In military settings, it has been well documented that soldiers are at risk of EHI during both times of war [2, 27] and peacetime [2, 27, 28], with the latter being more prevalent during training in the summer months [28] and of greater incidence among recruits/trainees versus seasoned enlistees and officers [2, 27]. Occupational work, particularly in agricultural [16, 29–32], forestry [29, 33], mining [34–36], and construction sectors [18, 37, 38], predisposes workers to an increased risk of EHI due to a combination of the environment (i.e., high ambient temperatures, high relative humidity, high solar loads, etc.) and other known risk factors afflicting this specific population. EHI in athletic settings is most common in American football and running events [22, 26, 39–43] due to (1) time of year in which these events are held (i.e., typically during warmer times of the year), (2) protective equipment that must be worn to participate in American football, (3) intensity and duration of the exercise that is performed, and (4) body size of the individual. However, the risk of

W. M. Adams (✉)
Department of Kinesiology, University of North Carolina at Greensboro, Greensboro, NC, USA
e-mail: wmadams@uncg.edu

J. F. Jardine
Korey Stringer Institute, University of Connecticut, Storrs, CT, USA

EHI in other sports must not be discounted due to the multifaceted etiologies of these conditions.

Given the complexities surrounding EHI relating to the etiologies of the various conditions and the diverse settings in which they occur, the purpose of this chapter is to provide an overview of the classification, nomenclature, and incidence of EHI and the specific conditions covered throughout this text. Gaining a better understanding of how these illnesses are classified and the incidence of these illnesses in military, athletic, and occupational settings will allow the reader to make appropriate, evidence-based decisions regarding the prevention, recognition, management, and care of EHIs.

Classification and Nomenclature

Prior to providing a thorough overview of the pathophysiology, etiology, and clinical management of the various EHIs, one must acknowledge the classification and nomenclature of the specific disorders that are encompassed within this broader term. To allow for uniformity, the World Health Organization has developed and published standards for classifying medical conditions; the International Classification of Diseases (ICD) serves as the source of this standardized method of reporting [44]. The medical disorders involving environmental heat, originally classified by the Medical Research Council's Climatic Physiology Committee of the United Kingdom and the US National Research Council's Subcommittee on Thermal Factors in the Environment in 1957 [45], are coded under T67 Effects of Heat and Light in the current 10th Revision of the ICD Clinical Modification document (ICD-10-CM). Within the T67 code of the ICD-10-CM, there are 10 subcategories that specify the individual heat-related disorders (Table 1.1) [44], which are universally applied when determining a clinical diagnosis.

While ICD-10-CM serves as the universal means of classifying medical conditions, some entities further classify heat-related illnesses for purposes of reporting and calculating incidence rates. For example, within the US Military, only hospitalizations, outpatient medical encounters, or records of reportable medical events with a primary or secondary diagnosis of the medical conditions that are considered heat illnesses (heat stroke [T67.0] and heat exhaustion [T67.3–5]) are classified as such [46]. The other taxonomies within code T67 do not qualify in the case definition of heat illnesses in this particular setting. Furthermore, issues related to the interpretability of the relevant ICD codes and/ or correctly classifying heat-related illnesses to the appropriate ICD code exist, particularly when attempting to discern between the various etiologies of heat exhaustion (T67.3–T67.5) or between heat stroke and heat exhaustion in a field-based setting [47, 48].

Table 1.1 Medical disorders involving environmental heat

ICD-10-CM code	ICD-10 category	Etiology	Signs and symptoms
T67.0	Heat stroke and sunstroke	Failure of body to dissipate heat	CNS dysfunction (e.g., irritability, confusion, coma, aggressive behavior) Extreme hyperthermia (>40.0 °C)
T67.1	Heat syncope	Circulatory instability	Fainting episode due to a reduction in central venous return
T67.2	Heat cramp (exercise-associated muscle cramp)	Water and electrolyte imbalance	Painful, involuntary muscle contractions
T67.3	Anhydrotic heat exhaustion (includes prostration due to water depletion)	Water and electrolyte imbalance	Nausea, anorexia, fatigue/weakness, tachycardia, loss of concentration, prominent sensation of thirst, decreased urine output Body temperature typically <40.0 °C
T67.4	Salt depletion heat exhaustion	Water and electrolyte imbalance	Nausea, anorexia, fatigue/weakness, tachycardia, loss of concentration, hemoconcentration, muscle cramps, vomiting Body temperature typically <40.0 °C
T67.5	Unspecified heat exhaustion	Unspecified causes: physical exertion (diagnosis of exclusion)	Nausea, anorexia, fatigue/weakness, tachycardia, loss of concentration, dizziness, confusion, pallor, profuse sweating, minimal CNS disturbances Body temperature typically <40.0 °C
T67.6	Transient heat fatigue	Psychological causes	Extreme tiredness, reluctance to perform physical work, deterioration of skilled performance in the absence of water and/or salt depletion
T67.7	Heat edema	Water and electrolyte imbalance	Pooling of fluid in interstitial spaces causes swelling in the extremities
T67.8	Other heat and light effects	Various causes	Signs and symptoms NOS
T67.9	Unspecified heat and light effects	Various causes	Signs and symptoms NOS

ICD-10-CM 10th revision of the international classification of diseases, *CNS* central nervous system, *NOS* not otherwise specified
CNS central nervous system, *NOS* not otherwise specified

Specific to heat stroke, it is classified by ICD-10-CM code T67.0. Heat stroke can be classified as either classic heat stroke (CHS), which typically occurs in the elderly or infants during times of excessive heat (e.g., heat waves), or exertional heat stroke (EHS) which is caused by the inability to dissipate metabolically produced body heat during physical activity. Although CHS and EHS demonstrate differing etiologies, they are classified under the same universal coding, which makes it difficult to distinguish in large-scale epidemiological data [49].

Epidemiology

To further understand the impact of EHI in a given population, acknowledging over-all and condition-specific epidemiological data is necessary. Examining emergency department (ED) data for treatment of heat illness in the United States shows that the annual incidence rate for heat illness is between 21.5 and 31.19 per 100,000 person-years and incidence rate for heat stroke is 1.34 per 100,000 person-years [21, 50–52]. These data also show that the incidence of heat illness and heat stroke is more likely to occur in men, during the summer months or during times of anomalously high temperatures for a given time of the year, and as age increases [21, 50–54].

Given that the aforementioned data reports cases across the lifespan, one must take into consideration the data points involving young children or elderly individuals. While these populations are at risk for heat illness, the injury insult is typically due to physiologic (e.g., incomplete development of thermoregulatory body systems in young children, decline in thermoregulatory capacity and/or presence of contributing comorbidities in the elderly) or external causes (e.g., no access to air conditioning or domiciles providing relief to extreme heat) that are exacerbated to exposure to extreme heat typically seen during heat waves [55–58] rather than physical exertion. When re-examining ED data on incidence of heat illness in age groups 15–34 and 35–64, ages that are most likely associated with recreational physical activity and/or occupational work, incidence rates increase to 41.8 and 32.8 per 100,000 person-years, respectively, with the former age group exhibiting a 39% higher incidence than the 35–64 age group [51]. This trend holds true when examining heat stroke incidence, in that of the 8,251 heat strokes treated in EDs in the United States from 2000 to 2010, 54% occurred in ages 20–59, which is typically more associated with recreational and occupational activities [21].

Heat Illness in Military Settings

EHI risk has been extensively studied within military operations due to the extent in which these injuries can affect the outcomes related to the preparation/training of warfighters and mission success during times of war. Research dating back to the late nineteenth century and early twentieth century began to characterize the factors responsible for the onset of EHI [4]. During World War I, while fighting in Mesopotamia, Macedonia, and South West Africa, British soldiers experienced heat-related hospital admissions rates of 0.1–77.39 per 1000 personnel, with the warmer summer months experiencing a larger rise of heat-related incidents [4]. Similar trends were also seen during World War II; higher incidence of heat illness occurring during hotter times of the calendar year and/or in geographical locations exposing the warfighters to thermal stress [4]. Following World War II,

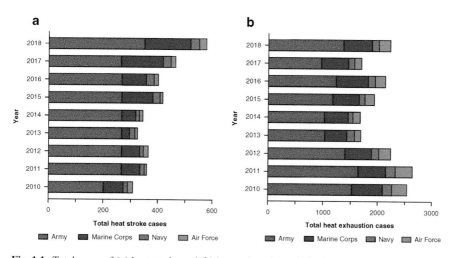

Fig. 1.1 Total cases of (**a**) heat stroke and (**b**) heat exhaustion within the separate branches of the US Armed Forces [27, 61–67]

the US Armed Forces still exhibited increased rates of EHI; this was most notably due to the expanded reach of the US Armed Forces around the world and the increased numbers of individuals going through basic training [5]. While the incidence rates for heat exhaustion and heat stroke varied between 16.0–56.8 and 1.5–9.1 per 100,000 per year, the advancements in the development of environmental-based activity modifications greatly reduced the incidence of training-related EHI [5].

As research into the epidemiology of EHI in military settings has expanded [2, 3, 8, 27, 48, 59–67], we have a better understanding of where, and to what extent these EHI events are occurring. Similar to what was seen during both World Wars, incidence rates for EHI are higher during hotter periods of the year and/or at geographical locations exhibiting more extreme environmental conditions [2, 3, 8, 27, 59, 61–67]. These data also suggest variations in total EHI cases and incidence based on branch of service (Fig. 1.1), enlistment status (Fig. 1.2), and gender (Fig. 1.3). While the total number of EHI events is lower in recruits (i.e., military personnel pursuing basic training and initial stages of training upon enlistment), the overall incidence is much greater when compared to the other enlistment groups. While this may be due to a number of factors, the geographical locations of basic training in the United States and physical demands of training may be greater contributors of EHI events in these specific populations. Other considerations on risk of EHI in military populations pertain to the overall fitness of military personnel, particularly in new recruits, where data shows an increased risk of EHI in individuals that are overweight and less cardiovascular fit than their more fit, less overweight counterparts [10, 68].

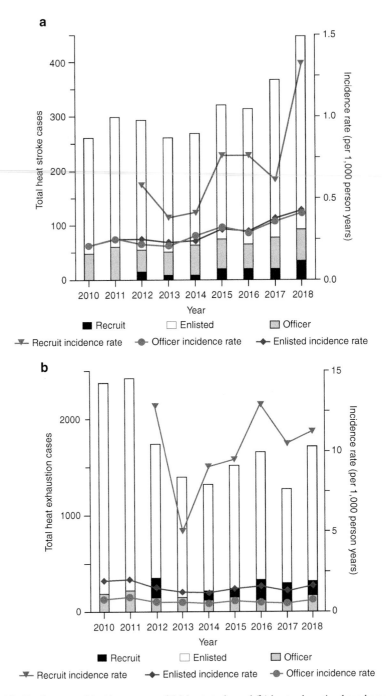

Fig. 1.2 Total cases and incidence rates of (**a**) heat stroke and (**b**) heat exhaustion based on enlistment status in the US Armed Forces. Recruit, which was not tracked until 2012, is defined as enlistee during the initial stages of training/preparation [E1–E4) [27, 61–67]

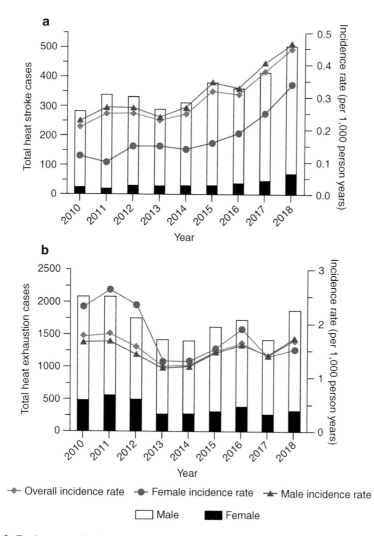

Fig. 1.3 Total cases and incidence rates of (**a**) heat stroke and (**b**) heat exhaustion between male and female enlisted members of the US Armed Forces [27, 61–67]

Heat Illness in Athletic Settings

Within the athletics setting, the risk of EHI is typically present in situations where athletes are performing intense exercise in hot environmental conditions or required to wear protective equipment as part of their sport's uniform. Sports such as American football, field hockey (particularly the goalie), and running events are sports where there is greatest risk. Within the United States, of the 54,983 EHIs treated in EDs from 1997 to 2006, 41,538 (75.5%) were sport related, with American football and recreational exercise (e.g., running) being the most common types of activity involved with EHI in men and women within the ≤19 and 20–39 age groups [52].

In-depth analyses of the incidence of EHI within secondary school and collegiate athletics have yielded a greater insight into where risk is greatest. Work by Kerr et al. [22] and Yard et al. [43] have shown the variability in EHI risk among secondary school athletics, with American football and girls' field hockey having the highest incidence rate (Fig. 1.4) [69]. This can be largely attributed to the time of year in which these sports begin (i.e., the later summer to early fall within the Northern Hemisphere) and the protective equipment worn by those participating; in girls' field hockey, only the goalie position wears protective equipment.

Recent work by Kerr et al. [23] expands on this previous work showing that American football and girls' field hockey remain the sports with highest risk of EHI among secondary school athletics. In addition, girls' cross-country also exhibited EHI incidence rates that are more than two times greater than all other secondary school sports aside from American football and field hockey [23]. Moreover, girls' (incidence rate [IR], 1.18 per 10,000 athlete exposures [AEs]) and boys' (0.52 per 10,000 AEs) cross-country and American football (0.61 per 10,000 AEs) EHI incidence rates are largest in competition than all other secondary school sports [23].

Risk of EHI within collegiate athletics exhibits similar trends of that observed within secondary school athletics. American football and men and women's

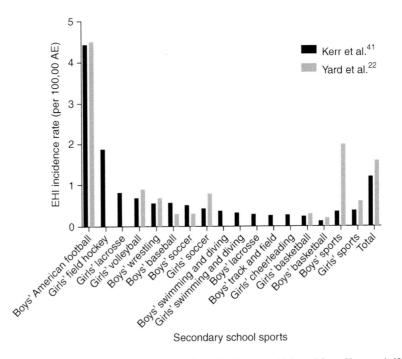

Fig. 1.4 EHS fatality incidence rates in secondary school sports. (Adapted from Kerr et al. [22] and Yard et al. [43]). (From Adams [69], with permission)

cross-country have higher overall EHI incidence rates (1.55, 0.48, 0.35 per 10,000 AEs, respectively) with men and women's cross-country having the largest EHI incidence rates during competition (4.01 and 3.69 per 10,000 AEs, respectively) [70] (Fig. 1.5). Most EHIs occurred during practices (72.8%) and during the pre-season (64.7%) portion of a sport's competitive seasons, with preseason practices having an EHI rate of 1.16 per 10,000 AEs compared with an EHI rate of 0.23 per 10,000 AEs during all other times of the season [70]. Furthermore, EHI rates were 2–4 times greater in warmer climates (1.05 per 10,000 AEs) than those of temperate (0.43 per 10,000 AEs) or cooler (0.26 per 10,000 AEs) climates [70].

American football is of particular concern for EHI given the construct of the sport; the sport requires individuals to don protective equipment covering roughly 75% of their body surface area, which is known to reduce the ability to dissipate body heat [71]. In addition, training for the competitive season begins in the late summer and early fall within the Northern Hemisphere and includes individuals of varying body size (i.e., amount of lean mass and fat mass), which may predispose the larger athletes to increased risk [25]. Over a 30-year period (1980–2009), there were 58 documented EHS-related deaths among American football athletes in the United States with a majority of these deaths involving athletes participating in this

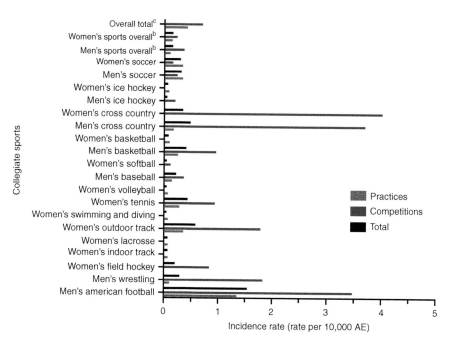

Fig. 1.5 Exertional heat illness incidence rates among National Collegiate Athletic Association sports from 2009 to 2010 through 2014 to 2015. [b]Only sex-comparable sports (baseball/softball, basketball, cross-country, ice hockey, indoor track, lacrosse, outdoor track, soccer, swimming and diving, tennis). [c]Exertional heat illnesses were not reported in women's gymnastics and men's indoor track, lacrosse, outdoor track, swimming and diving, and tennis [70]

sport in the southeastern portion of the United States (Fig. 1.6) where they were exposed to more extreme environmental conditions [25]. Data [72] support that there is an average of roughly three American football players that die each year due to EHS. Examining EHS-related American football deaths in 5-year blocks dating back to 1975, a greater number of annual deaths are occurring as time progresses (Fig. 1.7), which is particularly alarming given the advancements made in science and medicine surrounding the prevention, recognition, and treatment of EHS to optimize survivability.

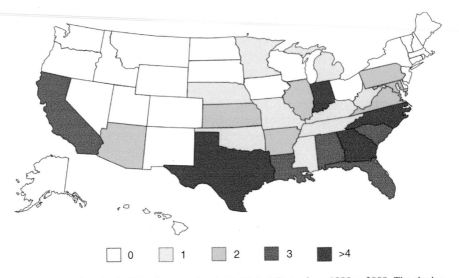

Fig. 1.6 American football deaths occurring in the United States from 1980 to 2009. The shades of color depict the total number of EHS deaths during the reported timeframe [25]

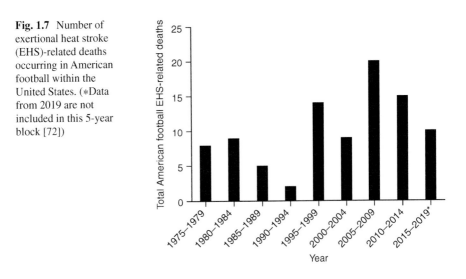

Fig. 1.7 Number of exertional heat stroke (EHS)-related deaths occurring in American football within the United States. (*Data from 2019 are not included in this 5-year block [72])

Aside from organized athletics, participation in recreational activities such as road running races of distances of 10–42 km [42, 73–78], cycling [79], and triathlon [80–82] events brings risk of EHI, particularly when events are held during warmer times of the year. The Falmouth Road Race, for example, an 11.3 km road running race that takes place in August in Cape Cod, MA, USA, increases the risk for EHI due to the warm environmental conditions that runners are exposed to. Epidemiological data [26, 83] from this race show that the incidence of EHS and heat exhaustion is 2.12–2.13 and 0.98 per 1000 finishers, respectively. Furthermore, as environmental conditions on race day become more extreme, the overall rate of EHS and EHI increases [42, 83]. Given that this race is shorter in duration, only 11.3 km, runners are able to compete at a higher intensity, which increases the rate of metabolic heat production. When coupled with increasing ambient temperature and relative humidity, the ability to dissipate stored body heat is reduced, thus increasing overall risk. However, it must be acknowledged that EHI can occur in events with cooler environmental conditions [84–86] and can be due to a number of factors including an increased exercise intensity (i.e., increased metabolic heat production) that may create an uncompensable heat load within the body [87].

Heat Illness in Occupational Settings

Exposure to excessive heat has raised concern of increased risk among occupational workers; prior literature has discussed the risks of EHI in occupations such as mining [34], agricultural [29, 30], firefighting [88–91], and construction [18, 37, 38]. In linking heat stress to EHI risk in occupational workers, a contextual understanding of the various factors (e.g., climate change, geographical locations, sociocultural factors, physical exertion, protective clothing, etc.) contributing to increased risk must be considered [92]. Current literature suggests that EHI incidence rates in occupational settings have been shown to be roughly 1.6–1.7 per 1,000,000 full-time equivalents [93] and the incidence rate for heat-related morality is approximately 0.22 per 1,000,000 workers.

While these numbers provide context into the extent of heat-related injuries occurring in the workforce, incidence rates of EHI vary across specific occupations. However, there are similar trends among published literature. EHI risk was greatest in younger men with shorter employment records during the summer months (June–August in the Northern Hemisphere) [14, 15, 17, 20, 30, 31, 34, 93–98]. Fortune et al. [93] found that men were 2.2 times more likely to succumb to EHI than women, while Gubernot et al. [20] found that men succumbed to heat-related death at a rate of 5.7 times greater than women. Furthermore, the months of June, July, and August exhibited greater incidence rates of EHI (4.2, 5.5, and 5.8 per 1,000,000 full-time equivalents) than all other months of the year [93].

Summary

Exertional heat illness, while rare in occurrence relative to the population as a whole, can be of considerable concern in athletes, soldiers, and laborers. Identifying the specific populations/settings, situations (e.g., athletic practice/training, military basic training, summer agricultural work), and risk factors responsible for EHI will allow for the strategic development of data-informed preventive strategies to enhance safety of the individuals performing physical activity in these settings.

References

1. A Roman experience with heat stroke in 24 B.C. Bull N Y Acad Med. 1967;43(8):767–8.
2. Armed Forces Health Surveillance Branch. Update: heat illness, active component, U.S. Armed Forces, 2018. MSMR. 2019;26(4):15–20.
3. Abriat A, Brosset C, Brégigeon M, Sagui E. Report of 182 cases of exertional heatstroke in the French Armed Forces. Mil Med. 2014;179(3):309–14.
4. Bricknell MC. Heat illness—a review of military experience (part 1). J R Army Med Corps. 1995;141(3):157–66.
5. Bricknell MC. Heat illness—a review of military experience (Part 2). J R Army Med Corps. 1996;142(1):34–42.
6. Gardner JW, Gutmann FD, Potter RN, Kark JA. Nontraumatic exercise-related deaths in the U.S. military, 1996–1999. Mil Med. 2002;167(12):964–70.
7. Hakre S, Gardner JW, Kark JA, Wenger CB. Predictors of hospitalization in male Marine Corps recruits with exertional heat illness. Mil Med. 2004;169(3):169–75.
8. Stacey MJ, Parsons IT, Woods DR, Taylor PN, Ross D, Brett SJ. Susceptibility to exertional heat illness and hospitalisation risk in UK military personnel. BMJ Open Sport Exerc Med. 2015;1(1):e000055.
9. Henderson A, Simon JW, Melia WM, Navein JF, Mackay BG. Heat illness. A report of 45 cases from Hong Kong. J R Army Med Corps. 1986;132(2):76–84.
10. Bedno SA, Li Y, Han W, Cowan DN, Scott CT, Cavicchia MA, et al. Exertional heat illness among overweight U.S. Army recruits in basic training. Aviat Space Environ Med. 2010;81(2):107–11.
11. Carter R, Cheuvront SN, Williams JO, Kolka MA, Stephenson LA, Sawka MN, et al. Epidemiology of hospitalizations and deaths from heat illness in soldiers. Med Sci Sports Exerc. 2005;37(8):1338–44.
12. Epstein Y, Moran DS, Shapiro Y, Sohar E, Shemer J. Exertional heat stroke: a case series. Med Sci Sports Exerc. 1999;31(2):224–8.
13. Rav-Acha M, Hadad E, Epstein Y, Heled Y, Moran DS. Fatal exertional heat stroke: a case series. Am J Med Sci. 2004;328(2):84–7.
14. Arbury S, Lindsley M, Hodgson M. A critical review of OSHA heat enforcement cases: lessons learned. J Occup Environ Med. 2016;58(4):359–63.
15. Arbury S, Jacklitsch B, Farquah O, Hodgson M, Lamson G, Martin H, et al. Heat illness and death among workers—United States, 2012–2013. MMWR Morb Mortal Wkly Rep. 2014;63(31):661–5.
16. Arcury TA, Summers P, Talton JW, Chen H, Sandberg JC, Spears Johnson CR, et al. Heat illness among North Carolina Latino farmworkers. J Occup Environ Med. 2015;57(12):1299–304.
17. Bonauto D, Anderson R, Rauser E, Burke B. Occupational heat illness in Washington state, 1995–2005. Am J Ind Med. 2007;50(12):940–50.

18. Dutta P, Rajiva A, Andhare D, Azhar GS, Tiwari A, Sheffield P, et al. Perceived heat stress and health effects on construction workers. Indian J Occup Environ Med. 2015;19(3):151–8.
19. Fortune M, Mustard C, Brown P. The use of Bayesian inference to inform the surveillance of temperature-related occupational morbidity in Ontario, Canada, 2004–2010. Environ Res. 2014;132:449–56.
20. Gubernot DM, Anderson GB, Hunting KL. Characterizing occupational heat-related mortality in the United States, 2000–2010: an analysis using the census of fatal occupational injuries database. Am J Ind Med. 2015;58(2):203–11.
21. Wu X, Brady JE, Rosenberg H, Li G. Emergency department visits for heat stroke in the United States, 2009 and 2010. Inj Epidemiol. 2014;1(1):8.
22. Kerr ZY, Casa DJ, Marshall SW, Comstock RD. Epidemiology of exertional heat illness among U.S. high school athletes. Am J Prev Med. 2013;44(1):8–14.
23. Kerr ZY, Yeargin SW, Hosokawa Y, Hirschhorn RM, Pierpoint LA, Casa DJ. The epidemiology and management of exertional heat illnesses in high school sports during the 2012/13–2016/17 academic years. J Sport Rehabil. 2019:1–7. https://doi.org/10.1123/jsr.2018-0364. [Epub ahead of print].
24. Yeargin SW, Kerr ZY, Casa DJ, Djoko A, Hayden R, Parsons JT, et al. Epidemiology of exertional heat illnesses in youth, high school, and college football. Med Sci Sports Exerc. 2016;48(8):1523–9.
25. Grundstein AJ, Ramseyer C, Zhao F, Pesses JL, Akers P, Qureshi A, et al. A retrospective analysis of American football hyperthermia deaths in the United States. Int J Biometeorol. 2012;56(1):11–20.
26. DeMartini JK, Casa DJ, Stearns R, Belval L, Crago A, Davis R, et al. Effectiveness of cold water immersion in the treatment of exertional heat stroke at the Falmouth Road Race. Med Sci Sports Exerc. 2015;47(2):240–5.
27. Armed Forces Health Surveillance Branch. Update: heat injuries, active component, U.S. Armed Forces, 2013. MSMR. 2014;21(3):10–3.
28. Barnes SR, Ambrose JF, Maule AL, Kebisek J, McCabe AA, Scatliffe K, et al. Incidence, timing, and seasonal patterns of heat illnesses during U.S. Army basic combat training, 2014–2018. MSMR. 2019;26(4):7–14.
29. Spector JT, Krenz J, Rauser E, Bonauto DK. Heat-related illness in Washington State agriculture and forestry sectors. Am J Ind Med. 2014;57(8):881–95.
30. Spector JT, Bonauto DK, Sheppard L, Busch-Isaksen T, Calkins M, Adams D, et al. A case-crossover study of heat exposure and injury risk in outdoor agricultural workers. PLoS One. 2016;11(10):e0164498.
31. Fuhrmann CM, Sugg MM, Ii CEK, Waller A. Impact of extreme heat events on emergency department visits in North Carolina (2007–2011). J Community Health. 2016;41(1):146–56.
32. Mirabelli MC, Quandt SA, Crain R, Grzywacz JG, Robinson EN, Vallejos QM, et al. Symptoms of heat illness among Latino farm workers in North Carolina. Am J Prev Med. 2010;39(5):468–71.
33. Biggs C, Paterson M, Maunder E. Hydration status of South African forestry workers harvesting trees in autumn and winter. Ann Occup Hyg. 2011;55(1):6–15.
34. Donoghue AM. Heat illness in the U.S. mining industry. Am J Ind Med. 2004;45(4):351–6.
35. Lambert GP. Intestinal barrier dysfunction, endotoxemia, and gastrointestinal symptoms: the "canary in the coal mine" during exercise-heat stress? Med Sport Sci. 2008;53:61–73.
36. Meshi EB, Kishinhi SS, Mamuya SH, Rusibamayila MG. Thermal exposure and heat illness symptoms among workers in Mara Gold Mine. Tanzania Ann Glob Health. 2018;84(3):360–8.
37. Acharya P, Boggess B, Zhang K. Assessing heat stress and health among construction workers in a changing climate: a review. Int J Environ Res Public Health. 2018;15(2) https://doi.org/10.3390/ijerph15020247.
38. El-Shafei DA, Bolbol SA, Awad Allah MB, Abdelsalam AE. Exertional heat illness: knowledge and behavior among construction workers. Environ Sci Pollut Res Int. 2018;25(32):32269–76.

39. Lyle DM, Lewis PR, Richards DA, Richards R, Bauman AE, Sutton JR, et al. Heat exhaustion in the Sun-Herald City to Surf fun run. Med J Aust. 1994;161(6):361–5.
40. Richards D, Richards R, Schofield PJ, Ross V, Sutton JR. Management of heat exhaustion in Sydney's the Sun City-to-Surf run runners. Med J Aust. 1979;2(9):457–61.
41. Brodeur VB, Dennett SR, Griffin LS. Exertional hyperthermia, ice baths, and emergency care at the Falmouth Road Race. J Emerg Nurs JEN Off Publ Emerg Dep Nurses Assoc. 1989;15(4):304–12.
42. DeMartini JK, Casa DJ, Belval LN, Crago A, Davis RJ, Jardine JJ, Stearns RL. Environmental conditions and the occurrence of exertional heat illnesses and exertional heat stroke at the Falmouth road race. J Athl Train. 2014;49(4):478–85.
43. Yard EE, Gilchrist J, Haileyesus T, Murphy M, Collins C, McIlvain N, et al. Heat illness among high school athletes—United States, 2005-2009. J Safety Res. 2010;41(6):471–4.
44. World Health Organization. International statistical classification of diseases and related health problems. 10th revision. Malta: WHO; 2011.
45. Weiner JS, Horne GO. A classification of heat illness. A memorandum prepared for the climatic physiology committee of the medical research council. Br Med J. 1958;1:1533–5.
46. Armed Forces Health Surveillance Branch. Armed forces reportable medical events guidelines and case definitions. 2017;39–40.
47. DeGroot DW, Mok G, Hathaway NE. International classification of disease coding of exertional heat illness in U.S. Army soldiers. Mil Med. 2017;182(9):e1946–50.
48. Dickinson JG. Heat illness in the services. J R Army Med Corps. 1994;140(1):7–12.
49. Casa D, Armstrong L. Exertional heatstroke: a medical emergency. In: Armstrong L, editor. Exertional heat illnesses. Champaign: Human Kinetics; 2003. p. 29–56.
50. Hess JJ, Saha S, Luber G. Summertime acute heat illness in U.S. emergency departments from 2006 through 2010: analysis of a nationally representative sample. Environ Health Perspect. 2014;122(11):1209–15.
51. Fechter-Leggett ED, Vaidyanathan A, Choudhary E. Heat stress illness emergency department visits in national environmental public health tracking states, 2005–2010. J Community Health. 2016;41(1):57–69.
52. Nelson NG, Collins CL, Comstock RD, McKenzie LB. Exertional heat-related injuries treated in emergency departments in the U.S., 1997–2006. Am J Prev Med. 2011;40(1):54–60.
53. Gifford RM, Todisco T, Stacey M, Fujisawa T, Allerhand M, Woods DR, et al. Risk of heat illness in men and women: a systematic review and meta-analysis. Environ Res. 2019;171:24–35.
54. Kazman JB, Purvis DL, Heled Y, Lisman P, Atias D, Van Arsdale S, et al. Women and exertional heat illness: identification of gender specific risk factors. US Army Med Dep J. 2015;10(2):58–66.
55. Naughton MP, Henderson A, Mirabelli MC, Kaiser R, Wilhelm JL, Kieszak SM, et al. Heat-related mortality during a 1999 heat wave in Chicago. Am J Prev Med. 2002;22(4):221–7.
56. Xu Z, Sheffield PE, Su H, Wang X, Bi Y, Tong S. The impact of heat waves on children's health: a systematic review. Int J Biometeorol Int J Biometeorol. 2014;58(2):239–47.
57. Sherbakov T, Malig B, Guirguis K, Gershunov A, Basu R. Ambient temperature and added heat wave effects on hospitalizations in California from 1999 to 2009. Environ Res. 2018;160:83–90.
58. Xu Z, Cheng J, Hu W, Tong S. Heatwave and health events: a systematic evaluation of different temperature indicators, heatwave intensities and durations. Sci Total Environ. 2018;630:679–89.
59. Moore AC, Stacey MJ, Bailey KGH, Bunn RJ, Woods DR, Haworth KJ, et al. Risk factors for heat illness among British soldiers in the hot collective training environment. J R Army Med Corps. 2016;162(6):434–9.
60. Ellis FP. Heat illness. I. Epidemiology. Trans R Soc Trop Med Hyg. 1976;70(5–6):402–11.
61. Armed Forces Health Surveillance Branch. Update: heat injuries, active component, U.S. Armed Forces, 2010. MSMR. 2011;18(3):6–8.
62. Armed Forces Health Surveillance Branch. Update: heat injuries, active component, U.S. Armed Forces, 2011. MSMR. 2012;19(3):14–6.

63. Armed Forces Health Surveillance Branch. Update: Heat injuries, active component, U.S. Armed forces, 2012. MSMR. 2013;20(3):17–20.
64. Armed Forces Health Surveillance Branch. Update: Heat injuries, active component, U.S. Armed Forces, 2014. MSMR. 2015;22(3):17–20.
65. Armed Forces Health Surveillance Branch. Update: heat injuries, active component, U.S. Army, Navy, Air Force, and Marine Corps, 2015. MSMR. 2016;23(3):16–9.
66. Armed Forces Health Surveillance Branch. Update: Heat illness, active component, U.S. Armed Forces, 2016. MSMR. 2017;24(3):9–13.
67. Armed Forces Health Surveillance Branch. Update: Heat illness, active component, U.S. Armed Forces, 2017. MSMR. 2018;25(4):6–12.
68. Bedno SA, Urban N, Boivin MR, Cowan DN. Fitness, obesity and risk of heat illness among army trainees. Occup Med Oxf Engl. 2014;64(6):461–7.
69. Adams WM. Exertional heat stroke within secondary school athletics. Curr Sports Med Rep. 2019;18(4):149–53.
70. Yeargin SW, Dompier TP, Casa DJ, Hirschhorn RM, Kerr ZY. Epidemiology of exertional heat illnesses in national collegiate athletic association athletes during the 2009–2010 through 2014–2015 academic years. J Athl Train. 2019;54(1):55–63.
71. Armstrong LE, Johnson EC, Casa DJ, Ganio MS, McDermott BP, Yamamoto LM, et al. The American football uniform: uncompensable heat stress and hyperthermic exhaustion. J Athl Train. 2010;45(2):117–27.
72. Kucera KL, Klossner D, Colgate B, Cantu RC. Annual survey of football injury research. Report no.: 2018–01. Chapel Hill: University of North Carolina Chapel Hill; 2018. p. 1–38.
73. Adams WM, Hosokawa Y, Huggins RA, Mazerolle SM, Casa DJ. An exertional heat stroke survivor's return to running: an integrated approach on the treatment, recovery, and return to activity. J Sport Rehabil. 2016;25(3):280–7.
74. Schwellnus M, Kipps C, Roberts WO, Drezner JA, D'Hemecourt P, Troyanos C, et al. Medical encounters (including injury and illness) at mass community-based endurance sports events: an international consensus statement on definitions and methods of data recording and reporting. Br J Sports Med. 2019; https://doi.org/10.1136/bjsports-2018-100092. [Epub ahead of print].
75. Roberts WO, Dorman JC, Bergeron MF. Recurrent heat stroke in a runner: race simulation testing for return to activity. Med Sci Sports Exerc. 2016;48(5):785–9.
76. Sloan BK, Kraft EM, Clark D, Schmeissing SW, Byrne BC, Rusyniak DE. On-site treatment of exertional heat stroke. Am J Sports Med. 2015;43(4):823–9.
77. Hostler D, Franco V, Martin-Gill C, Roth RN. Recognition and treatment of exertional heat illness at a marathon race. Prehosp Emerg Care. 2014;18(3):456–9.
78. Noakes T, Mekler J, Pedoe DT. Jim Peters' collapse in the 1954 Vancouver Empire Games marathon. South Afr Med J. 2008;98(8):596–600.
79. Rae DE, Knobel GJ, Mann T, Swart J, Tucker R, Noakes TD. Heatstroke during endurance exercise: is there evidence for excessive endothermy? Med Sci Sports Exerc. 2008;40(7):1193–204.
80. Johnson EC, Kolkhorst FW, Richburg A, Schmitz A, Martinez J, Armstrong LE. Specific exercise heat stress protocol for a triathlete's return from exertional heat stroke. Curr Sports Med Rep. 2013;12(2):106–9.
81. Gosling CM, Forbes AB, McGivern J, Gabbe BJ. A profile of injuries in athletes seeking treatment during a triathlon race series. Am J Sports Med. 2010;38(5):1007–14.
82. Gosling CM, Gabbe BJ, McGivern J, Forbes AB. The incidence of heat casualties in sprint triathlon: the tale of two Melbourne race events. J Sci Med Sport. 2008;11(1):52–7.
83. Hosokawa Y, Adams WM, Belval LN, Davis RJ, Huggins RA, Jardine JF, et al. Exertional heat illness incidence and on-site medical team preparedness in warm weather. Int J Biometeorol. 2018;62(7):1147–53.
84. Weaving EA, Berro VE, Kew MC. Heat stroke during a "run for fun": a case report. South Afr Med J. 1980;57(18):753–4.

85. Smith R, Jones N, Martin D, Kipps C. "Too much of a coincidence": identical twins with exertional heatstroke in the same race. BMJ Case Rep. 2016;2016 https://doi.org/10.1136/bcr-2015-212592.
86. Roberts WO. Exertional heat stroke during a cool weather marathon: a case study. Med Sci Sports Exerc. 2006;38(7):1197–203.
87. Hanson PG, Zimmerman SW. Exertional heatstroke in novice runners. JAMA. 1979;242(2):154–7.
88. McEntire SJ, Suyama J, Hostler D. Mitigation and prevention of exertional heat stress in firefighters: a review of cooling strategies for structural firefighting and hazardous materials responders. Prehosp Emerg Care. 2013;17(2):241–60.
89. Petruzzello SJ, Gapin JI, Snook E, Smith DL. Perceptual and physiological heat strain: examination in firefighters in laboratory- and field-based studies. Ergonomics. 2009;52(6):747–54.
90. Cheung SS, Petersen SR, McLellan TM. Physiological strain and countermeasures with firefighting. Scand J Med Sci Sports. 2010;20(Suppl 3):103–16.
91. Hollowell DR. Perceptions of, and reactions to, environmental heat: a brief note on issues of concern in relation to occupational health. Glob Health Action. 2010;3:5632. https://doi.org/10.3402/gha.v3i0.5632.
92. Lucas RAI, Epstein Y, Kjellstrom T. Excessive occupational heat exposure: a significant ergonomic challenge and health risk for current and future workers. Extreme Physiol Med. 2014;3:14.
93. Fortune MK, Mustard CA, Etches JJC, Chambers AG. Work-attributed illness arising from excess heat exposure in Ontario, 2004–2010. Can J Public Health. 2013;104(5):e420–6.
94. Riley K, Wilhalme H, Delp L, Eisenman DP. Mortality and morbidity during extreme heat events and prevalence of outdoor work: an analysis of community-level data from Los Angeles County, California. Int J Environ Res Public Health. 2018;15(4):E580.
95. Petitti DB, Harlan SL, Chowell-Puente G, Ruddell D. Occupation and environmental heat-associated deaths in Maricopa county, Arizona: a case-control study. PLoS One. 2013;8(5):e62596.
96. Xiang J, Hansen A, Pisaniello D, Bi P. Extreme heat and occupational heat illnesses in South Australia, 2001–2010. Occup Environ Med. 2015;72(8):580–6.
97. Harduar Morano L, Watkins S, Kintziger K. A comprehensive evaluation of the burden of heat-related illness and death within the Florida Population. Int J Environ Res Public Health. 2016;31:13(6).
98. Tustin AW, Lamson GE, Jacklitsch BL, Thomas RJ, Arbury SB, Cannon DL, et al. Evaluation of occupational exposure limits for heat stress in outdoor workers—United States, 2011–2016. MMWR Morb Mortal Wkly Rep. 2018;67(26):733–7.

Chapter 2
Physiological Response to Heat Stress

Luke N. Belval and Margaret C. Morrissey

Introduction

Humans, as homeothermic endotherms, regulate their body heat storage within narrow limits through internal physiologic control. The hallmark of this physiologic control in *Homo sapiens* is the profound ability to generate heat through skeletal muscle metabolism and in turn dissipate that heat to the environment, all while maintaining a relatively stable internal body temperature in a variety of situations. While exercise in the heat is particularly taxing to these systems responsible for homeothermy, humans possess unique adaptations to adapt and manage thermal stressors.

Successful thermoregulation during exercise fundamentally relies on two components: physical dissipation of heat to the external environment and physiological mechanisms that facilitate the transfer of heat from muscles and internal organs to the skin surface. While these two aspects of homeothermy are often discussed separately, biophysical and physiological phenomenon must occur in concert to successfully sustain exercise and life in the presence of exercise and heat stress.

This chapter will first examine the physical methods of heat dissipation as they are responsible for ultimately transferring heat from the body to the external environment. From there, we will discuss the body's physiological responses that facilitate (or impede) internal control of body temperature. Finally, the physical and physiological responses to exercise in the heat will be integrated as we survey the modifiable aspects of human's responses to exercise heat stress. This chapter will provide information on the normal function of the thermoregulatory and supporting body systems, so that future chapters can illuminate the dysfunctions that manifest as exertional heat illnesses.

L. N. Belval (✉) · M. C. Morrissey
Korey Stringer Institute, Department of Kinesiology, University of Connecticut, Storrs, CT, USA
e-mail: luke.belval@uconn.edu

© Springer Nature Switzerland AG 2020
W. M. Adams, J. F. Jardine (eds.), *Exertional Heat Illness*,
https://doi.org/10.1007/978-3-030-27805-2_2

Classification of Heat Stress

While there are many ways to classify the extent of thermal stress on the human body, it is perhaps easiest to classify stressors by the capability to sustain physiological thermoregulation and performance in a given environment or exercise stress. Lind identified three such classifications that correspond to human tolerance to heat stress: (1) prescriptive zones, (2) compensatory zones, and (3) intolerable zones [1]. In this paradigm the interaction between the environment and internal metabolism is considered as to whether they permit achievement of a thermal equilibrium or a stable body temperature within safe limits [2].

In the prescriptive zone, thermal equilibrium is achieved independent of environmental conditions, representing metabolic workloads that can be sustained in even the warmest conditions [1]. These metabolic workloads in the prescriptive zone allow the body to maintain heat balance resulting in no changes in core temperature. The compensatory zone, meanwhile, allows for thermal equilibrium dependent on the severity of environmental conditions [1]. Modern classifications of heat stress further simplify these categories into a singular term, compensable heat stress, characterizing the situations where athletes, laborers, and soldiers can maintain workloads without thermoregulatory limitations [3]. As environmental temperature rises, metabolic heat production exceeds heat dissipation, which may cause an increase in body temperature.

On the other end of the spectrum, intolerable zones or uncompensable heat stress represents the limits of human exercise in the heat, as individuals will only be able to sustain performance or safety in these environments for a limited period of time [1, 3]. It is important to note that the exact determination of uncompensable or compensable heat stress is dynamic and individual. For example, American football uniforms or other protective gear can easily create situations of uncompensable heat stress when compared to similar bouts of exercise in similar environmental conditions without the equipment [4]. These theoretical constructs are useful in the context of examining exertional heat illnesses, as the determination of compensable or uncompensable heat stress depends on the individual, exercise, and environment. Figure 2.1 demonstrates the connection between metabolic heat production and total heat loss in both compensable (light, moderate, and high) and uncompensable (very high) exercise conditions [5]. The nature of the environment and stress will change the nature of this relationship as described in future sections. What is easily sustainable and safe for one individual may be strenuous and dangerous for another based upon the biophysical and physiological circumstances.

Biophysical Determinants of Thermoregulation

The properties of thermal exchange between the human body and environment are presented by the general heat balance equation:

$$S = (M - W) \pm K \pm R \pm C - E$$

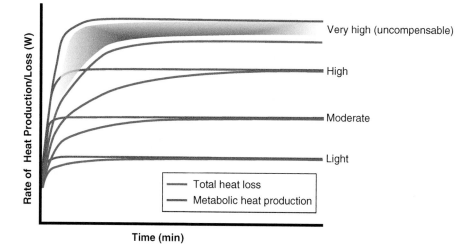

Fig. 2.1 Theoretical whole-body heat loss (dry + evaporative) responses to rapid increases in metabolic heat production associated with exercise at fixed rates of heat production in the heat (30 °C/86 °F, 20% relative humidity). (From Wingo et al. [5], with permission)

where S is heat storage, M is metabolic heat production, W is work, K is conduction, R is radiation, C is convection, and E is evaporation. Positive S represents heat gain, and negative S represents heat loss. Internal body temperature will rise if heat gain exceeds heat loss (+S), and internal body temperature will fall if heat loss exceeds heat gain (–S). To maintain heat balance (S = 0), heat gain and heat loss must be equivalent. It should be noted that the heat exchange interaction between the environment and the body occurs across both the skin surface and respiratory tract. During exercise the magnitude of heat exchange across the skin surface is increased such that the skin factors can be considered the primary mechanisms of heat loss and gain from the body.

Metabolic Heat Production

Skeletal muscle metabolism yields two products, locomotion and heat. The amount of heat generated is directly proportional to the intensity of exercise with net heat gain being calculated by accounting for work (W) [6, 7]. Humans are relatively inefficient during exercise, with ~90% of energy being transformed to heat during treadmill exercise, yielding a mechanical efficiency of 10% [6, 7]. While this endothermy is necessary in many situations, during exercise in warm environments this heat can be excessive and lead to heat storage, resulting in increases in body temperature. The specific values for the heat production that results from metabolic energy expenditure can be calculated using calorimetry, which is estimated by rate of oxygen consumption [8]. Estimating metabolic heat production indicates how much heat must be lost to the environment to maintain heat balance and limit an increase in core temperature.

Radiation

Radiation is characterized as heat exchange in the form of electromagnetic waves between objects of different temperatures. Mean radiant temperature for the human body is dependent on the temperature of surrounding surfaces and changes with respect to the location of the heat source from the body [9]. This suggests that the orientation of the body from a radiant heat source, such as the sun, can greatly impact rate of radiant heat exchange. Some authors have suggested that ancestors of *Homo sapiens* adopted bipedalism to help mitigate thermal stress by reducing total body surface area exposed to the sun [10]. Limiting surface area exposure to the sun in other ways would also decrease heat gain via radiant heat but may inhibit other heat loss mechanisms.

Conduction

Conduction, as the direct transfer of heat through two solid objects in contact, generally plays a negligible role in exercise thermoregulation [11]. However, it should be noted that some cooling modalities, such as cooling vests, rely on conduction into a thermal medium for their cooling potential [12]. In the same fashion, direct contact with a heat source, more commonly seen in occupational settings (e.g., hot ovens, metal objects), can also contribute to heat gain.

Convection

Convective means of heating or cooling are the most intuitive aspects of human heat balance. For the purposes of human thermoregulation, we can consider our most common interaction with a fluid medium or air, as our primary convective interface [9]. In this sense, the gradient that dictates the rate of heat transfer is a function of the difference between skin temperature and ambient temperature [6]. As long as the temperature of the skin is greater than the surrounding air, heat loss can occur. This means that in most situations where ambient temperature is less than ~36 °C, convective cooling naturally occurs [13]. However, as soon as ambient temperature exceeds skin temperature, convective heating results in increasing thermal stress.

It is important to distinguish that convective heat exchange occurs on a local basis. Ambient temperature as reported by a weather station may not be representative of the local environment being experienced by an individual. Wet Bulb Globe Temperature (WBGT) reported by a weather station underestimates local athletic surfaces approximately 45% of the time [14]. A key consideration in this aspect is the concept of forced convection. In situations where there is no air movement, such as indoor exercise, convective cooling can decrease fairly rapidly due to the transfer of heat to the environment directly surrounding the individual [11]. Without air movement created by wind or a fan, the local temperature gradient between the skin and the environment can rapidly decrease.

This lack of forced convection is important to note in situations where individuals must exercise in enclosed environments. This most commonly manifests through the microenvironments created by protective equipment worn. While full body enclosures like nuclear, biological, and chemical warfare equipment fundamentally limit capacity for exercise in warm environments [15], even American football equipment covering some of the body surface can drastically increase heat stress [4].

Evaporation

Evaporative heat loss is a result of the eccrine sweating response. A sympathetic cholinergic activation of eccrine sweat glands results in sweat production on the skin surface for evaporation. Eccrine gland sweat secretion is an important avenue of heat dissipation as a result of the energy released through vaporization. For every gram of sweat evaporated from the body's surface, the body loses 0.580 kcal or 2426 J of heat [16]. This results in a potent mechanism for dissipating heat in a variety of situations. In hot environmental conditions when ambient temperature exceeds skin temperature, evaporation is the only mechanism of heat loss to prevent further increases in body temperature. As a result, human thermoregulation is dependent on the appropriate dissipation of heat through evaporative cooling. Situations where evaporative cooling capacity is lower than the required demands of an environment and exercise combination are considered uncompensable heat stress, severely limiting the duration of time that an individual can perform a task.

Maximum evaporative heat loss (E_{max}) is dependent on the vapor pressure gradient between sweat on the skin surface and ambient air; which is a function of humidity, ambient temperature, and barometric pressure [6]. Unfortunately, when ambient temperature and relative humidity are high, the potential for evaporation is low, greatly diminishing the capacity of humans' most powerful heat dissipation mechanism. In a simplified fashion, to maintain thermal equilibrium, E_{max} must be greater or equal to the evaporative requirements (E_{req}) of the environment at a given metabolic rate. Exceeding the E_{req} of the environment results in heat storage and uncompensable heat stress [17].

E_{max} is also dictated by skin wettedness (ϖ_{max}) which is the proportion of total skin surface area of the body that is covered with sweat [18]. The more skin surface that is covered with sweat, the greater the E_{max}. Increased skin wettedness is acquired by recurrent exposure to increased thermal loads, which directly elicits alterations in sudomotor responses (typically occurring as part of heat acclimatization) [19]. ϖ_{max} typically ranges from 0.85 to 1.0 (i.e., 85–100% body surface coverage of sweat). A heat-acclimatized individual is theoretically capable of attaining a ϖ_{max} of 1.0, whereas non-heat-acclimatized individuals are considered to be unable to attain equivalent levels of skin wettedness [9]. Therefore, an acclimatized individual can theoretically cover a greater proportion of their skin surface area in sweat, increasing the area over which evaporation can occur. This alone will lead to increases in evaporative capacity independent of other mechanisms.

Biophysical Factors that Affect Heat Stress

Just as environmental conditions can dictate the individual factors of heat gain or loss, physical characteristics of an individual can dictate relative responses to a given heat stress. Most commonly, the units of energy for the heat balance equation are expressed as W/m^2 to normalize responses on the basis of body surface area (BSA) [11]. On the basis of the DuBois equation, this primarily allows for interindividual differences in stature (as an adjunct for BSA) to account for the amount of skin surface capable of interacting with the environment for heat exchange.

The other key demographic considerations in the determination of biophysical heat stress are body mass and body composition. Increased body mass not only increases the thermal inertia of an individual, it also increases the metabolic demand of a given exercise [20]. While theoretically the relationship between increases in body mass and body surface ratios is important, laboratory findings on the topic appear equivocal [21]. Similarly, body composition or increased body fat percentage can hypothetically influence the nature of heat exchange within the body. However, controlled laboratory work has found limited evidence for an independent effect of adiposity [22].

As nude exercise is not as popular as it used to be, the thermal properties of clothing and equipment must be considered alongside cutaneous factors. In addition to the microenvironments created between clothing and the body, clothing and equipment itself interact with the environment [23]. Fabrics and materials possess thermal and evaporative properties that interact in conjunction with human responses in proportion to the skin surface area covered [9]. Generally speaking, the greater surface area covered by a less "breathable" fabric, the greater heat stress [24].

Physiological Control of Heat Stress

Physiologic control of heat stress relies on the principles of heat balance discussed above and the integration of a neurologic autonomic control. This control, like many physiologic systems, can be divided into afferent and efferent responses, the former acting as a sensor and the latter acting as a regulator of the mechanisms the body employs. As in the cases of most diseases, exertional heat illnesses are often underpinned by either an inadequate or inappropriate physiological response.

Peripheral sensation of thermal stress is primarily believed to be mediated through the activation of temperature-specific transient receptor potential (TRP) channels [25]. These diffuse signaling pathways allow for region specific sensation of temperature and are primarily influenced by ambient temperature [26]. This afferent information is likely responsible for not only thermoeffector responses but also the perception of temperature and thermal comfort [27]. The abdomen also contains thermosensory neurons that proceed to the spinal column as a method of detecting deep body temperature [28].

The integration of human thermoregulatory information occurs in the hypothalamus, specifically the preoptic area [29]. Information from skin temperature sensors is integrated with temperature signals from the brain, spinal cord, and viscera alongside pyrogenic mediators (i.e., PGE_2, which is activated as part of the immune response) [28]. It should be noted that this temperature information is obtained across the skin surface, viscera, and nervous system; therefore, no single anatomical point serves as a physiologic representation of internal body temperature.

In the context of hyperthermia, warm-activated neurons in the hypothalamus stimulate a GABAergic response which results in the activation of thermoeffector circuits and the body's physiological mechanisms for heat dissipation [28]. The efferent responses of the thermoregulatory system during exercise in the heat are primarily eccrine sweating and cutaneous vasodilation. Both of these responses are sympathetically activated proportionally to afferent stimuli.

Sweating is the cholinergically activated result of sweat glands being activated via neural pathways descending from the sympathetic ganglia. This results in the activation of aquaporin channels that facilitate the entry of fluid into the sweat gland [30]. From there a hormone-mediated reabsorption of ions occurs as the fluid proceeds through the gland and onto the skin surface where it can be released for vaporization [31]. Since the vaporization of sweat liberates body fluid, prolonged or intense sweating has the ability to affect total body water and osmolality. Hypohydration has also been observed to diminish the sweating response at a given body temperature, demonstrating the compounding nature of hypohydration and heat stress [32].

During heat stress, the autonomic nervous system facilitates the delivery of blood to the skin's surface to dissipate heat. As internal body temperature rises, relaxation of vasoconstrictor tone in non-glabrous (hair bearing) skin occurs to increase skin blood flow [33]. If convective heat loss via relaxation of vasoconstrictor tone cannot maintain heat balance, acetylcholine or other transmitters are released from sympathetic nerve endings to increase skin blood flow through active vasodilation [33]. The extent of this vasodilation, coupled with vasoactive effects of exercising muscle and the dehydrating effect of sweat, can limit the ability of the cardiovascular system to adequately perfuse tissues, resulting in cardiovascular drift [33, 34].

In glabrous (non-hair bearing) skin, withdrawal of sympathetic nervous activity increases blood flow through passive vasodilation [35]. Glabrous skin contains arteriovenous anastomoses (AVA), which directly connect small arteries and veins without capillaries in between. AVA can be found on the palms of hands, soles of feet, and lips. AVA primary function are to transfer heat from the skin's surface to the environment since it does not contain capillaries for transportation of oxygen, nutrients, or waste products between blood and other tissues [35].

Acclimatization

Heat acclimatization (or acclimation in artificial environments) refers to the physiological adaptations that occur in response to repeated exposure to heat stress. Increasing exercise intensity in the heat exacerbates thermal strain (i.e., increased core temperature, heart rate, skin temperature), which can reduce exercise or work capacity. Heat acclimatization attenuates thermal strain through frequent heat exposures and produces positive adaptations that can preserve or improve performance [36]. HA induction over the course of 7–14 days can improve exercise performance in hot and temperate conditions through increased plasma volume, reduced core/skin temperature, improved thermal comfort, decreased heart rate, and improved sweating response [37]. The magnitude of changes that occur during and after HA is dependent on environmental conditions, exercise duration, exercise intensity, and HA induction method. Chapter 3, *Predisposing Factors for Exertional Heat Illness*, will discuss heat acclimatization in more detail.

Behavioral Thermoregulation

Control of body temperature through biological mechanisms carries a physiologic cost. Many species, including humans, employ behavioral thermoregulation as means to control body temperature more efficiently. This process is underpinned by temperature and thermal comfort infromation integrated in the nervous system, however, instead of an afferent physiological response, a behavior change occurs in its stead [38]. Figure 2.2 outlines the differences in common autonomic and behavioral responses to warm and cold stimuli [39].

The physiological connection that behavioral thermoregulation shares with autonomic thermoregulation is that both utilize peripheral thermosensors to detect changes [40]. While autonomic signals terminate in the hypothalamus, the sensory aspects of thermal sensation and comfort synapse to the brainstem [41]. The proximal nature of these structures further supports an intertwined relationship between autonomic and behavioral responses for appropriate thermoregulation.

The most common behavioral action that contributes to thermoregulation is the voluntary reduction in exercise work rate during exercise in the heat [40]. During self-paced exercise, this can be a very potent means of maintaining safety and per-

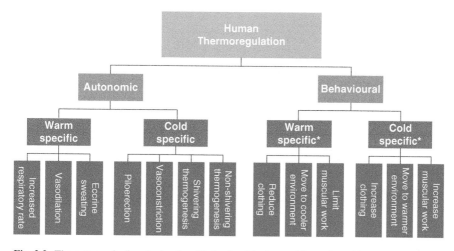

Fig. 2.2 The autonomic (involuntary) and behavioral (voluntary) branches of human thermoregulation together with warm- and cold-specific thermoeffector responses. The asterisks denote that the provided responses are some examples of the multitude of behavioral response options. (From Flouris [39], with permission)

formance [42]. However, in studies of exertional heat stroke, forced or mandated exercise beyond abilities is typically found as a common risk factor, indicating behavioral limits can be overridden through motivation [43]. Furthermore rating of perceived exertion during exercise seems to be the key predictor of volitional fatigue during exercise in the heat; thermal comfort may modulate this response, particularly when body temperature is lower [40].

Other common examples of behavioral thermoregulation in humans include exercising in cooler parts of the day, wearing fewer layers of clothing, or increasing the number of breaks during exercise, all of which do not require physiological adaptations to occur [44]. In the discussion of prevention of exertional heat illnesses, note that most acute primary methods of prevention rely on behavioral rather than physiologic thermoregulation.

Conclusion

Hot environmental conditions, intense workloads, and wearing insulating clothing result in heat storage causing body core temperature to rise. Temperature regulation in the preoptic area of the hypothalamus signals thermoregulatory effector and behavioral responses such as skin vasodilation and sweating to facilitate heat transfer from the body to the environment. Conditions that hinder heat loss or contribute to heat gain can lead to heat illness.

References

1. Lind AR. Human tolerance to hot climates. Compr Physiol. 2011, Suppl. 26: Handbook of physiology, reactions to environmental agents: 93–109. First published in print 1977. https://doi.org/10.1002/cphy.cp090106.
2. Lind AR. A physiological criterion for setting thermal environmental limits for everyday work. J Appl Physiol. 1963;18:51–6.
3. Cheung SS, McLellan TM, Tenaglia S. The thermophysiology of uncompensable heat stress. Physiological manipulations and individual characteristics. Sports Med. 2000;29(5):329–59.
4. Armstrong LE, Johnson EC, Casa DJ, Ganio MS, McDermott BP, Yamamoto LM, et al. The American football uniform: uncompensable heat stress and hyperthermic exhaustion. J Athl Train. 2010;45(2):117–27.
5. Wingo JE, Crandall CG, Kenny GP. Human heat physiology. In: Casa DJ, editor. Sport and physical activity in the heat: maximizing performance and safety. Cham: Springer; 2018. p. 15–30.
6. Gagge AP, Gonzalez RR. Mechanisms of heat exchange: biophysics and physiology. Compr Physiol. 2011, Suppl. 14: Handbook of physiology, environmental physiology: 45–84. First published in print 1996. https://doi.org/10.1002/cphy.cp040104.
7. Whipp BJ, Wasserman K. Efficiency of muscular work. J Appl Physiol. 1969;26(5):644–8.
8. Cramer MN, Jay O. Partitional calorimetry. J Appl Physiol (1985). 2019;126(2):267–77.
9. Parsons K. Human thermal environments: the effects of hot, moderate and cold environments on human health, comfort and performance. 3rd ed. Boca Raton: CRC Press; 2014.
10. Bramble DM, Lieberman DE. Endurance running and the evolution of Homo. Nature. 2004;432(7015):345–52.
11. Cramer MN, Jay O. Biophysical aspects of human thermoregulation during heat stress. Auton Neurosci. 2016;196:3–13.
12. Ross M, Abbiss C, Laursen P, Martin D, Burke L. Precooling methods and their effects on athletic performance. Sports Med. 2013;43(3):207–25.
13. Gagge AP, Nishi Y. Heat exchange between human skin surface and thermal environment. Compr Physiol. 2011, Suppl. 26: Handbook of physiology, reactions to environmental agents: 69–92. First published in print 1977. https://doi.org/10.1002/cphy.cp090105.
14. Pryor JL, Pryor RR, Grundstein A, Casa DJ. The heat strain of various athletic surfaces: a comparison between observed and modeled wet-bulb globe temperatures. J Athl Train. 2017;52(11):1056–64.
15. Muza SR, Banderet LE, Cadarette BS. Protective uniforms for nuclear, biological, and chemical warfare: metabolic, thermal, respiratory, and psychological issues. In: Pandoff KB, Re B, editors. Medical aspects of harsh environments. Washington, DC: Office of the Surgeon General, United States Army; 2002. p. 1095–138. https://ke.army.mil/bordeninstitute/published_volumes/harshEnv2/HE2ch36.pdf. Accessed 21 Mar 2019.
16. Wenger CB. Heat of evaporation of sweat: thermodynamic considerations. J Appl Physiol. 1972;32(4):456–9.
17. Gagnon D, Jay O, Kenny GP. The evaporative requirement for heat balance determines whole-body sweat rate during exercise under conditions permitting full evaporation. J Physiol. 2013;591(11):2925–35.
18. Candas V, Libert JP, Vogt JJ. Human skin wettedness and evaporative efficiency of sweating. J Appl Physiol Respir Environ Exerc Physiol. 1979;46(3):522–8.
19. Ravanelli N, Coombs GB, Imbeault P, Jay O. Maximum skin wettedness after aerobic training with and without heat acclimation. Med Sci Sports Exerc. 2018;50(2):299–307.
20. Passmore R, Durnin JVGA. Human energy expenditure. Physiol Rev. 1955;35(4):801–40.
21. Jay O, Cramer MN. A new approach for comparing thermoregulatory responses of subjects with different body sizes. Temperature (Austin). 2015;2(1):42–3.

22. Adams JD, Ganio MS, Burchfield JM, Matthews AC, Werner RN, Chokbengboun AJ, et al. Effects of obesity on body temperature in otherwise-healthy females when controlling hydration and heat production during exercise in the heat. Eur J Appl Physiol. 2015;115(1):167–76.
23. McLellan TM, Daanen HA, Cheung SS. Encapsulated environment. Compr Physiol. 2013;3(3):1363–91.
24. Pascoe DD, Bellingar TA, McCluskey BS. Clothing and exercise. II. Influence of clothing during exercise/work in environmental extremes. Sports Med. 1994;18(2):94–108.
25. Filingeri D. Neurophysiology of skin thermal sensations. Compr Physiol. 2016;6(3):1429–91. https://doi.org/10.1002/cphy.c150040.
26. Schlader ZJ, Stannard SR, Mündel T. Human thermoregulatory behavior during rest and exercise – a prospective review. Physiol Behav. 2010;99(3):269–75.
27. Kingma BR, Frijns AJ, Schellen L, van Marken Lichtenbelt WD. Beyond the classic thermoneutral zone: including thermal comfort. Temperature (Austin). 2014;1(2):142–9.
28. Morrison SF, Nakamura K. Central mechanisms for thermoregulation. Annu Rev Physiol. 2019;81(1):285–308.
29. Abbott SBG, Saper CB. Role of the median preoptic nucleus in the autonomic response to heat-exposure. Temperature (Austin). 2018;5(1):4–6.
30. Shibasaki M, Crandall CG. Mechanisms and controllers of eccrine sweating in humans. Front Biosci (Schol Ed). 2010;2(1):685–96.
31. Low PA. Evaluation of sudomotor function. Clin Neurophysiol. 2004;115(7):1506–13.
32. Kenefick RW, Cheuvront SN. Physiological adjustments to hypohydration: impact on thermoregulation. Auton Neurosci. 2016;196:47–51.
33. Gonzalez-Alonso J, Crandall CG, Johnson JM. The cardiovascular challenge of exercising in the heat. J Physiol. 2008;586(1):45–53.
34. Coyle EF, Gonzalez-Alonso J. Cardiovascular drift during prolonged exercise: new perspectives. Exerc Sport Sci Rev. 2001;29(2):88–92.
35. Walloe L. Arterio-venous anastomoses in the human skin and their role in temperature control. Temperature (Austin). 2016;3(1):92–103.
36. James CA, Richardson AJ, Watt PW, Willmott AG, Gibson OR, Maxwell NS. Short-term heat acclimation improves the determinants of endurance performance and 5-km running performance in the heat. Appl Physiol Nutr Metab. 2017;42(3):285–94.
37. Périard JD, Racinais S, Sawka MN. Adaptations and mechanisms of human heat acclimation: applications for competitive athletes and sports. Scand J Med Sci Sports. 2015;25(Suppl 1):20–38.
38. Flouris AD. Functional architecture of behavioural thermoregulation. Eur J Appl Physiol. 2011;111(1):1–8.
39. Flouris AD. Human thermoregulation. In: Périard J, Racinais S, editors. Heat stress in sport and exercise: thermophysiology of health and performance. Cham: Springer; 2019. p. 3–28.
40. Flouris AD, Schlader ZJ. Human behavioral thermoregulation during exercise in the heat. Scand J Med Sci Sports. 2015;25(Suppl 1):52–64.
41. Craig AD. Significance of the insula for the evolution of human awareness of feelings from the body. Ann N Y Acad Sci. 2011;1225:72–82.
42. Schlader ZJ, Stannard SR, Mündel T. Evidence for thermoregulatory behavior during self-paced exercise in the heat. J Therm Biol. 2011;36(7):390–6.
43. Rav-Acha M, Hadad E, Epstein Y, Heled Y, Moran DS. Fatal exertional heat stroke: a case series. Am J Med Sci. 2004;328(2):84–7.
44. Belval LN, Armstrong LE. Comparative physiology of thermoregulation. In: Casa D, editor. Sport and physical activity in the heat. Cham: Springer; 2018. p. 3–14.

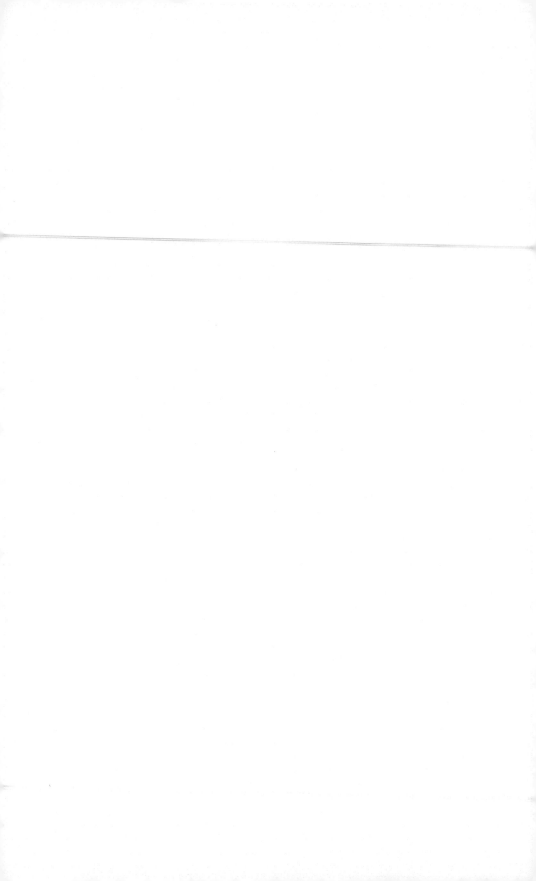

Chapter 3
Predisposing Factors for Exertional Heat Illness

J. Luke Pryor, Julien D. Périard, and Riana R. Pryor

Introduction

Exertional heat illnesses (EHI) represent a continuum of medical conditions with potentially deadly consequences that can affect physically active individuals in hot and cool environments. The severity of EHI can range from heat syncope, exercise-associated muscle cramps, heat exhaustion, and on to exertional heat stroke (EHS). Unlike classic heat stroke, which is primarily observed in vulnerable (e.g., very young and elderly) and immunocompromised populations during seasonal heat waves, EHS often occurs in healthy young individuals considered low risk and performing routine physical activities (e.g., exercise or occupational and military tasks) in cool or hot environmental conditions. Since EHS is the most catastrophic EHI, this chapter will focus on EHS risk factor identification and prevention. By and large, prevention strategies aimed at mitigating EHS risk will also attenuate other EHIs.

Individual EHS susceptibility is multifactorial, with the highest probability of occurrence when several risk factors coalesce in time creating the "perfect storm" [1]. Best practice approaches to preventing EHI begin with an awareness of and pre-participation screening for predisposing risk factors. Once risk factors have been determined, prevention strategies addressing these factors can be employed. It is crucial to implement all available prevention strategies when EHI risk is greatest. Research has shown EHI risk is greatest during summer conditioning sessions, fall

J. L. Pryor (✉) · R. R. Pryor
Exercise and Nutrition Sciences, University at Buffalo, Buffalo, NY, USA
e-mail: lpryor@buffalo.edu

J. D. Périard
Research Institute for Sport and Exercise, University of Canberra, Bruce, ACT, Australia

© Springer Nature Switzerland AG 2020
W. M. Adams, J. F. Jardine (eds.), *Exertional Heat Illness*,
https://doi.org/10.1007/978-3-030-27805-2_3

preseason sports, midday activity, early season heat waves, and when traveling to unaccustomed oppressive climates [2–6].

Predisposing factors for EHI can be categorized into two classifications: *modifiable* or those that are within an individual's control and *non-modifiable* which are innate or unchangeable. While excellent reviews on EHI risk factors and mitigation strategies have been published [7–10], this chapter aims to serve as an updated evidence-based guide for practitioners and clinicians. After a primer on human thermoregulation, we divide this chapter into three sections discussing (a) non-modifiable risk factors, (b) modifiable risk factors, and (c) risk mitigation strategies that lower EHI potential.

Overview of Human Thermoregulation

Humans are homeotherms. We aim to regulate core body temperature within a narrow homeostatic range at rest and during exercise. This heat storage balance is accomplished through consistent modifications in autonomic (skin blood flow and sweating) and behavioral heat loss effectors in an effort to offset heat gain produced by metabolic processes and/or environmental stress [11]. See Chap. 2 *Physiological Response to Heat Stress* for further discussion on human thermoregulation. Germane to this section is the understanding that EHI risk stems from factors within and outside an individual's control which influence skin blood flow, sweating, metabolism, and physical activity within an environment (Fig. 3.1). In turn, these predisposing factors influence fluid balance, cardiovascular stability, heat storage, and ultimately EHI potential.

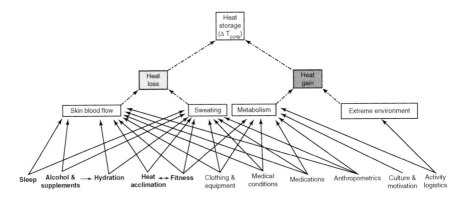

Fig. 3.1 Relationships among variables that influence heat storage and ultimately exertional heat illness (EHI) risk. Activity logistics include time of day, location, and activity programming (e.g., work/rest cycles, duration, etc.). Authors assume activity logistics remain outside of an individual's control (e.g., military and sporting activities). **Bolded**, modifiable EHI risk factors; unbolded, non-modifiable EHI risk factors; T_{core}, core body temperature; $T_{ambient}$, ambient temperature; T_{skin}, skin temperature

Non-modifiable Risk Factors

Many non-modifiable risk factors have been identified, with these factors falling into intrinsic or extrinsic categories. Some of these factors cannot be modified due to individual demographics and morphology, while others are limiting due to the environment and circumstances surrounding physical activity. While direct prevention strategies cannot be implemented to mitigate risk of developing EHI in individuals with non-modifiable risk factors, identification of these individuals is key. Medical providers can better prepare for potential EHI and differentially diagnose an individual with EHI when risk factors are identified through pre-participation screening.

A pre-participation examination provides vital information about an athlete's EHI risk and should include questions and a physical exam to evaluate factors known to influence an individual's ability to tolerate heat stress. These factors include recent exercise history, environmental conditions in which the athlete exercises to estimate heat acclimation status, previous history of EHI, medications and supplements, medical conditions, body composition, and demographic characteristics. Pre-participation examination forms including these questions have been created and successfully implemented (see Pre-participation Examination section). This screening may also include genetic screening for conditions known to elevate EHI occurrence such as sickle cell trait and malignant hyperthermia. A number of other non-modifiable risk factors exist (environmental conditions, motivation and risk tolerance, team culture, and programmed exercise demands) that may not apply to a pre-participation examination but must be considered when assessing overall EHI risk.

Programmed Clothing and Exercise Demands

There are many times in sport and physical activity during which the external demands of the activity limit individual freedom to modify activity or clothing/equipment parameters. For example, lacrosse, American football, and field hockey goalies are required to wear protective equipment such as helmets and shoulder pads. Likewise, hazardous material workers and firefighters wear fully encapsulated personal protective equipment, while law enforcement officers and military members wear extensive protective body armor to prevent physical harm. This equipment impairs heat dissipation by creating a microclimate of hot, moist air between the skin and equipment limiting evaporative cooling. Metabolically generated heat is also increased due to the added equipment mass. In these circumstances, uncompensable heat stress is more likely resulting in rapidly increasing thermal strain and EHI risk due to greater heat production and lower heat dissipation [12–14].

Work intensity is usually self-regulated during recreational activities such as running and cycling; however, this may not be true in competitive or more structured sports and physical activity. In athletics, coaches set the physical activity parameters such as exercise intensity, frequency, duration, and rest and hydration breaks. During structural fire suppression, firefighters complete standard 15–30-minute shifts before recovering. During military marches, all soldiers must complete activities in a given period to ensure a successful mission. These strict limitations leave little ability for individualization of activity parameters to meet differing thermoregulatory needs when completed in hot conditions.

The standardization of activity across all individuals completing the same tasks leads to equal absolute workload across individuals but unequal relative workloads and heat production. Less fit individuals must exercise at a relatively greater intensity, leading to unmatched workload to fitness. This discrepancy leads to greater core temperatures in unfit individuals compared to fit individuals completing the same absolute work and can be attributed to greater metabolic heat production in less fit individuals [15], possibly increasing EHI risk in these individuals. Similarly, individual hydration needs are typically not addressed by individualizing hydration breaks, leading to variable levels of dehydration, a known risk factor of EHI [8]. Rest breaks provide an opportunity to dissipate heat and consume water. Without proper work-to-rest cycles, the risk of dehydration during exercise and continual body temperature rise (uncompensable heat stress) with concurrent performance decrements exist [16].

The frequency and duration of activity in the heat represent other programmed exercise variables which influence EHI risk. During August preseason football practices, 37% of EHI occurred after 2 h of practice [3], and when practice continued beyond 3 h in length, individuals were nine times more likely to experience EHI [5]. Multiple exercise sessions on the same day and consecutive days of exercise in the heat exacerbate heat strain during the subsequent exercise session [17, 18]. While physiological mechanisms of this phenomenon warrant further investigation, epidemiological evidence indicates greater rates of EHI on the second day of exercise in the heat compared to the first day in unacclimatized football athletes [19].

Environmental Conditions

Air temperature, relative humidity, solar radiation, and wind each impact an individual's ability to thermoregulate. Environmental conditions exacerbate heat strain by either diminishing the effectiveness of heat loss mechanisms (e.g., reduced evaporation due to high humidity, reduced convection due to low wind speed) or directly promoting heat gain which occurs when ambient temperature surpasses skin temperature. To better predict when an individual is at greater risk of developing EHI, the wet-bulb globe temperature (WBGT) can be measured, which incorporates air temperature, relative humidity, solar radiation, and wind into one numerical value. A retrospective study determined that a high WBGT (>75 °F) the day prior to an EHI was more predictive of the EHI in Marine Corps recruits than the WBGT on the day of the incident [20]. In collegiate football athletes, the greatest number of heat illnesses occurred on the second day of August preseason practice, not on the first day [19].

Fatal exertional heat stroke cases in American football athletes competing in cooler parts of the United States most commonly occurred when the WBGT was higher than average for that region [21]. Both epidemiological [19–21] and lab studies [17, 18] indicate that environmental conditions are a risk factor for EHI and that there is a residual effect of the environment among consecutive days of exercise in the heat.

To offset the impact of environmental stress on thermoregulation, behavioral responses such as reducing exercise intensity or duration, removing clothing/equipment, and moving indoors or to a shaded area are effective heat stress mitigation strategies [11]. Unfortunately, certain populations such as occupational workers, military personnel in forward deployment, and athletes during competition or practice may not be able to respond in these manners increasing EHI risk.

The autonomic heat loss mechanisms of skin blood flow (convective) and sweat evaporation are effective at transferring heat to the environment provided there is a favorable gradient between skin and air temperature and water vapor pressure (i.e., ambient temperature is lower than skin temperature). Convective heat loss becomes negligible when ambient temperature surpasses skin temperature, and under these conditions sweat evaporation is the primary means of heat loss [22]. When the amount of moisture in the air increases, more sweat must be present on the skin to increase water vapor pressure around the skin enabling sweat evaporation. If fluid intake is not matched with sweat rate, this higher sweat production requirement results in fluid and electrolyte loss leading to dehydration-induced cardiovascular strain [23], impairments in thermoregulation [24, 25], and challenges blood pressure regulation [23, 26]. In particularly humid conditions, maximal sweating rates may be insufficient to overcome the water vapor pressure gradient such that evaporative cooling requirements are not met yielding uncompensable heat stress. Consequently, body temperature continually rises, and EHI risk is extremely high. Interestingly, even at 100% relative humidity, the body has some evaporative potential as long as air temperature remains below that of the skin and there is airflow across the skin.

Air movement created naturally, artificially (e.g., fan), or by activity (e.g., running, cycling) enhances the ability to cool via convection and evaporation. In the absence of adequate sweat production, air movement increases heat storage in extreme heat in older individuals with lower sweat evaporation [27, 28].

Age

There is a wealth of knowledge on the impact of age on heat balance during exercise in the heat. Middle aged and older men have reduced sweat rates compared to younger men exercising in the heat [29]. Older adults also exhibit reduced skin blood flow possibly stemming from lower stroke volume and cardiac output compared to young individuals [30, 31]. Unsurprisingly during exercise in the heat, older men and women have greater heat storage than their younger counterparts [31–33]. The decrement in evaporative heat loss exists even when age-matched for aerobic fitness and physical characteristics [33]. In older men, this reduced evaporative heat loss is even greater in untrained individuals, but this reduction can be minimized by improving aerobic fitness [34]. Combined, these studies indicate that older individuals gain heat at a faster rate than younger individuals, likely due to reduced evaporative ability. Considering that evaporation accounts for the majority of heat loss during exercise in a hot environment, older individuals are likely more susceptible to EHI when completing equal work to their younger peers.

Contrary to previous beliefs, children are not at a greater EHI risk than adults due to physical characteristics. When hydration is properly maintained, and accounting for differences in body size and exercise intensity, thermoregulatory ability [35, 36], cardiovascular capacity, exercise economy [37], and tolerance between adults and children are similar [38]. The greater body surface area to mass ratio of children is expected to be advantageous to heat loss during exercise except when environmental conditions are extremely hot. Aside from poor hydration practices, the incidence of EHI in youth sport [6] is thought to be related to other modifiable risk factors. These include improper programmed exercise and clothing/equipment requirements, unmatched physical activity to fitness, undue exercise duration, use of exercise as punishment, and insufficient recovery from activity (improper work-to-rest cycles or rest between exercise sessions [two-a-day practices]) during activity in the heat [38].

Sex

Differences in temperature regulation between men and women do not stem from inherent differences between sexes but instead are attributed to differences in aerobic fitness (modifiable) and physical characteristics including body mass and surface area (non-modifiable) [39]. The impact of anthropometrics and aerobic fitness on the predisposition of developing EHI will be discussed later in this chapter. However, because females typically have lower absolute VO_2max than men, when exercising at a similar absolute work intensity (e.g., 7.5 mph), females will have a greater metabolic heat production, leading to a greater core temperature increase. In situations such as military drills or occupational tasks when men and women must complete work at the same absolute work intensity, this could possibly predispose women to EHI.

Most published research on EHS patients involves men which may be due to a variety of factors. First, many cases of EHI occur in the military, causing this population to be greatly studied, most of whom are men (males represent 79–86% of enlistees across the Army, Navy, and Air Force, and 92% in the Marines). Secondly, men more often than women elect activities that result in EHI (e.g., American football, military, occupational work). Lastly, in situations with high EHI potential, men may more likely push themselves to greater levels of hyperthermia due to greater work intensities, although this is yet to be fully explored. When studied more systematically through epidemiological research, accounting for all sports, US high school male athletes have a greater rate of developing EHI than female athletes [3]. However, when football-related EHI were excluded and only those sports in which both girls and boys participate were included, EHI rates were similar between sexes.

Anthropometrics

Differences in body size and composition affect thermoregulation by way of affecting the physical process of heat exchange. This is accomplished by differences in body fat, body surface area to mass ratio, and body weight [3, 40–42]. Body surface area determines the heat exchange area with the environment for both dry (convective and radiative) and wet (sweat evaporation) heat loss and thus contributes to overall heat storage. A high body surface area to mass ratio is usually beneficial except when environmental conditions are extreme and impede heat loss.

As body weight increases, so does the metabolic demand involved in weight-bearing locomotion. In other words, greater metabolic heat is generated by heavier athletes completing the same absolute workload as lighter athletes. Body mass and body composition also determine heat storage capacity as the specific heat of fat mass (2.97 kJ·kg^{-1} °C^{-1}) is 20% less than the specific heat of fat free mass (3.66 kJ·kg^{-1} °C^{-1}) due to water content differences. This means that fat-free mass can store more heat than fat mass. This is relevant with passive heat exposures, or when heat loss is limited and body temperature increase is determined by storage capacity. Also, at fixed metabolic heat production rates, those with equal mass but higher body fat percentage will gain heat faster possibly because of lower mean specific heat capacity or impaired sweat gland function [41]. It is also documented that larger individuals produce lower self-generated airflow [43], decreasing the potential for heat loss. While body fat usually adds to body mass increasing metabolically generated heat, cutaneous fat is well perfused and in weight-matched subject's whole body and local sweating responses as well as skin surface, heat dissipation is not affected by body composition [41]. In summary, anthropometric differences in heat production, heat storage, and self-generated airflow may explain why larger individuals (males/females, BMI $\geq$ 29.5/25.7 kg/m^2, body fat $\geq$28.8%/34.9%, body surface area $\geq$2.0/1.7 m^2) are at greater EHI risk [3, 6, 40, 42, 44].

Motivation, Culture, and Risk Tolerance

The willingness to succumb to intense discomfort in anticipation of an achievement or reward is an acknowledged EHI risk factor. For example, the psychological and physiological feedback of exercise (e.g., pain, discomfort, sensations of hotness, or dehydration) may be overshadowed by intrinsic or extrinsic motivators or some combination of both. Regardless of the motivator(s), the desire to complete a task or obtain an achievement or award drives metabolic heat production which may exceed heat loss capacity and increase heat storage, especially when environmental conditions are warm to hot.

It may be initially difficult to identify overzealousness as motivators among individuals vary widely. For example, a strong internal motivation to "make the team" or secure a starting position may be present in transfer or underclassmen athletes, whereas top-performing athletes may push themselves to achieve new personal bests. Others may be highly influenced by external motivators such as peers, rivals, coaches, or an audience. In the military, never married cadets had a greater incidence of severe EHI compared to married counterparts [42]. While the reason(s) for this relationship is unknown, it may be due to the differences in risk tolerance between married and single cadets.

In recent years, a number of American EHS deaths have occurred resulting in litigious investigations. A culture of not reporting EHI signs or symptoms, inaction upon knowledge of EHI symptomology, and/or using physical activity as punishment have been commonalities among many lawsuits representing risk factors associated with EHI and EHS. If modification of these risk factors is to occur, administration, coach, and athlete EHI education, communication expectations, and cultural awareness are necessary.

Peer, Coach, and Organization Pressure

Individuals may feel perceived pressure to continue exercising to keep up with their peers or opponents, particularly when they are competing to make the team, secure a starting position, finish in a certain time, or win a race. This may lead to unmatched exercise intensity to fitness levels and/or a reluctance to report symptoms of EHI to their coaches or superiors. These issues further exacerbate the risk of developing EHI. Similarly, youth athletes may perceive pressure to impress parents or coaches and not "let them down," a phenomenon reported in youth hockey, wrestling, and soccer [45–47]. This thought process leads to the athletes continuing to exercise at a relatively greater intensity than peers with a higher fitness level or for a longer duration, leading to greater thermal strain and risk of EHI.

Medications

The majority of information regarding the impact of medication on the risk of EHI comes from case series or case-control studies of heat stroke patients, many times investigating classic heat stroke during heat waves [48–50]. Medications can affect thermoregulation, and therefore may exacerbate heat strain during physical activity, by preventing heat loss to the environment or by increasing metabolic heat gain during activity. Impaired sweat gland function reduces evaporative heat loss and is affected by medications such as anticholinergics, antihistamines, phenothiazines,

Table 3.1 Selected medical and recreational drugs that may alter exertional heat illness risk

Drug class	Proposed mechanism
Anticholinergics	Impaired sweat gland function
Antidepressants	Increased heat production
Antihistamine	Impaired sweat gland function
Beta-blockers and calcium channel blockers	Impaired CO increases
Diuretics (antihypertensive)	Depletion of fluid and electrolytes
Phenothiazines	Impaired sweat gland function Altered hypothalamic function
NSAIDs	Increased gut and liver toxicity
Sympathomimetics	Increased heat production Impaired sweat gland function Increased heart rate and blood pressure
Tricyclic antidepressants	Increased heat production
Recreational drugs	
Alcohol	Diuretic Peripheral vasodilation
Ephedrine	Increased heat production Impaired sweating
Ecstasy (MDMA)	Increased heart rate and blood pressure Increased muscle tension Increased sweating or chills
Cocaine	Decreased sweating threshold Decreased skin blood flow threshold Attenuated perception of thermal sensation

Modified from Leon and Bouchema [7], with permission

CO cardiac output, *POAH* posterior optic anterior hypothalamus, *NSAIDs* nonsteroidal anti-inflammatory drug, *MDMA* 3,4-methylenedioxy-methamphetamine

and other stimulants. Cardiac function is affected by medications such as beta-blockers, calcium channel blockers, and sympathomimetics such as methylphenidate (i.e., Ritalin). Other medications may lead to increased heat production such as antidepressants and stimulants. Medications with a diuretic effect deplete the body of fluid and electrolytes, potentially reducing sweat rate and increasing resting and exercising body temperature and increasing heart rate. Table 3.1 presents medical and recreational drug or drug classes and their respective proposed mechanism(s) influencing EHI risk [7].

Medical Conditions

Certain medical conditions influence the physiological mechanisms for cooling (cutaneous vasodilation and sweat production), impairing heat loss, and/or altering metabolism resulting in a net EHI risk increase (Table 3.2) [51]. Other medical conditions increase EHI risk by altering fluid-electrolyte balance and cardiovascular stability. This section provides succinct discussion of the pathophysiology connecting medical conditions most common in an active population with EHI risk. It is important to note that the medications to treat certain medical conditions may also contribute to EHI risk (see Table 3.1).

Febrile Events　Current or unresolved illness (cold, fever, infection, etc.) may predispose an individual to EHI, especially EHS, and can be rationalized from three perspectives. First, pyrokines such as IL-1 and TNF increase the hypothalamic core temperature set point to fight infection [52]. The elevated resting body temperature means there is less capacity to increase core temperature before reaching dangerously high internal temperatures (>104 °F) [8]. Second, the risk of dehydration is higher due to excessive fluid loss (diarrhea) or lack of fluid replacement resulting in dehydration or hypohydration-induced impairments in cardiovascular and thermoregulatory function (see Hydration). Third, an individual may reside in an immunocompromised state limiting their ability to rapidly resolve the systemic inflammatory response characteristic of EHS [7]. A prodromal viral illness leading to altered gene expression and unchecked inflammatory pathways has also been purported [53]. Exercise in the heat should be avoided until an individual is fully recovered from febrile events.

Previous History of Heat Illness　In a recent epidemiological study of military cadets examining 427,922 person-years, the risk of heat-related cramping, syncope, or exhaustion was fourfold higher in cadets with a previous EHI [42]. Alarmingly, the risk of EHS was almost doubled when cadets reported a previous EHI [42]. The occurrence of an EHI may underscore the inability of certain biological systems (thermoregulation, fluid-electrolyte, cardiovascular, inflammation) to manage the additive stressors of exercise and heat. On the other hand, after EHS, cellular damage may precipitate impaired biological responses to exercise in the heat eliciting a heat-intolerant individual which may be transient or persistent [54].

Whether heat intolerance is a within-lifetime maladaptation or genetically founded (e.g., malignant hyperthermia, TLR4 polymorphisms) is debated [55].

Table 3.2　Medical conditions that increase exertional heat illness (EHI) risk [51]

Skin disorders	Sweat gland disorders	Cardiovascular diseases	Metabolic disorders	Thermoregulatory disorders
Sunburn Ectodermal dysplasia Psoriasis Miliaria rubra Substantial scarring Therapeutic radiation	Cystic fibrosis Chronic anhidrosis Substantial scarring Diabetes I and II	Heart failure Cardiomyopathy Myocarditis Hypertension	Hyperthyroidism	Malignant hyperthermia Insomnia Febrile events (fever, streptococcal pharyngitis, mononucleosis, etc.) Previous EHI

Medications to treat these disorders also influence EHI risk mainly by effects on fluid balance, vasoconstrictor/dilator activity, and/or cardiac function (see Medications section)

Associational but not causal links between malignant hyperthermia and EHS are published [56, 57]. A small percentage of the population is thought to be heat intolerant, but through heat acclimation, tolerance to exercise-heat stress is markedly improved [58]. Thus, while previous EHI may indicate genetic predisposition or inefficient biological functioning in response to exercise-heat stress and increase EHI risk [55], adaptation to exercise-heat stress (heat acclimation) improves thermoregulation, fluid-electrolyte, cardiovascular, and cellular (heat shock protein) function leading to a more heat-tolerant individual [59].

Sickle Cell Trait Sickle cell trait afflicts 8% of African-Americans and increases exertional collapse risk, a primary cause of which is thought to be heat-related injury and death. The strength of this association varies across studies with some reporting no association [42], while others show a strong relationship in military (33% increased EHI risk) [60] and athletic populations [61]. The exact link between sickle cell trait and EHI risk is unclear. It is likely that environmental conditions are a mediating variable in this relationship as 87% of sickle cell trait deaths occurred when ambient temperature exceeded 80 ° F [61]. Environmental heat stress can exacerbate sweat-induced dehydration increasing the potential for sickle cell vaso-occlusion and exertional collapse.

Spinal Cord Injury As wheelchair sports continue to grow in popularity, understanding heat exchange and EHI potential in the paraplegic and quadriplegic athlete is crucial. As a consequence of spinal cord injury, heat production (muscle mass) and loss (blood redistribution and sweating capacity) are reduced below the level of the spinal cord lesion. However, heat balance remains a function of heat gain vs. loss as in able-bodied athletes. In both cool (15–25 °C) and warm-to-hot (25–40 °C) conditions, paraplegic athletes demonstrate similar core body temperature responses as able-bodied athletes [62]. However, it is consistently observed that lower body heat storage was greater in wheelchair athletes, possibly due to reduced lower body and, therefore, whole-body sweat rates. Quadriplegic athletes consistently show exacerbated heat gain due to the severe reduction or absence of sweat evaporation to dissipate environmental and metabolic heat stress during continuous exercise. Taken as a whole, wheelchair athletes present with potentially greater EHI risk due to elevated heat storage and reduced sweat rates below the level of the lesion.

Skin and Sweat Gland Disorders Healthy skin contains a vast network of capillary beds and eccrine sweat glands. Damage to the skin from direct trauma or scarring could result in the inability to create sweat (anhidrosis) or adequate perfusion to dissipate heat through evaporation and convection. Chronic inflammation, genetic, neurologic, medicinal, and idiopathic etiologies underscore most disorders of the skin and sweating. Trauma may be mild and transitory such as a grade 1 sunburn, but even a mild sunburn has been shown to diminish local sweat production [63]. On the other hand, severe burns result in scarring and fibrotic tissue absent of sweat glands. The risk of EHI increases with the amount of scarring as sweat evaporation is negligible. Importantly, well-healed skin grafts can effectively increase blood flow and sweat production during exercise-heat stress [64]. Inflammatory skin disorders such as large rashes, psoriasis, and eczema disrupt skin vasodilation and potentially heat exchange.

A common complication of diabetes is peripheral neuropathy which could impair neural control of vasomotor and sudomotor function. Early research has shown that in type 1 diabetics, local cutaneous vasodilation [65] and sweating [66] were impaired at rest without neuropathy. However, recent work demonstrated only at moderate-to-intense cycling in the heat was whole-body sweat rate reduced in type 1 diabetics [67] and whole-body heat loss lower in type 2 diabetics [68]. In both studies greater exercising body temperature, thermal strain, and EHI risk were noted, largely due to reductions in evaporative heat loss.

Cystic fibrosis is an autosomal recessive trait disease that alters sweat gland transmembrane ion trafficking resulting in difficulty regulating sweat sodium losses. The risk of cramping and hyponatremia is elevated during exercise in the heat as greater sweat evaporation is necessary to regulate body temperature, at the expense of excessive sodium loss [69]. Mutations in genes coding calcium channels such as ryanodine receptor 1 responsible for calcium trafficking during skeletal muscle contraction underscore the life-threatening phenomena known as malignant hyperthermia [70]. This condition occurs in operating rooms when exposed to certain anesthetic agents resulting in unregulated calcium cycling causing muscle rigidity, rhabdomyolysis, and extreme hyperthermia. Death occurs without rapid dantrolene administration. While malignant hyperthermia and EHS are both deadly and arise as a result of excessive metabolic heat production, evidence to suggest a causal link between the two conditions is nonexistent.

Modifiable Risk Factors

Lack of Heat Acclimation

Heat acclimation, or the lack thereof, is arguably one of the most influential predisposing factors for EHI. Growing evidence from lab, field, and climatology studies demonstrate that EHI risk is greatest during unseasonably hot weather [71] and the initial 1–3 days of exercise-heat exposure [2, 17, 19] when heat acclimation adaptations have yet to be established. The first day of work in the heat appears to exacerbate next-day fatigue, thermal sensation, and body temperature increases [17, 18], possibly leading to greater EHI risk. Heat acclimation diminishes EHI risk due to enhancements in fluid-electrolyte balance (conserved sweat electrolytes, higher sweat rate and sensitivity), cardiovascular stability (expanded plasma volume, lower exercising heart rate), increased skin blood flow, and lower resting and exercising core body temperature, summating in a more heat-tolerant individual [72–74]. Several practical reviews outline best practices for heat acclimation induction [72, 75] and maintenance [73] in athletes. The effectiveness of heat acclimation in lowering EHI occurrence was recently demonstrated in high school American football. In schools that implemented preseason heat acclimatization guidelines [76], 55% less EHI were observed [77].

Low Physical Fitness

Low physical fitness has been cited in EHI/EHS case reports [1] and epidemiological studies [42, 78] as a predisposing risk factor. Conversely, developing physical fitness and increasing VO_2max are associated with reduced physiological and thermal strain during exercise-heat stress [79–82]. Trained athletes exercising at the same relative intensity as untrained individuals do so at a higher metabolic rate (i.e., absolute workload) generating more heat [83], even in cool environments. Thermoeffectors respond to dissipate the metabolically generated heat stress and over time result in key adaptations. Adaptions observed in well-trained individuals include lower resting and exercising HR and core temperature, expanded blood volume, greater sweat rate and sensitivity, and greater exercise-heat tolerance among others [59, 84], consummate with a "quasi-heat-acclimated state." However, to optimize thermal tolerance, performance, and safety in the hot conditions, heat acclimation is required. It should be noted that VO_2max is partially genetically determined [85] and a moderate-to-high VO_2max may occur in the absence of robust physical training. Therefore, it is believed that recent aerobic training and the environment of this training, rather than VO_2max alone, are more informative when relating aerobic fitness, the quasi-heat-acclimated state, and EHI risk.

Hydration

Water is essential for life, serving as a cell volume regulator, transport and chemical reaction medium, and mediator of thermoregulatory and cardiovascular function. Regarding EHI risk, fluid balance is implicated as a major predisposing factor [7]. Progressively greater levels of hypohydration or dehydration result in proportionately faster increases in body temperature and heart rate [86, 87]. For every 1% body mass loss due to dehydration, body temperature and heart rate increase 0.16–0.4 °C and 3 bpm, respectively, faster than euhydrated counterparts in hot environments [88–90].

The greater rise in body temperature is a function of dehydration-induced impairments in dry (skin blood flow) and evaporative (sweat) heat loss mechanisms. Specifically, as the degree of dehydration increases, progressive decrements in sweat rate, sensitivity, and onset are observed during exercise in the heat [91, 92]. Similarly, skin blood flow volume and sensitivity are diminished when dehydrated [93]. Shunting blood from thermoeffectors serves to limit further (a) fluid losses from sweating and (b) reductions in central blood volume to sustain mean arterial pressure [23, 26], at the expense of heat loss productivity.

From a performance viewpoint, dehydration (>2% body mass loss) consistently yields impaired cognition, sporting skills, aerobic, strength, power, and repetitive high-intensity performance [94–97]. Importantly, the aforementioned thermoregulatory, cardiovascular, and performance impairments demonstrate a dose (dehydration)-dependent response suggesting interventions to minimize dehydration are crucial not only to prevent dangerously high body temperature and EHI but also to maximize performance in hot environments.

Alcohol, Sleep, and Supplements

Alcohol, sleep, and supplements are factors that influence EHI risk through modulation of heat loss, hydration status, and metabolic rate, for which we know very little. Among the available evidence, it appears that alcohol influences autonomic thermoregulation (impaired vasomotor reflexes, core temperature set point) and perceptions of hotness during heat exposure [98, 99]. Beverages containing ≥4% alcohol by volume elicit diuretic effects by inhibiting vasopressin activity in active populations and should be discouraged for fluid replacement [100, 101]. Diuretics (alcohol, hypertensive medications, weight loss supplement, etc.) pose severe consequences to individuals engaging in exercise in the heat due to the potential of dehydration-induced impairments in thermoregulatory and cardiovascular functioning (see Hydration section).

Whether altered sleep (deprivation or interrupted) leads to impaired thermoregulation and increased EHI risk is unclear. In two case series, 5/6 fatal EHS [1] and 7/10 EHS [54] patients experienced some degree of sleep disturbance the nights preceding the event. Beyond case series, lab studies show conflicting evidence regarding the effects of sleep on thermoregulation. Some sleep deprivation studies (27–60 h awake) show lower sweat sensitivity [102] resulting in higher exercising core temperature [103]. Decrements in sweat rate and peripheral vasodilation have also been reported following sleep deprivation, albeit this observation is not consistently seen across the literature [103–105]. Moreover, there is evidence indicating disturbed sleep results in lower pre-exercise body temperatures and does not affect exercise-induced body temperature responses [106–108].

Markers of systemic inflammation [109] and the stress hormone cortisol [110] are greater after sleep disturbance and long sleep duration, but not short sleep duration. This sleep-induced pro-inflammatory state may compromise an individual's ability to quickly resolve the systemic inflammatory response characteristic of EHS [7]. Altered sleep increases submaximal heart rate up to 5%, demonstrating a reduction in cardiovascular efficiency and capacity to adjust to exercise-heat stress [107, 111]. The interrelationships among sleep modification, thermoregulation, and overall health warrant future research given the frequency of interrupted, restricted, and deprived sleep in today's society. Whether altered sleep is conclusively linked to

EHI risk is debatable. However, considering altered sleep appears to affect some more than others, for those wishing to optimize safety during physical activity in the heat, attention to adequate sleep quality and quantity is warranted.

The use of recreational drugs and some supplements before or during exercise in the heat are cause for caution due to the lack of FDA oversight and questionable business practices of some manufacturers. While many individuals consume supplements for purported ergogenic effects, some supplements could influence thermoregulatory effectors and fluid balance elevating EHI risk (see Table 3.1). When consumed within reported ergogenic ranges, the popular supplements creatine and caffeine do not impair fluid balance or thermoregulation during exercise [112, 113]. It has been purported that creatine may actually improve thermoregulation by increasing the water content of fat-free mass and therefore heat storage capacity [113]. In military enlistees, tobacco, opioid, and NSAID use increased relative risk of mild and severe heat-related injury [42]. Cocaine was shown to diminish the onset of skin blood flow and sweating leading to elevations in core body temperature while also attenuating the perception of thermal discomfort [114]. Heavy use of over-the-counter medications, recreational drugs, and certain supplements should be cautioned and individualized when exercising in the heat. Medicinal substances should be taken with oversight from trained healthcare providers to ensure safety.

Heat Illness Mitigation Strategies

There is great inter- and intraindividual variation in EHI risk factors that modify an individual's physiological and psychological tolerance to heat stress. Implementing prevention strategies addressing every foreseeable risk factor is very challenging in team-based sports but may be warranted on an individual basis in those with the highest EHI risk. Importantly, EHS risk may be mitigated by using evidenced-based approaches that can be modified at the team and individual level to address specific athlete concerns. These interventions include heat acclimation, increasing fitness level, ensuring proper hydration, cooling before and during exercise, as well as modifying the physical activity or exercise setting.

Heat Acclimation

Acute exposure to hot and/or humid ambient conditions results in the development of thermal strain (i.e., elevated skin, muscle, and core temperatures) during prolonged exercise, which impairs performance and increases the risk of EHI. However, when repeatedly exposed to conditions that elicit profuse sweating and elevate whole-body temperature, adaptations develop that reduce the deleterious effects of heat stress. Heat acclimation and acclimatization, which refer to periods of heat exposure undertaken in artificial (i.e., laboratory) or natural (i.e., outdoor) settings, respectively, lead to improved submaximal exercise performance, increased VO_{2max}, and improved thermal comfort in the heat, as well as reduced susceptibility to EHI. These benefits are achieved through enhanced sweating and skin blood flow responses, plasma volume expansion, better fluid balance (i.e., hydration) and cardiovascular stability, eliciting acquired thermal tolerance [72, 73, 115].

Adaptations to the heat are generally achieved through five main induction pathways: self-paced exercise, constant work rate exercise, passive heating, controlled hyperthermia (i.e., isothermic heat acclimation), and controlled heart rate heat acclimation (Fig. 3.2). Although these approaches have all been shown to induce adaptations, exercise-heat acclimatization has been suggested to provide more specific adaptations in response to heat exposures being specific to the conditions encountered during competition (i.e., exercise task, solar radiation, wind speed, and terrain/ geography) [72]. The time course of heat acclimation/acclimatization is relatively rapid, with a significant fraction of the adaptations developing during the first week of heat exposure and 10–14 days being optimal for complete or near-complete acclimation/acclimatization. The rate of decay for the main adaptive responses (i.e., lowered heart rate and core temperature during exercise) is ~2.5% per day without heat exposure [74]. Training regularly has been suggested to aid in maintaining heat adaptations, as high core temperatures and sweat rates can be achieved when training vigorously, even in cooler climates [73]. It is therefore advisable to complete an acclimation or acclimatization regimen as close as possible to the competition being held in the heat. If heat acclimation takes place well in advance of competition (e.g., 6–8 weeks), then regular top-up heat training sessions (e.g., 1–3 per week) may be warranted [73, 116, 117]. These top-up sessions might include performing non-key workouts in the heat (e.g., running for ≥60 min in 40 °C and 40% RH), undertaking a controlled heat rate protocol session (e.g., maintaining 85% of maximum heart rate

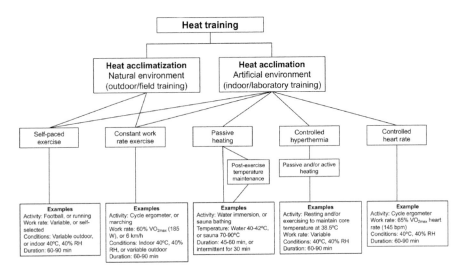

Fig. 3.2 Five main heat acclimation induction pathways

for ≥60 min in 40 °C and 40% RH), or passive heating session following a workout in cool conditions (e.g., 20–45 min in a sauna at ~80 °C or hot bath at 40 °C). In a military or occupational context, it is advisable to undertake passive heating sessions as these may be more logistically feasible. Alternatively, occupation-specific heat interventions may be developed (e.g., marching in the heat at 40 °C and 40% RH).

Fitness

Endurance-trained athletes exhibit several characteristics that heat-acclimated individuals acquire when heat training (e.g., lowered core temperature and heart rate, greater sweat rate, less sweat sodium loss). As such, endurance training, even in temperate climates, reduces physiological strain and increases exercise capacity in the heat [84]. For example, trained athletes exercising at the same relative intensity as untrained individuals, but at a higher metabolic rate (i.e., absolute workload), experience a higher rate of heat storage [83] but fatigue at a similar or higher core temperature [15, 118, 119]. This suggests that adaptations related to training may allow for greater rates of body heat storage to occur before exercise capacity in the heat is compromised [80].

Aerobically trained athletes may also adapt to the heat more rapidly than unfit individuals [79, 120] and exhibit less susceptibility to heat injury/illness [78]. However, an elevated VO_2max per se does not necessarily confer improved heat tolerance [121]. For endurance training in temperate climates, to improve thermoregulatory capacity, either strenuous interval training or continuous training at an elevated exercise intensity (e.g., >50% VO_2max) should be employed. Lesser training intensities produce questionable effects on performance during exercise-heat stress [84]. Although some suggest that endurance training must last at least 1 week [122], others have demonstrated that the best improvements require a minimum of 8–12 weeks of training [84]. Ultimately, while aerobic fitness by virtue of the thermoregulatory strain incurred during high-intensity training can impart benefits similar to those of heat acclimation, endurance training does not fully replace heat acclimation and the adaptations stemming from repeated heat exposure.

Hydration

Hydration in hot/humid conditions is critical for maximizing safety and performance during training and competition. Athletes should therefore undertake endurance events in a rested, well-fed, and well-hydrated state [9]. Consuming 5–6 ml of water per kg of body mass every 2–3 h prior to training or competing in the heat is advisable; however, this strategy should be tested and practiced prior to competition in order to establish individual volume needs [9]. This strategy may also be implemented several days in advance of competition, so as not to promote dehydration via frequent urination. A daily water intake target based on the European Food Safety Authority of 2.0 L/day for females and 2.5 L/day for males [123] is an adequate starting point for athletes, as well as those in the military or occupational work force, with exercise-related water losses added to these minimum guidelines.

During physical activity, it is advisable to minimize body mass losses induced via sweating while using caution to avoid overdrinking as this may lead to hyponatremia. From a practical perspective, it has recently been highlighted that high-intensity exercise in which sweat rate is elevated, along with activities lasting >90 min in the heat, should be accompanied by a planned hydration strategy [124]. Matching fluid intake to sweat losses is necessary for those wishing to optimize performance in the heat, heavy sweaters, or during prolonged exercise leading to excessive dehydration [8, 125]. In contrast, drinking to thirst may be sufficient to offset fluid losses during low-intensity exercise of shorter duration (<90 min), particularly in cool climates [124]. Sodium is the main electrolyte lost in sweat, and if a deficit is not compensated, it may prompt muscle cramping when reaching 20–30% of the exchangeable sodium pool [126]. Other risk factors linked to exercise-associated muscle cramping include a history of cramping, faster performance times, and prior muscle, tendon, or ligament injury [8]. Chapter 6 contains a comprehensive overview of the mechanisms mediating exercise-associated muscle cramping. Those that sweat profusely may therefore require supplementing their fluids with additional sodium. During exercise lasting longer than 1 h, athletes may aim to consume a solution containing 0.5–0.7 g/L of sodium [127]. It is worth noting that the Institute of Medicine [128] highlighted that public health recommendations regarding sodium ingestion do not apply to individuals that lose large volumes of sodium in sweat, such as those training or competing in the heat. Athletes should also aim to include 30–60 g/h of carbohydrates in their hydration regimen for exercise lasting longer than 1 h and up to 90 g/h for events lasting over 2.5 h [129]. This can be achieved through a combination of fluids and solid foods. Finally, fluid should always be available and never restricted during physical activity in the heat regardless of setting (military, industry, athletics, etc.).

Rehydration following work, training, or competing in the heat is important for the optimization of recovery. If a large fluid deficit needs to be urgently replenished, it is suggested to replace 150% of body mass losses within 1 h following the cessation of exercise [127, 130]. From a practical perspective, this may not be achievable (e.g., time, gastrointestinal discomfort), and so this time frame may be extended. Recovery of significant fluid loss after exercise is assisted by the simultaneous replacement of electrolyte losses, particularly sodium, as it helps retain ingested fluids and stimulate thirst [127]. Sports drinks (e.g., flavored drinks consisting of water, some salt and sugar) allow more complete hydration than drinking plain water or soft drinks as they have optimal sugar concentrations to maximize the uptake of water by the body. A drink containing protein (e.g., milk) may allow to better restore fluid balance after exercise than a standard carbohydrate-electrolyte sport drink. Combining protein (0.2–0.4 g/kg/h) to carbohydrate (0.8 g/kg/h) has also been reported to maximize protein synthesis rates [131]. Consuming a combination of fluids and solid foods is also advisable for rehydration and electrolyte replacement.

Pre and Per Cooling

Reducing body temperature prior to competition or its rate of rise during an athletic event in the heat has the benefit of lessening the impact of heat stress on aerobic performance and decreasing the risk of EHI. Pre (before competition) and per (during competition) cooling interventions have thus become a staple for many athletes competing in the heat. Indeed, pre-cooling may benefit sporting activities involving sustained exercise in warm-hot environments, whereas cooling during exercise may be an approached used in sports with regular breaks or opportunities to access cooling solutions. The most effective cooling modalities depend on the sport, timing of cooling, and feasibility based on the constraints of the particular rules and regulations of a sport [132]. Several cooling interventions exist, ranging from internal (e.g., cold fluid or ice slurry ingestion) to external (e.g., cold-water immersion, cooling garments) methods. The effectiveness of these methods is varied however, and prior use and practice are recommended. It must also be acknowledged that laboratory-based cooling interventions generally improve exercise capacity in the heat but that they may overestimate the effectiveness of cooling relative to outdoor scenarios, where a warm-up generally occurs and airflow is commensurate with that of the activity [9].

The most impactful external cooling method is that of cold-water immersion, with a range of protocols available. The most common techniques are whole-body cold-water immersion (22–30 °C for ~30 min) or body segment (e.g., legs) immersion (10–18 °C) [9]. While effective, it is noteworthy that the cooling of segments and locomotor muscles in particular via whole-body immersion decreases nerve conduction and muscle contraction velocities, which may lead to athletes having to re-warm-up before competition. As such, other techniques have been developed to selectively cool the torso and legs to prevent the excessive cooling of locomotor muscles. One particular example is the use ice towels, which is an easy and low-cost strategy to implement. It involves a container (e.g., cooler) filled with water and ice, along with 2–3 towels. The towels are submerged in the ice water and then placed over the shoulders and/or legs of the athlete, rotating between towels every 2–3 min for maximal cooling effect. Based on the use of iced towels, different ice-cooling garments or vests have also been developed. Although not as effective cold-water immersion, cooling garments offer the potential advantage of lowering skin temperature and reducing cardiovascular strain. Cooling garments may therefore be a practical approach to adopt during the warm-up or recovery breaks, as long as the cooling benefits outweigh any loss of evaporative capacity stemming from the torso being covered.

The ingestion of cold fluids is a method that can potentially enhance endurance performance when consumed before exercise. Ice slurry ingestion is more efficient than cold-water ingestion at cooling the body, as ice requires substantially more heat energy (334 J/g) to cause a phase change from solid to liquid (at 0 °C) compared with the energy required to increase the temperature of water (4 J/g/°C). Several reports therefore support the consumption of an ice slurry beverage (~1 L crushed ice at ≤4 °C) prior to [133] and during exercise [134]. The ingestion of ice slurry may be a practical complement or alternative approach to external cooling methods as well as an additional hydration strategy, although more studies are required to identify its effects during actual outdoors competitions. Interestingly, water dousing is a method that can be implemented during competition in conjunction with fluid ingestion. Indeed, athletes may wish to consume some fluid (e.g., water) and douse themselves with the remainder. This approach has been suggested to yield a greater level of heat dissipation, via evaporation, than drinking cold or ice water [135]. For this to occur optimally, however, environmental conditions should be dry with a high wind velocity, so as to favor evaporation.

A mixed-method cooling strategy approach appears to be the most effective. Indeed, combining techniques by using both external and internal cooling strategies has a higher cooling capacity than the same techniques used in isolation, allowing for greater benefit on exercise performance [133]. The mixed methods approach can be achieved by combining simple strategies, such as the ingestion of ice slurry, wearing cooling vests, and providing fanning.

Activity Modifications Based on WBGT Monitoring

The most common set of recommendations followed by athletic event organizers to modify (e.g., reschedule or cancel) an event is based on the WBGT index developed by the US Military and popularized by the American College of Sports Medicine [136]. These athletic activity recommendations were recently extended in the United States to include regional heat safety thresholds based on geographical variations in heat exposure and acclimatization status (Table 3.3) [137]. The majority of the recommendations are centered on activity modifications to undertake during training, based on adjusting exercise intensity and duration, work-to-rest ratios, and clothing or equipment worn [55]. These guidelines are supported by epidemiological EHI data

Table 3.3 Regional heat safety guidelines for low-risk acclimatized individuals based on American College of Sports Medicine guidelines. Values are wet-bulb globe temperatures (°C)

Category 3	Category 2	Category 1	Activity guidelines
≤10.0	≤8.7	≤6.7	Normal activity
10.1–18.3	8.8–17.0	6.8–15.0	Normal activity
18.4–22.2	17.1–20.9	15.1–18.9	Normal activity
22.3–25.6	21.0–24.3	19.0–22.3	Normal activity, monitor fluids
25.7–27.8	24.4–26.5	22.4–24.5	Normal activity, monitor fluids
27.9–30.0	26.6–28.7	24.6–26.7	Plan intense or prolonged exercise with discretion
30.1–32.2	28.8–30.9	26.8–28.9	Limit intense exercise and total daily exposure to heat and humidity
>32.3	>31.0	>29.0	Cancel exercise

From Grundstein et al. [137], with permission

[3, 4, 138, 139]. As such, heat-specific activity recommendations for individual sports that take into consideration competition rules and protective equipment are limited.

Moreover, it is important to recognize that the WBGT is a climatic index and cannot directly predict heat dissipation. As such, environmental indices should be viewed as recommendations for event organizers to develop and implement specific preventive countermeasures in order to offset the potential risk of EHI. This includes the Universal Thermal Climate Index (UTCI), which provides an alternative to the WBGT by integrating predictive formulas of heat strain based on activities conducted in different temperatures, at varying constant metabolic heat productions, and in different clothing [140]. Despite the introduction of procedures to adjust the UTCI to higher metabolic activities, the level of physical activity tested within the new model was only equivalent to moderate intensity exercise [141], which may not accurately represent a sporting event undertaken at a high intensity.

Recommended countermeasures based on the prevailing environmental conditions include adapting the rules and regulations with regard to cooling breaks and the availability of fluids (e.g., time and locations), as well as providing active cooling during rest periods. It is also recommended that medical response protocols and facilities to deal with cases of EHI/EHS be in place. Other approaches include forward planning and appropriately scheduling an event at the coolest part of the day [139] or even stopping practice/competition when the thermal environment becomes physiologically uncompensable. The environmental conditions under which this occurs depend on several factors, including metabolic heat production (e.g., workload and efficiency/economy), athlete morphology (e.g., body surface area to mass ratio), acclimatization state (e.g., sweat rate), and clothing. It is therefore difficult to establish universal activity guidelines and cutoff values for the cancellation or modification of exercise across different sports. In sum, EHI may seem predictable in hot, humid weather or particularly unexpectedly hot and humid environmental conditions. However, EHI may occur in any environment, even in seemingly ideal conditions for exercise [142]. Activity must be modified based upon environmental heat stress.

Pre-participation Examination

Organizers of athletics events that are likely to be held in hot and/or humid environmental conditions should pay particular medical attention to populations potentially at a greater risk of EHI. This includes participants currently unwell or recovering from a recent infection, with diarrhea, recently vaccinated, with limited heat dissipation capacity due to medical conditions (e.g., Paralympic athletes), or involved in sports with rules restricting heat dissipation capacity (e.g., protective clothing/equipment). Unacclimatized participants should also be considered at risk. Indeed, when comparing two triathlon races in similar environmental conditions (WBGT, 22–27 °C) but 2 months apart, it was noted that 15 cases of EHI (including 3 EHS) occurred in the first race held at the start of summer, whereas no cases were reported in the second race later on during summer [143]. This suggests that the risk of EHI is increased in individuals that are not seasonally heat acclimatized and supports earlier epidemiological studies regarding the increased risk of EHI early in July/August and unseasonably hot weather (e.g., heat wave) [19, 20]. Although it is impractical to screen every athlete during large events, organizers are encouraged to provide information, possibly in registration kits, advising all athletes of the risks associated with participation in a compromised state and suggesting potential countermeasures. Efforts to identify individuals at greatest risk, and what type of risk factors, are worthwhile since these are the individuals most likely to succumb to EHI. This information can also inform practitioners as to the most effective preventative strategies to implement. A heat illness screening instrument is available [144]. Another screening tool is available using utilizing established EHI risk factors to identify at-risk individuals defined as meeting ≥ 2 thresholds: for males ≥ 53 years old, BMI ≥ 29.5 kg/m^2, body fat $\geq 28.8\%$, body surface area ≥ 2.0 m^2, and peak oxygen consumption less than VO$_2$peak <48.3 ml/kg/min. Female thresholds are ≥ 55.8 years old, BMI ≥ 25.7 kg/m^2, body fat $\geq 34.9\%$, body surface area ≥ 1.7 m^2, and VO$_2$peak <41.4 ml/kg/min [44].

Education and Communication

Education and communication regarding how heat stress can impact the health and performance of athletes may represent a novel and important approach in the prevention of EHI, particularly during mass participation events. Event organizers could provide basic information in registration packets regarding the effects of heat stress on performance during intermittent and continuous exercise. Information about how the environment in combination with exercise can lead to EHI could also be communicated, perhaps in the form of infographics. These could include a list of factors that increase the risk of EHI such as recent illness, unseasonably hot weather, high humidity, a lack of heat acclimatization, and poor hydration practices. Given the conflicting messages regarding exercise hydration originating from different sources, sport-specific recommendations about what, when, and how much to drink are certainly warranted. In military and occupational contexts, several initiatives have already been introduced to ensure the safety of personnel and of the workforce. For example, heat acclimation protocols were used in South African mines at the turn of the nineteenth century. Military personnel have guidelines and operating procedures to ensure adequate preparation to heat stress. Notwithstanding, educating those that may be exposed to extreme conditions is a key component to preventing EHI.

Conclusion

Understanding and screening for predisposing EHI risk factors inform sports medicine staff and healthcare professionals when and in whom EHI risk is greatest. EHI risk is derived from several factors including the weather and inter- and intraindividual factors which may be within or outside a person's control. Preventative strategies should be employed whenever EHI risk is present.

References

1. Rav-Acha M, Hadad E, Epstein Y, Heled Y, Moran DS. Fatal exertional heat stroke: a case series. Am J Med Sci. 2004;328(2):84–7.
2. Wallace RF, Kriebel D, Punnett L, Wegman DH, Wenger CB, Gardner JW, et al. The effects of continuous hot weather training on risk of exertional heat illness. Med Sci Sports Exerc. 2005;37(1):84–90.
3. Kerr ZY, Casa DJ, Marshall SW, Comstock RD. Epidemiology of exertional heat illness among U.S. high school athletes. Am J Prev Med. 2013;44(1):8–14.
4. Grundstein AJ, Ramseyer C, Zhao F, Pesses JL, Akers P, Qureshi A, et al. A retrospective analysis of American football hyperthermia deaths in the United States. Int J Biometeorol. 2012;56(1):11–20.
5. Tripp BL, Eberman LE, Smith MS. Exertional heat illnesses and environmental conditions during high school football practices. Am J Sports Med. 2015;43(10):2490–5.
6. Yeargin SW, Kerr ZY, Casa DJ, Djoko A, Hayden R, Parsons JT, et al. Epidemiology of exertional heat illnesses in youth, high school, and college football. Med Sci Sports Exerc. 2016;48(8):1523–9.
7. Leon LR, Bouchama A. Heat stroke. Compr Physiol. 2015;5(2):611–47.
8. Casa DJ, DeMartini JK, Bergeron MF, Csillan D, Eichner ER, Lopez RM, et al. National Athletic Trainers' Association position statement: exertional heat illnesses. J Athl Train. 2015;59(9):986–1000.
9. Racinais S, Alonso JM, Coutts AJ, Flouris AD, Girard O, Gonzalez-Alonso J, et al. Consensus recommendations on training and competing in the heat. Scand J Med Sci Sports. 2015;25(Suppl 1):6–19.
10. Pryor RR, Casa DJ, Adams WM, Belval LN, DeMartini JK, Huggins RA, et al. Maximizing athletic performance in the heat. Strength Cond J. 2013;35(6):24–33.
11. Flouris AD, Schlader ZJ. Human behavioral thermoregulation during exercise in the heat. Scand J Med Sci Sports. 2015;25(Suppl 1):52–64.
12. Armstrong LE, Johnson EC, Casa DJ, Ganio MS, McDermott BP, Yamamoto LM, et al. The American football uniform: uncompensable heat stress and hyperthermic exhaustion. J Athl Train. 2010;45(2):117–27.
13. Johnson EC, Ganio MS, Lee EC, Lopez RM, McDermott BP, Casa DJ, et al. Perceptual responses while wearing an American football uniform in the heat. J Athl Train. 2010;45(2):107–16.
14. Montain SJ, Sawka MN, Cadarette BS, Quigley MD, McKay JM. Physiological tolerance to uncompensable heat stress: effects of exercise intensity, protective clothing, and climate. J Appl Physiol (1985). 1994;77(1):216–22.
15. Selkirk GA, McLellan TM. Influence of aerobic fitness and body fatness on tolerance to uncompensable heat stress. J Appl Physiol (1985). 2001;91(5):2055–63.
16. Maresh CM, Sokmen B, Armstrong LE, Dias JC, Pryor JL, Creighton BC, et al. Repetitive box lifting performance is impaired in a hot environment: implications for altered work-rest cycles. J Occup Environ Hyg. 2014;11(7):460–8.
17. Schlader ZJ, Colburn D, Hostler D. Heat strain is exacerbated on the second of consecutive days of fire suppression. Med Sci Sports Exerc. 2017;49(5):999–1005.
18. Meade RD, D'Souza AW, Krishen L, Kenny GP. The physiological strain incurred during electrical utilities work over consecutive work shifts in hot environments: a case report. J Occup Environ Hyg. 2017;14(12):986–94.
19. Cooper ER, Ferrara MS, Casa DJ, Powell JW, Broglio SP, Resch JE, et al. Exertional heat illness in American football players: when is the risk greatest? J Athl Train. 2016;51(8):593–600.
20. Wallace RF, Kriebel D, Punnett L, Wegman DH, Wenger CB, Gardner JW, et al. Risk factors for recruit exertional heat illness by gender and training period. Aviat Space Environ Med. 2006;77(4):415–21.
21. Grundstein AJ, Hosokawa Y, Casa DJ. Fatal exertional heat stroke and American football players: the need for regional heat-safety guidelines. J Athl Train. 2018;53(1):43–50.

22. Gagnon D, Jay O, Kenny GP. The evaporative requirement for heat balance determines whole-body sweat rate during exercise under conditions permitting full evaporation. J Physiol. 2013;591(11):2925–35.
23. Senay LC Jr. Effects of exercise in the heat on body fluid distribution. Med Sci Sports. 1979;11(1):42–8.
24. Sawka MN, Toner MM, Francesconi RP, Pandolf KB. Hypohydration and exercise: effects of heat acclimation, gender, and environment. J Appl Physiol Respir Environ Exerc Physiol. 1983;55(4):1147–53.
25. Brengelmann GL. Circulatory adjustments to exercise and heat stress. Annu Rev Physiol. 1983;45:191–212.
26. Rowell LB, Brengelmann GL, Blackmon JR, Twiss RD, Kusumi F. Splanchnic blood flow and metabolism in heat-stressed man. J Appl Physiol. 1968;24(4):475–84.
27. Ravanelli NM, Hodder SG, Havenith G, Jay O. Heart rate and body temperature responses to extreme heat and humidity with and without electric fans. JAMA. 2015;313(7):724–5.
28. Gagnon D, Romero SA, Cramer MN, Kouda K, Poh PYS, Ngo H, et al. Age modulates physiological responses during fan use under extreme heat and humidity. Med Sci Sports Exerc. 2017;49(11):2333–42.
29. Larose J, Boulay P, Sigal RJ, Wright HE, Kenny GP. Age-related decrements in heat dissipation during physical activity occur as early as the age of 40. PLoS One. 2013;8(12):e83148.
30. Kenny GP, Flouris AD, Dervis S, Friesen BJ, Sigal RJ, Malcolm J, et al. Older adults experience greater levels of thermal and cardiovascular strain during extreme heat exposures. Med Sci Sports Exerc. 2015;47(5s):497.
31. Kenny GP, Poirier MP, Metsios GS, Boulay P, Dervis S, Friesen BJ, et al. Hyperthermia and cardiovascular strain during an extreme heat exposure in young versus older adults. Temperature. 2017;4(1):79–88.
32. Stapleton JM, Poirier MP, Flouris AD, Boulay P, Sigal RJ, Malcolm J, et al. At what level of heat load are age-related impairments in the ability to dissipate heat evident in females? PLoS One. 2015;10(3):e0119079.
33. Larose J, Wright HE, Stapleton J, Sigal RJ, Boulay P, Hardcastle S, et al. Whole body heat loss is reduced in older males during short bouts of intermittent exercise. Am J Physiol Regul Integr Comp Physiol. 2013;305(6):R619–29.
34. Stapleton JM, Poirier MP, Flouris AD, Boulay P, Sigal RJ, Malcolm J, et al. Aging impairs heat loss, but when does it matter? J Appl Physiol. 2014;118(3):299–309.
35. Armstrong LE, Maresh CM. Exercise-heat tolerance of children and adolescents. Pediatr Exerc Sci. 1995;7(3):239–52.
36. Drinkwater B, Kupprat I, Denton J, Crist J, Horvath S. Response of prepubertal girls and college women to work in the heat. J Appl Physiol. 1977;43(6):1046–53.
37. Maliszewski AF, Freedson PS. Is running economy different between adults and children? Pediatr Exerc Sci. 1996;8(4):351–60.
38. Bergeron M, Devore C, Rice S. Policy statement—climatic heat stress and exercising children and adolescents. Pediatrics. 2011;128(3):e741–7.
39. Gagnon D, Kenny GP. Does sex have an independent effect on thermoeffector responses during exercise in the heat? J Physiol. 2012;590(Pt 23):5963–73.
40. Havenith G. Individualized model of human thermoregulation for the simulation of heat stress response. J Appl Physiol (1985). 2001;90(5):1943–54.
41. Dervis S, Coombs GB, Chaseling GK, Filingeri D, Smoljanic J, Jay O. A comparison of thermoregulatory responses to exercise between mass-matched groups with large differences in body fat. J Appl Physiol (1985). 2016;120(6):615–23.
42. Nelson DA, Deuster PA, O'Connor FG, Kurina LM. Timing and predictors of mild and severe heat illness among new military enlistees. Med Sci Sports Exerc. 2018;50(8):1603–12.
43. Deren TM, Coris EE, Casa DJ, DeMartini JK, Bain AR, Walz SM, et al. Maximum heat loss potential is lower in football linemen during an NCAA summer training camp because of lower self-generated air flow. J Strength Cond Res. 2014;28(6):1656–63.

44. Flouris AD, McGinn R, Poirier MP, Louie JC, Ioannou LG, Tsoutsoubi L, et al. Screening criteria for increased susceptibility to heat stress during work or leisure in hot environments in healthy individuals aged 31–70 years. Temperature (Austin, Tex). 2018;5(1):86–99.
45. Vallance JK, Dunn JG, Dunn JLC. Perfectionism, anger, and situation criticality in competitive youth ice hockey. J Sport Exerc Psychol. 2006;28(3):383–406.
46. Scanlan TK, Lewthwaite R. Social psychological aspects of competition for male youth sport participants: I. predictors of competitive stress. J Sport Exerc Psychol. 1984;6(2):208–26.
47. Ommundsen Y, Roberts GC, Lemyre P-N, Miller BW. Parental and coach support or pressure on psychosocial outcomes of pediatric athletes in soccer. Clin J Sport Med. 2006;16(6):522–6.
48. Jones TS, Liang AP, Kilbourne EM, Griffin MR, Patriarca PA, Wassilak SGF, et al. Morbidity and mortality associated with the July 1980 heat wave in St Louis and Kansas City, Mo. JAMA. 1982;247(24):3327–31.
49. Dematte JE, O'mara K, Buescher J, Whitney CG, Forsythe S, McNamee T, et al. Near-fatal heat stroke during the 1995 heat wave in Chicago. Ann Intern Med. 1998;129(3):173–81.
50. Kilbourne EM, Choi K, Jones TS, Thacker SB. Risk factors for heatstroke: a case-control study. JAMA. 1982;247(24):3332–6.
51. Casa DJ, editor. Sport and physical activity in the heat: maximizing performance and safety. Cham: Springer; 2018.
52. Stitt JT. Fever versus hyperthermia. Fed Proc. 1979;38(1):39–43.
53. Sonna LA, Wenger CB, Flinn S, Sheldon HK, Sawka MN, Lilly CM. Exertional heat injury and gene expression changes: a DNA microarray analysis study. J Appl Physiol (1985). 2004;96(5):1943–53.
54. Armstrong LE, De Luca JP, Hubbard RW. Time course of recovery and heat acclimation ability of prior exertional heatstroke patients. Med Sci Sports Exerc. 1990;22(1):36–48.
55. Hosokawa Y, Stearns RL, Casa DJ. Is heat intolerance state or trait? Sports Med. 2019;49(3):365–70.
56. Reske-Nielsen C, Schlosser K, Pascucci RC, Feldman JA. Is it exertional heatstroke or something more? A case report. J Emerg Med. 2016;51(2):e1–5.
57. Hosokawa Y, Casa DJ, Rosenberg H, Capacchione JF, Sagui E, Riazi S, et al. Round table on malignant hyperthermia in physically active populations: meeting proceedings. J Athl Train. 2017;52(4):377–83.
58. Dresoti A. The results of some investigations into the medical aspects of deep mining on the Witwatersrand. J Chem Metal Mining Soc S Afr. 1935;6:102–29.
59. Taylor NA. Human heat adaptation. Compr Physiol. 2014;4(1):325–65.
60. Singer DE, Byrne C, Chen L, Shao S, Goldsmith J, Niebuhr DW. Risk of exertional heat illnesses associated with sickle cell trait in U.S. Military. Mil Med. 2018;183(7–8):e310–e7.
61. Harris KM, Haas TS, Eichner ER, Maron BJ. Sickle cell trait associated with sudden death in competitive athletes. Am J Cardiol. 2012;110(8):1185–8.
62. Price MJ. Thermoregulation during exercise in individuals with spinal cord injuries. Sports Med. 2006;36(10):863–79.
63. Pandolf KB, Gange RW, Latzka WA, Blank IH, Kraning KK 2nd, Gonzalez RR. Human thermoregulatory responses during heat exposure after artificially induced sunburn. Am J Phys. 1992;262(4 Pt 2):R610–6.
64. Cramer MN, Moralez G, Huang MU, Crandall CG. No thermoregulatory impairment in skin graft donor sites during exercise-heat stress. Med Sci Sports Exerc. 2019;51(5):868–73.
65. Wilson SB, Jennings PE, Belch JJ. Detection of microvascular impairment in type I diabetics by laser Doppler flowmetry. Clin Physiol. 1992;12(2):195–208.
66. Hoeldtke RD, Bryner KD, Hoeldtke ME, Christie I, Ganser G, Hobbs G, et al. Sympathetic sudomotor disturbance in early type 1 diabetes mellitus is linked to lipid peroxidation. Metabolism. 2006;55(11):1524–31.
67. Carter MR, McGinn R, Barrera-Ramirez J, Sigal RJ, Kenny GP. Impairments in local heat loss in type 1 diabetes during exercise in the heat. Med Sci Sports Exerc. 2014;46(12):2224–33.

68. Kenny GP, Stapleton JM, Yardley JE, Boulay P, Sigal RJ. Older adults with type 2 diabetes store more heat during exercise. Med Sci Sports Exerc. 2013;45(10):1906–14.
69. Smith HR, Dhatt GS, Melia WM, Dickinson JG. Cystic fibrosis presenting as hyponatraemic heat exhaustion. BMJ. 1995;310(6979):579–80.
70. Poussel M, Guerci P, Kaminsky P, Heymonet M, Roux-Buisson N, Faure J, et al. Exertional heat stroke and susceptibility to malignant hyperthermia in an athlete: evidence for a link? J Athl Train. 2015;50(11):1212–4.
71. Roberts WO. Determining a "do not start" temperature for a marathon on the basis of adverse outcomes. Med Sci Sports Exerc. 2010;42(2):226–32.
72. Periard JD, Racinais S, Sawka MN. Adaptations and mechanisms of human heat acclimation: applications for competitive athletes and sports. Scand J Med Sci Sports. 2015;25(Suppl 1):20–38.
73. Pryor JL, Pryor RR, Vandermark LW, Adams EL, VanScoy RM, Casa DJ, et al. Intermittent exercise-heat exposures and intense physical activity sustain heat acclimation adaptations. J Sci Med Sport. 2019;22(1):117–22.
74. Daanen HAM, Racinais S, Periard JD. Heat acclimation decay and re-induction: a systematic review and meta-analysis. Sports Med. 2018;48(2):409–30.
75. Guy JH, Deakin GB, Edwards AM, Miller CM, Pyne DB. Adaptation to hot environmental conditions: an exploration of the performance basis, procedures and future directions to optimise opportunities for elite athletes. Sports Med. 2015;45(3):303–11.
76. Casa DJ, Csillan D, Armstrong LE, Baker LB, Bergeron MF, Buchanan VM, et al. Preseason heat-acclimatization guidelines for secondary school athletics. J Athl Train. 2009;44(3):332–3.
77. Kerr ZY, Register-Mihalik JK, Pryor RR, Pierpoint LA, Scarneo SE, Adams WM, et al. The Association between mandated preseason heat acclimatization guidelines and exertional heat illness during preseason high school American football practices. Environ Health Perspect. 2019;127(4):47003.
78. Gardner JW, Kark JA, Karnei K, Sanborn JS, Gastaldo E, Burr P, et al. Risk factors predicting exertional heat illness in male Marine Corps recruits. Med Sci Sports Exerc. 1996;28(8):939–44.
79. Pandolf KB, Burse RL, Goldman RF. Role of physical fitness in heat acclimatisation, decay and reinduction. Ergonomics. 1977;20(4):399–408.
80. Mora-Rodriguez R. Influence of aerobic fitness on thermoregulation during exercise in the heat. Exerc Sport Sci Rev. 2012;40(2):79–87.
81. Piwonka RW, Robinson S, Gay VL, Manalis RS. Preacclimatization of men to heat by training. J Appl Physiol. 1965;20(3):379–83.
82. Lamarche DT, Notley SR, Poirier MP, Kenny GP. Fitness-related differences in the rate of whole-body total heat loss in exercising young healthy women are heat-load dependent. Exp Physiol. 2018;103(3):312–7.
83. Mora-Rodriguez R, Del Coso J, Hamouti N, Estevez E, Ortega JF. Aerobically trained individuals have greater increases in rectal temperature than untrained ones during exercise in the heat at similar relative intensities. Eur J Appl Physiol. 2010;109(5):973–81.
84. Armstrong LE, Pandolf KB. Physical training, cardiorespiratory physical fitness and exercise-heat tolerance. In: Pandolf KB, Sawka MN, Gonzalez RR, editors. Human performance physiology and environmental medicine at terrestrial extremes. Indianapolis: Benchmark Press; 1988. p. 199–226.
85. Williams CJ, Williams MG, Eynon N, Ashton KJ, Little JP, Wisloff U, et al. Genes to predict VO2max trainability: a systematic review. BMC Genomics. 2017;18(Suppl 8):831.
86. Montain SJ, Coyle EF. Influence of graded dehydration on hyperthermia and cardiovascular drift during exercise. J Appl Physiol (1985). 1992;73(4):1340–50.
87. Gonzalez-Alonso J. Separate and combined influences of dehydration and hyperthermia on cardiovascular responses to exercise. Int J Sports Med. 1998;19(Suppl 2):S111–4.
88. Buono MJ, Wall AJ. Effect of hypohydration on core temperature during exercise in temperate and hot environments. Pflugers Arch. 2000;440(3):476–80.

89. Gisolfi CV, Copping JR. Thermal effects of prolonged treadmill exercise in the heat. Med Sci Sports. 1974;6(2):108–13.
90. Adams WM, Ferraro EM, Huggins RA, Casa DJ. Influence of body mass loss on changes in heart rate during exercise in the heat: a systematic review. J Strength Cond Res. 2014;28(8):2380–9.
91. Sawka MN, Young AJ, Francesconi RP, Muza SR, Pandolf KB. Thermoregulatory and blood responses during exercise at graded hypohydration levels. J Appl Physiol (1985). 1985;59(5):1394–401.
92. Armstrong LE, Maresh CM, Gabaree CV, Hoffman JR, Kavouras SA, Kenefick RW, et al. Thermal and circulatory responses during exercise: effects of hypohydration, dehydration, and water intake. J Appl Physiol (1985). 1997;82(6):2028–35.
93. Gonzalez-Alonso J, Mora-Rodriguez R, Coyle EF. Stroke volume during exercise: interaction of environment and hydration. Am J Physiol Heart Circ Physiol. 2000;278(2):H321–30.
94. Judelson DA, Maresh CM, Anderson JM, Armstrong LE, Casa DJ, Kraemer WJ, et al. Hydration and muscular performance: does fluid balance affect strength, power and high-intensity endurance? Sports Med. 2007;37(10):907–21.
95. Kenefick RW, Cheuvront SN. Hydration for recreational sport and physical activity. Nutr Rev. 2012;70(Suppl 2):S137–42.
96. Goodman SPJ, Moreland AT, Marino FE. The effect of active hypohydration on cognitive function: a systematic review and meta-analysis. Physiol Behav. 2019;204:297–308.
97. Baker LB, Dougherty KA, Chow M, Kenney WL. Progressive dehydration causes a progressive decline in basketball skill performance. Med Sci Sports Exerc. 2007;39(7):1114–23.
98. Yoda T, Crawshaw LI, Nakamura M, Saito K, Konishi A, Nagashima K, et al. Effects of alcohol on thermoregulation during mild heat exposure in humans. Alcohol. 2005;36(3):195–200.
99. Kalant H, Lê AD. Effects of ethanol on thermoregulation. Pharmacol Ther. 1983;23(3):313–64.
100. Hobson RM, Maughan RJ. Hydration status and the diuretic action of a small dose of alcohol. Alcohol Alcohol. 2010;45(4):366–73.
101. Shirreffs SM, Maughan RJ. Restoration of fluid balance after exercise-induced dehydration: effects of alcohol consumption. J Appl Physiol (1985). 1997;83(4):1152–8.
102. Dewasmes G, Bothorel B, Hoeft A, Candas V. Regulation of local sweating in sleep-deprived exercising humans. Eur J Appl Physiol Occup Physiol. 1993;66(6):542–6.
103. Tokizawa K, Sawada S, Tai T, Lu J, Oka T, Yasuda A, et al. Effects of partial sleep restriction and subsequent daytime napping on prolonged exertional heat strain. Occup Environ Med. 2015;72(7):521–8.
104. Muginshtein-Simkovitch E, Dagan Y, Cohen-Zion M, Waissengrin B, Ketko I, Heled Y. Heat tolerance after total and partial acute sleep deprivation. Chronobiol Int. 2015;32(5):717–24.
105. Kolka MA, Stephenson LA. Exercise thermoregulation after prolonged wakefulness. J Appl Physiol (1985). 1988;64(4):1575–9.
106. Vaara J, Kyrolainen H, Koivu M, Tulppo M, Finni T. The effect of 60-h sleep deprivation on cardiovascular regulation and body temperature. Eur J Appl Physiol. 2009;105(3):439–44.
107. Oliver SJ, Costa RJ, Laing SJ, Bilzon JL, Walsh NP. One night of sleep deprivation decreases treadmill endurance performance. Eur J Appl Physiol. 2009;107(2):155–61.
108. Moore JP, Harper Smith AD, Di Felice U, Walsh NP. Three nights of sleep deprivation does not alter thermal strain during exercise in the heat. Eur J Appl Physiol. 2013;113(9):2353–60.
109. Irwin MR, Olmstead R, Carroll JE. Sleep disturbance, sleep duration, and inflammation: a systematic review and meta-analysis of cohort studies and experimental sleep deprivation. Biol Psychiatry. 2016;80(1):40–52.
110. Wolkow A, Aisbett B, Reynolds J, Ferguson SA, Main LC. The impact of sleep restriction while performing simulated physical firefighting work on cortisol and heart rate responses. Int Arch Occup Environ Health. 2016;89(3):461–75.
111. Mougin F, Simon-Rigaud ML, Davenne D, Renaud A, Garnier A, Kantelip JP, et al. Effects of sleep disturbances on subsequent physical performance. Eur J Appl Physiol Occup Physiol. 1991;63(2):77–82.

112. Ely BR, Ely MR, Cheuvront SN. Marginal effects of a large caffeine dose on heat balance during exercise-heat stress. Int J Sport Nutr Exerc Metab. 2011;21(1):65–70.
113. Twycross-Lewis R, Kilduff LP, Wang G, Pitsiladis YP. The effects of creatine supplementation on thermoregulation and physical (cognitive) performance: a review and future prospects. Amino Acids. 2016;48(8):1843–55.
114. Crandall CG, Vongpatanasin W, Victor RG. Mechanism of cocaine-induced hyperthermia in humans. Ann Intern Med. 2002;136(11):785–91.
115. Sawka MN, Leon LR, Montain SJ, Sonna LA. Integrated physiological mechanisms of exercise performance, adaptation, and maladaptation to heat stress. Compr Physiol. 2011;1(4):1883–928.
116. Pryor JL, Johnson EC, Roberts WO, Pryor RR. Application of evidence-based recommendations for heat acclimation: individual and team sport perspectives. Temperature. 2019;6(1):37–49.
117. Saunders PU, Garvican-Lewis LA, Chapman RF, Periard JD. Special environments: altitude and heat. Int J Sport Nutr Exerc Metab. 2019;29(2):210–9.
118. Periard JD, Caillaud C, Thompson MW. The role of aerobic fitness and exercise intensity on endurance performance in uncompensable heat stress conditions. Eur J Appl Physiol. 2012;112(6):1989–99.
119. Sawka MN, Young AJ, Latzka WA, Neufer PD, Quigley MD, Pandolf KB. Human tolerance to heat strain during exercise: influence of hydration. J Appl Physiol (1985). 1992;73(1):368–75.
120. Shvartz E, Shapiro Y, Magazanik A, Meroz A, Birnfeld H, Mechtinger A, et al. Heat acclimation, physical fitness, and responses to exercise in temperate and hot environments. J Appl Physiol Respir Environ Exerc Physiol. 1977;43(4):678–83.
121. Avellini BA, Shapiro Y, Fortney SM, Wenger CB, Pandolf KB. Effects on heat tolerance of physical training in water and on land. J Appl Physiol Respir Environ Exerc Physiol. 1982;53(5):1291–8.
122. Nadel ER, Pandolf KB, Roberts MF, Stolwijk JA. Mechanisms of thermal acclimation to exercise and heat. J Appl Physiol. 1974;37(4):515–20.
123. EFSA Panel on Dietetic Prfoducts, Nutrition, and Allergies (NDA). Scientific opinion on dietary reference values for water. EFSA J. 2010;8(3):1459. https://doi.org/10.2903/j.efsa.2010.1459.
124. Kenefick RW. Drinking strategies: planned drinking versus drinking to thirst. Sports Med. 2018;48(Suppl 1):31–7.
125. McDermott BP, Anderson SA, Armstrong LE, Casa DJ, Cheuvront SN, Cooper L, et al. National Athletic Trainers' Association position statement: fluid replacement for the physically active. J Athl Train. 2017;52(9):877–95.
126. Bergeron MF. Muscle cramps during exercise-is it fatigue or electrolyte deficit? Curr Sports Med Rep. 2008;7(4):S50–S5.
127. Sawka MN, Burke LM, Eichner ER, Maughan RJ, Montain SJ, Stachenfeld NS. American College of Sports Medicine position stand. Exercise and fluid replacement. Med Sci Sports Exerc. 2007;39(2):377–90.
128. Panel on Dietary Reference Intakes for Electrolytes and Water. Institute of Medicine Dietary reference intakes for water, potassium, sodium, chloride, and sulfate: National Academies Press; 2005. https://www.nap.edu/read/10925/chapter/1. Accessed 15 May 2019.
129. Burke LM, Hawley JA, Wong SH, Jeukendrup AE. Carbohydrates for training and competition. J Sports Sci. 2011;29(Suppl 1):S17–27.
130. Shirreffs SM. Restoration of fluid and electrolyte balance after exercise. Can J Appl Physiol. 2001;26(Suppl):S228–35.
131. Beelen M, Burke LM, Gibala MJ, van Loon LJ. Nutritional strategies to promote postexercise recovery. Int J Sport Nutr Exerc Metab. 2010;20(6):515–32.
132. Adams WM, Hosokawa Y, Casa DJ. Body-cooling paradigm in sport: maximizing safety and performance during competition. J Sport Rehabil. 2016;25(4):382–94.

133. Bongers CC, Thijssen DH, Veltmeijer MT, Hopman MT, Eijsvogels TM. Precooling and per-cooling (cooling during exercise) both improve performance in the heat: a meta-analytical review. Br J Sports Med. 2015;49(6):377–84.
134. Stevens CJ, Taylor L, Dascombe BJ. Cooling during exercise: an overlooked strategy for enhancing endurance performance in the heat. Sports Med. 2017;47(5):829–41.
135. Morris NB, Jay O. To drink or to pour: How should athletes use water to cool themselves? Temperature (Austin, Tex). 2016;3(2):191–4.
136. Armstrong LE, Casa DJ, Millard-Stafford M, Moran DS, Pyne SW, Roberts WO. American College of Sports Medicine position stand. Exertional heat illness during training and competition. Med Sci Sports Exerc. 2007;39(3):556–72.
137. Grundstein A, Williams C, Phan M, Cooper E. Regional heat safety thresholds for athletics in the contiguous United States. Appl Geogr. 2015;56:55–60.
138. Kark JA, Burr PQ, Wenger CB, Gastaldo E, Gardner JW. Exertional heat illness in Marine Corps recruit training. Aviat Space Environ Med. 1996;67(4):354–60.
139. Grundstein A, Cooper E, Ferrara M, Knox JA. The geography of extreme heat hazards for American football players. Appl Geogr. 2014;46:53–60.
140. Fiala D, Havenith G, Brode P, Kampmann B, Jendritzky G. UTCI-Fiala multi-node model of human heat transfer and temperature regulation. Int J Biometeorol. 2012;56(3):429–41.
141. Bröde P, Fiala D, Kampmann B. Considering varying clothing, activities and exposure times with the Universal Thermal Climate Index UTCI. Proceedings 21st International Congress of Biometeorology, 3–7 Sept, 2017, Durham University, UK.
142. Roberts WO. Exertional heat stroke during a cool weather marathon: a case study. Med Sci Sports Exerc. 2006;38(7):1197–203.
143. Gosling CM, Gabbe BJ, McGivern J, Forbes AB. The incidence of heat casualties in sprint triathlon: the tale of two Melbourne race events. J Sci Med Sport. 2008;11(1):52–7.
144. Eberman LE, Cleary MA. Development of a heat-illness screening instrument using the Delphi panel technique. J Athl Train. 2011;46(2):176–84.

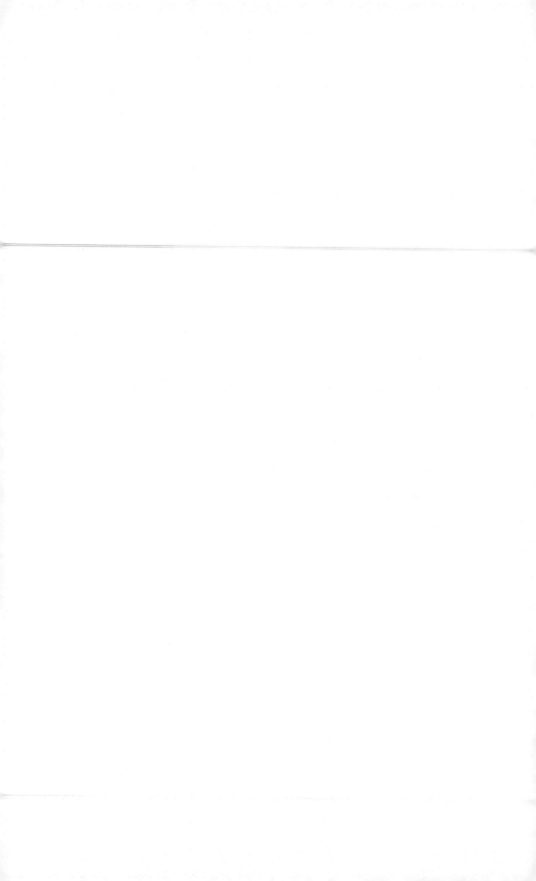

Chapter 4
Exertional Heat Stroke

William M. Adams, Rebecca L. Stearns, and Douglas J. Casa

An American football athlete collapsing during a strenuous preseason training session, a military recruit exhibiting obvious cognitive impairment during the first few days of basic training, a railroad worker dispatched to repair a section of railway in the middle of the summer in the southeastern portion of North America, and a recreational runner competing in a summer time road running race. These examples depict common scenarios in which individuals in these settings succumb to exertional heat illness (EHI).

Exertional heat stroke (EHS) is the most severe of the EHIs, with this medical emergency being fatal or leading to long-term morbidity if not properly managed. Defined as extreme hyperthermia with accompanying altered mental status, EHS represents a failure of one's thermoregulatory capacity and is a prominent concern in athletic, military, and occupational settings, particularly when physical activity is occurring in hot environmental conditions. This chapter will provide readers with an in-depth review of EHS from the perspectives of etiology and pathophysiology, recognition, management and care, and return to physical activity considerations.

Etiology

EHS is caused by an overwhelming of the body's ability to maintain thermal balance. When metabolic heat production exceeds the rate at which heat dissipation occurs, the

W. M. Adams (✉)
Department of Kinesiology, University of North Carolina at Greensboro,
Greensboro, NC, USA
e-mail: wmadams@uncg.edu

R. L. Stearns · D. J. Casa
Korey Stringer Institute, Department of Kinesiology, University of Connecticut,
Storrs, CT, USA

© Springer Nature Switzerland AG 2020
W. M. Adams, J. F. Jardine (eds.), *Exertional Heat Illness*,
https://doi.org/10.1007/978-3-030-27805-2_4

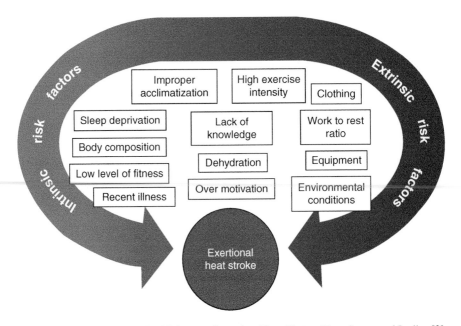

Fig. 4.1 Extrinsic and intrinsic risk factors of exertional heat illness. (From Lopez and Jardine [2], with permission. Figure courtesy Douglas J. Casa, PhD and Miwako Suzuki, KSI Summer Fellow; Korey Stringer Institute)

body enters a state of uncompensable heat stress, and if the continued rise in body temperature is left unabated, EHS ensues. The cause of EHS is multifactorial, with the risk factors responsible encompassing aspects that are both extrinsic (factors outside of one's control) and intrinsic (factors within one's control) (Fig. 4.1) [1, 2]. Interestingly, the onset of EHS is rather individualized where a constellation of risk factors may or may not be present to cause the condition. Figure 4.2 depicts the presence of various risk factors in a case series of fatal and nonfatal EHS patients [3], which supports the notion that a varying number and combination of EHS risk factors may cause an event in any one individual on any given day.

Typically, extrinsic risk factors (e.g., required clothing/protective equipment, environmental conditions, peer and/or organizational pressure, etc.) are non-modifiable in that these risk factors may not be avoidable during physical activity, particularly in hot environmental conditions. For example, in forward deployment in military operations or road construction work, it may not be possible to alter the amount of clothing worn or perform physical activity during cooler parts of the day depending on the objectives at hand. Intrinsic risk factors (e.g., acclimatization status, cardiorespiratory fitness, hydration status, etc.), on the other hand, are those that are typically modifiable in that these risk factors can be addressed to reduce overall risk. Implementation of a heat acclimatization protocol at the outset of athletic/military training and occupational work that allows progressive and gradual exposure to thermal stress to improve thermal tolerance is an example of one method to address one of the intrinsic risk factors associated with EHS. The latter example has been shown to be extremely effective in reducing EHI risk; data examining the incidence

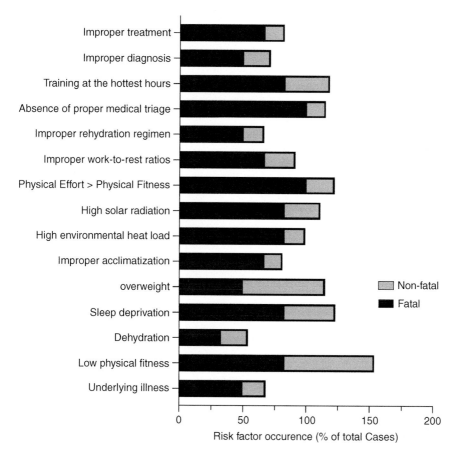

Fig. 4.2 Predisposing factors associated with fatal ($n = 6$) and nonfatal ($n = 128$) cases of exertional heat stroke. (From Rav-Acha et al. [3], with permission)

of EHI in secondary school athletics in the United States that have mandated heat acclimatization into preseason training has shown a 55% reduction in EHI risk, which provides compelling evidence on the effectiveness of such measures [4].

Pathophysiology

Homeostatic control of body temperature is tightly controlled by the preoptic portion of the anterior hypothalamus; afferent input from thermoreceptors in the skin via the spinal cord directs the appropriate efferent signals to the body to maintain the body's set point of approximately 37 °C. During exercise, metabolic activity produces body heat (additional body heat is gained if environmental conditions exceed skin temperature), prompting the stimulation of sympathetic cutaneous vasodilation and visceral vasoconstriction which permits an increased skin blood flow, cardiac output, and sweating responses for evaporation of sweat from the skin's surface to dissipate body heat [5, 6]. At the cellular level, the physiological response to thermal stress involves various cytokines (e.g., tumor necrosis factor (TNF) α, interleukin-1 (IL-1), and interleukin-6 (IL-6)), heat shock proteins (HSPs), endothelial cells, leukocytes, and epithelial cells that act to protect the body from injury, mediate the body's inflammatory response, promote tissue repair, and mitigate the leakage of endotoxins across the intestinal barrier [7–14].

In EHS, there is a breakdown in the homeostatic control of internal body temperature, setting off a cascade of events leading to thermoregulatory failure (Fig. 4.3)

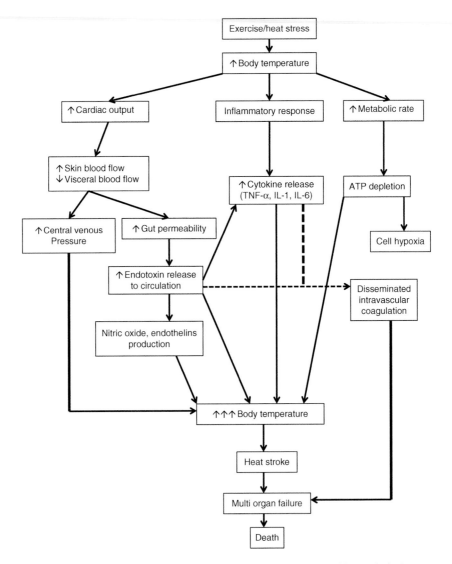

Fig. 4.3 Pathophysiology of heat stroke. (From Vandermark et al. [17], with permission)

that is triggered by endotoxemia originating in the gut [5, 6, 15–17]. The cardiovascular response to thermal stress, the redistribution of blood from the visceral organs to the skin, permits the hyperpermeability of the tight junctions of the endothelium in the intestines as a result of increased levels of hypoxia, thus allowing the infiltration of endotoxins into the systemic circulation [16, 18]. The ensuing systemic inflammatory response promotes a further increase in body temperature mediated by the increase in circulating cytokines and release of nitric oxide and endothelins [5, 6, 12]. Combined with the systemic inflammatory response and cytotoxicity, disseminated intravascular coagulation, a common occurrence in EHS, can contribute to prolonged tissue damage causing multiorgan failure and oftentimes death when prompt care is not provided [5, 6, 12, 19]. (This is similar to what occurs in sepsis and may be a clinical pearl for our medical readers.)

Recognition and Assessment

Timely recognition of EHS is of utmost importance, and is the first step, in ensuring survival and recovery from the condition [20]. Observation of altered mental status (e.g., combativeness, agitation, confusion, unresponsive, etc.) in anyone performing physical activity warrants prompt attention. If EHS is suspected (i.e., prolonged and intense exercise or physical activity in hot conditions, situations where heat dissipation may be impeded [e.g., warfighter wearing an impermeable chemical and biological warfare ensemble], etc.), confirmation of one's internal body temperature is warranted in order to rule out other potential medical conditions causing altered mental status such as heat exhaustion (see Chap. 5, *Heat Exhaustion*), exertional hyponatremia, exertional sickling, head injury, cardiac event, respiratory event, or shock (Table 4.1) [21].

Obtaining an accurate internal body temperature measure is essential for an accurate diagnosis of EHS. Prior literature [22–27] has extensively examined methods of temperature assessment during exercise, whereby rectal temperature prevails as the only valid measure of internal body temperature in exercising individuals. While assessment of rectal temperature is standard of care in the diagnosis of EHS [1, 20, 28–32], some data suggests that there are inconsistencies with utilizing best practices, including taking a rectal temperature in patients suspected of EHS, among the medical community [33, 34]. While there are a number of reasons that may explain these aforementioned inconsistencies (Table 4.2), a common misconception pertains to maintaining patient privacy during assessment of an individual's rectal temperature. The issue of patient privacy can be avoided if proper steps are taken by the on-site medical provider to minimize the risk of exposure (Fig. 4.4). Nonetheless, if EHS is suspected, observation and recognition of obvious central nervous system dysfunction, followed by an assessment of internal body temperature using rectal thermometry, permits the on-site medical provider to determine an accurate diagnosis, which will guide the treatment plan.

Table 4.1 Preventing sudden death in sport: a potentially complex overlap of signs and symptoms of common causes of death[a]

	EHS	Heat cramp[b]	Heat syncope[b]	Exercise heat exhaustion[b]	Exertional hyponatremia	Exertional sickling	Head injury	Cardiac[c]	Respiratory[d]	Shock
CNS dysfunction[e]	X		X	X	X	X	X	X	X	X
Dizziness	X		X	X	X		X	X	X	
Drowsiness	X				X		X			X
Fatigue	X	X	X	X	X	X	X	X	X	X
Headache	X		X		X		X			
Light-headedness			X	X	X		X	X		X
Staggering	X		X	X	X	X	X	X	X	
Syncope	X		X	X				X	X	
Tunnel vision			X					X		
Personality changes[f]	X			X	X		X	X	X	X
Lethargy				X	X		X	X	X	X
Core body temperature usually <40 °C		X	X	X	X	X	X	X	X	X
Core body temperature usually >40 °C	X									
Cool, clammy skin			X	X	X	X		X		X
Hot and wet or dry skin	X	X	X	X	X	X		X		X
Pale skin			X	X				X		X
Cerebral edema				X	X		X			
Chills				X				X		X
Bradycardia			X					X	X	X
Decreased urine output	X			X	X	X				
Dehydration	X	X	X	X						
Diarrhea	X			X						
Hyperventilation	X			X				X	X	X

	EHS	Heat cramp[b]	Heat syncope[b]	Exercise heat exhaustion[b]	Exertional hyponatremia	Exertional sickling	Head injury	Cardiac[c]	Respiratory[d]	Shock
Hypotension	X							X		X
Low blood sodium concentrations (<130 mEq Na+L−1)					X					
Nausea/vomiting	X			X	X		X	X		X
Muscle cramps/pain		X				X				
Pulmonary edema					X				X	
Seizures	X				X					
Swelling of hands and feet					X					
Tachycardia (100–120 bpm)	X							X	X	X

From Casa et al. [21], with permission

bpm beats per minute, *CNS* central nervous system, *EHS* exertional heat stroke

[a]This table is not meant to be inclusive of all signs and symptoms of the conditions listed or of all conditions that could cause sudden death in sport. Nor is the table implying that all the signs and symptoms indicated for a particular condition would be present on each occasion

[b]Heat cramps (i.e., exercise associated muscle cramps), heat syncope, and heat exhaustion are not life threatening but are included due to similarity of these conditions with other conditions that could cause sudden death and the potential for confusion with acute recognition

[c]Cardiac conditions could be heart attack, hypertrophic cardiomyopathy, commotio cordis, etc.

[d]Respiratory could be asthma, pneumothorax, pulmonary edema, etc.

[e]CNS dysfunction could include altered consciousness, coma, confusion, disorientation, collapse, etc.

[f]Personality changes could include hysteria, irrational behavior, combativeness, aggressiveness, irritability, apathy, decreased mental acuity, etc.

Table 4.2 Common misconceptions surrounding the assessment of rectal temperature in exercising individuals to diagnose exertional heat stroke (EHS)

Misconception	Dispelling misconception
1. Assessing an individual's rectal temperature when EHS is suspected will expose the patient and create a concern for patient privacy	1. The on-site medical provider can ensure the patient's privacy with proper patient positioning, draping the patient with a sheet/towels, and being cognizant of surroundings (see Fig 4.4)
2. A qualified medical provider would risk legal liability issues in assessing a rectal temperature in a patient suspected of EHS who is a minor (under the legal age of consent in their respective geographical locale)	2. A qualified medical provider, an individual that is board certified and licensed within their respective jurisdiction that is acting within their scope of practice and training, is fully qualified and authorized to assess rectal temperature in a patient suspected of EHS
3. Administrator (e.g., athletic director) will not permit the use of rectal temperature by on-site qualified medical providers	3. This is oftentimes a concern within an athletics setting (e.g., secondary school athletics in the United States). Administrators making these decisions often have zero medical expertise or training and should not be permitted to make medical decisions that overrule the on-site medical provider. The on-site medical provider (e.g., athletic trainer), in conjunction with the overseeing sports medicine physician, should be permitted to be the sole decision-makers for the policies and procedures pertaining to the medical care of the patients they are employed to care for
4. Qualified medical providers lack the training and education in assessing rectal temperature	4. Some medical professions (e.g., athletic training) require education and hands-on training in assessment of rectal temperature as part of the standards required for these degree-granting programs to maintain their accreditation standards as of 2012. Medical providers certified prior to that date are expected to become proficient in these standards of care to remain current in medical practices within the scope of practice of their profession
5. An invalid measure (e.g., tympanic, temporal, oral, axillary) can be taken, with the resulting measure being used in an algorithm that translates to rectal temperature	5. External variables such as ambient temperature, skin temperature, presence of sweat on the skin, and presence of solar radiation confound the assessment of body temperature using external methods (tympanic, temporal, oral, and axillary temperature). As such, attempting to apply a normalized algorithm reduces the sensitivity and specificity of assessing an individual's internal body temperature
6. The organization/institution/entity does not have the financial means to purchase a thermometer to assess rectal temperature	6. The financial burden of purchasing a thermometer capable of assessing rectal temperature (range $15–$300 USD for a rigid device to one utilizing a flexible thermistor for continuous temperature assessment, respectively) should not deter any organization/institution/entity from purchasing this diagnostic tool. In the event of an EHS-related death and ensuing litigation for negligent care of the patient, those associated costs would far outweigh the cost of purchasing a thermometer

Table 4.2 (continued)

Misconception	Dispelling misconception
7. Assessment of rectal temperature is not needed in order to successfully treat EHS; assessment of CNS dysfunction is sufficient to diagnose EHS	7. Without an assessment of rectal temperature, the medical provider is unable to discern between EHS and other medical conditions exhibiting CNS dysfunction (see Table 4.1). Furthermore, the medical provider would be unable to gauge the length of cooling, which may cause a premature removal from the cooling source and prohibit reducing body temperature below the critical threshold for cell damage within 30 minutes to ensure survival

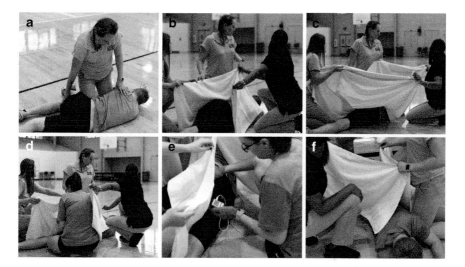

Fig. 4.4 Procedures to properly assess rectal temperature. (**a**) Position the patient on their side with the superior leg flexed. *Note*: If possible, the patient should be brought as close to the immersion tub as possible with the posterior aspect of their body positioned away from anyone in eyesight. The patient should be draped with either towels (**b**) or a sheet (**c**) to further limit the risk of exposure. Other medical providers (if available) or those educated and trained (e.g., athletics coaches, fellow military soldiers, occupational first responders/managers) can assist in maintaining patient privacy (**d**). (**e**) The on-site medical provider will position themselves behind the patient, lower their clothing to expose the buttocks, and insert the thermometer 15 cm past the anal sphincter to ensure an accurate measure. *Note*: If possible, a flexible thermistor should be used to gather a continuous measure of body temperature. (**f**) Once the thermistor is inserted, the patient's clothing can be returned to its original position prior to transporting the patient to the nearest CWI tub. *CWI* cold water immersion

Management and Care

Once a diagnosis of EHS has been confirmed by verification of internal body temperature >40 °C using rectal thermometry with associated altered mental status, immediate and aggressive whole-body cooling must ensue to optimize the patient's outcome. Prolonged hyperthermia >40.83 °C [105.5 °F], the critical threshold in humans for cell and tissue damage, precipitates an increased risk of morbidity and mortality, thus prompting expedient treatment. Support for this has been previously

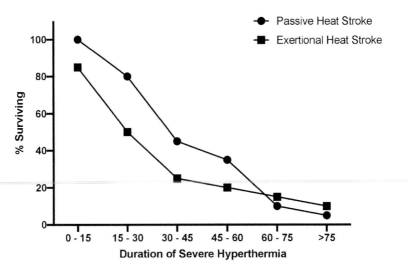

Fig. 4.5 Survivability rates in a rat model of heat stroke based on the duration and severity of thermal stress. Duration of severe hyperthermia = Σ time interval (min) × ½ [°C above 40.4 °C at start of interval + °C above 40.4 °C at end of interval]. (Adapted from Casa et al. [35], with permission)

shown in a rat model in that the duration of severe hyperthermia dictates survival rates (Fig. 4.5) [35]. In humans, evidence chronicling 274 EHS patients participating in a summer road running race has shown a 100% survival rate with no known sequelae when patients are cooled below the critical threshold for cell damage within 30 minutes [36].

Using the mantra "cool first, transport second," the goal of whole-body cooling in the treatment of EHS is to reduce the patient's rectal temperature below 40.0 °C within 30 minutes of collapse before transporting the patient to more advanced care [36–38]. Given the timeframe that clinicians must work with to reduce an EHS patient's body temperature to a safe level requires an expedient cooling modality that produces an ideal cooling rate of ≥0.155 °C/min [39]. Given water's 24-fold greater potential for thermal conductivity than air (630.5 mW/m²/°K versus 26.2 mW/m²/°K, respectively) [40], the current gold standard for EHS treatment is cold water immersion (Fig. 4.6) [1, 28–30, 36, 41].

To guarantee success as it relates to achieving optimal cooling rates, maximizing the amount of body surface area submersed in the cold water is imperative. In the event that the submersion tank/tub is small and/or the patient is large (e.g., American football lineman), covering any exposed body areas with rotating ice towels will assist in mitigating any declines in cooling rates of the patient (Fig. 4.7). Cooling an EHS patient must continue until the rectal temperature reaches 38.89 °C [102 °F] to prevent a subsequent rise in body temperature above the critical threshold once cooling has ceased as well as prevent the patient from becoming hypothermic [1, 20, 28, 29].

Other considerations that must be made regarding cooling an EHS patient are water temperature, physical characteristics, clothing/protective equipment, and alternative methods of body cooling if CWI is unavailable.

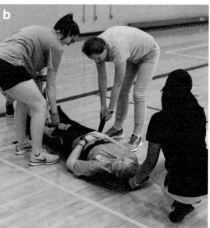

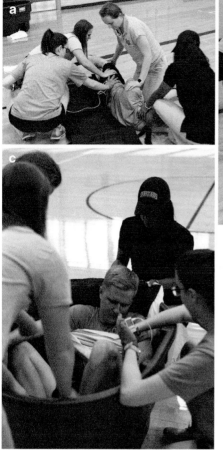

Fig. 4.6 Step-by-step procedure for implementing cold water immersion (CWI). (**a**) Once the rectal thermistor is inserted, the patient can be rolled into a supine position. If there is access to a porous, poleless stretcher, roll the patient onto the stretcher to assist in transporting the patient. (**b**) Once the patient is in a supine position and placed on the porous stretcher, the medical personnel and staff can transport the patient to the CWI tub. *Note*: If there is not access to a porous stretcher, utilizing a 4–6-person lift is an effective and safe alternative for transporting the patient. Caution must be made to ensure that the rectal thermistor remains in place during transport. (**c**) Place the patient in the CWI tub with as much of their body being immersed in the cold water as possible. Cover any exposed surface area, including the head, with cold, wet towels to assist in the cooling process. The medical provider at the patient's head should place a sheet and/or towels under the patient's arms to ensure their head remains above water. *Note*: The cold water must be continuously stirred to maximize the convective properties of water

Water Temperature

Water temperature of 2–20 °C has been shown to produce ideal cooling rates (≥0.155 °C/min) within scientific literature [39]. Other literature has shown that temperate water temperatures (21–26 °C) can produce acceptable cooling rates

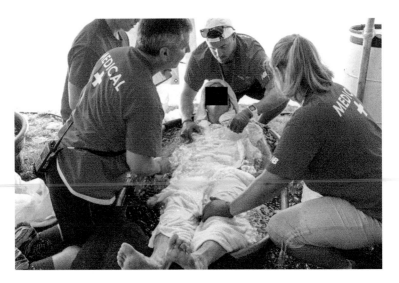

Fig. 4.7 An example of CWI treatment in an EHS patient. With large patients, utilizing ice towels to cover exposed body surface areas aids in optimizing cooling rates

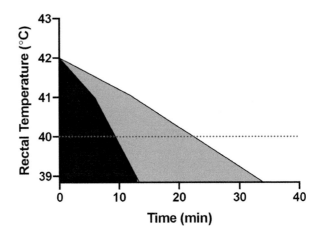

Fig. 4.8 Hypothetical model of EHS patient (initial rectal temperature of 42 °C) cooling time utilizing cold water immersion with water temperature of 2 °C (shaded in black) or 26 °C (shaded in gray). The dotted red line at $y = 40.0$ °C dictates the threshold that clinicians should aim to reduce rectal temperature under within 30 minutes of collapse with cooling ceasing once rectal temperature reaches 38.89 °C. (Redrawn using cooling rate data from Friesen et al. [43])

(0.078–0.154 °C/min) [42, 43], which would have the ability to reduce rectal temperature to <40 °C within 30 minutes (if initial rectal temperature is ≤42 °C) (Fig. 4.8); however, the goal is to keep water temperature <15 °C to ensure ideal cooling rates.

Physical Characteristics

Physical characteristics such as body size, shape, and composition may influence whole-body cooling rates with CWI. Prior literature has shown that those with a low body surface area-to-lean body mass ratio exhibit reduced cooling rates and longer cooling times than those with a high body surface area-to-lean body mass ratio [43]. In addition, individuals with larger amounts of subcutaneous fat and/or small body surface area to mass ratios tend to exhibit reduced cooling rates in normothermic conditions [44]. It must be acknowledged, however, that these latter findings do not depict cooling of hyperthermic individuals; when CWI is applied to hyperthermic individuals, differences in body fat and body surface area to mass on cooling rates are negligible [45, 46], thus supporting the efficiency of CWI in effectively cooling individuals with severe hyperthermia.

Clothing/Protective Equipment

Confirmation of EHS in an individual donning protective equipment (e.g., military soldier, American football uniform, etc.) necessitates removal of protective equipment prior to cooling to maximize body surface area. In some instances, it may not be feasible to remove the protective equipment immediately, such as when an EHS patient may be combative or the time it would take to remove the protective equipment would impede on the overall cooling time. In situations such as these, it is recommended that patients be immersed in a CWI tub, with removal of protective equipment occurring once cooling has commenced [47, 48].

Alternative Methods of Body Cooling

Some settings (e.g., military operations, wilderness firefighting, etc.) may not be conducive to having a CWI tub on-site in the event of an EHS. In these instances, alternative cooling methods must be implemented to ensure cooling takes place. Tarp-assisted cooling, a portable cooling modality that mimics CWI, has been shown to produce ideal cooling rates (>0.155 °C/min) that can be easily utilized in remote settings when access to a large tub is absent [49–51]. Rotating ice water towels (cooling rates, 0.11 °C/min) can also be easily implemented and may be another alternative method of cooling if CWI is not available; however, the clinician must determine the time to cool the patient to ensure timely treatment.

Lastly, once the EHS patient has been treated on-site (body temperature < 38.89 °C), the patient must be transported to a higher care medical facility to have follow-up laboratory work performed to ensure normal physiologic function [20]. In some instances, there may not be appropriate on-site medical personnel and/or appropriate cooling modalities. In these situations, immediate transport to the hospital is warranted; however, it is prudent that attempts to cool the patient en route to the hospital and once the patient arrives at the hospital continue to minimize the length of time spent in hyperthermia.

Return to Physical Activity

While clear guidelines have been established for the successful treatment of EHS, the process of returning individuals who have survived EHS is much more ambiguous. A lack of evidence due to an inability to systematically research this topic in a human population coupled with the relatively low number of occurrences when compared to other major causes of death limits the evidence on return to play/duty/work guidelines. Return decisions must also take into context the activity and situation the individual wishes to participate in. The military, for example, must be much more stringent on its qualifications for an individual to return to duty due to the potential for unregulated and unpredictable scenarios they may be placed in. A sport athlete, in comparison, may have more flexibility and the ability to have safety precautions, like individual athlete monitoring, in place.

Typically, immediately following an EHS, blood markers will be used to monitor organ function and recovery status. Traditional markers include those related to liver function (aspartate aminotransferase, AST; alanine aminotransferase, ALT), kidney function (blood urea nitrogen, BUN), and muscle damage, most notably creatine kinase (CK). It is important to note that these markers are not necessarily specific to EHS as they may also be altered by a variety of factors [52]. While recommendations call for these biomarkers to return to normal values, followed by a progressive return to activity, these steps do not guarantee one's ability to return to exercise in the heat safely [52]. Unfortunately today's current biomarkers remain as supporting values to aid in determining progression back to activity and are not diagnostically sound tools for determining future risk for subsequent heat illness. Currently, consensus remains that the following progression is the best approach for the assessment of an individual's ability to return to activity following EHS [1, 28, 53]:

- Monitor athlete until normal blood work is obtained; ensure that kidney and liver function returns to baseline levels.
- Wait at least 7–21 days before any activity is performed.
- Obtain physician clearance before any activity or progression for return to activity starts in conjunction with the first two bullets.
- Initiate activity with low-intensity exercise in a cool environment to progressively increase to higher intensity exercise in a cool environment.
- Begin exercise progression within a warm environment once exercise in a cool environment is successfully achieved.
- Begin a period of heat acclimatization prior to full return to activity.
- Have a medical professional monitor for signs and symptoms of exertional heat illness.

Ideally, body temperature (either via rectal or gastrointestinal temperature) should be monitored during the initial return to exercise and during the initial 7–10 exposures to exercise in warm to hot environments. If progression is stalled due to inability to thermoregulate, reoccurrence of symptoms, and/or an inability to recover from a previous day's training session, a heat tolerance test (HTT) should be considered. Two other circumstances may automatically call for a HTT to be performed. First, if the individual has not received the standard of care for EHS (if the individual was not completely cooled to a rectal temperature of 38.89 °C or lower within 30 minutes of the onset of EHS), a HTT should be considered prior to any exercise with heat exposure. Second, a HTT should also be considered when the person has had a previous episode of EHS as this could suggest other underlying pathology (e.g., malignant hyperthermia) [54, 55] or incomplete recovery from the previous EHS (Fig. 4.9).

While there is no validated, objective measure or procedure that can evaluate the body's ability to handle exercise heat stress (generally termed heat tolerance) following an EHS, the HTT has been a highly successful tool within the military to determine if a soldier is prepared to return to duty. This was the original purpose of the heat tolerance test (HTT), which was first developed by the Israel Defense Forces [56, 57]. Recently, a publication by Shermann [58] demonstrated the HTT had a specificity of 77.7%, demonstrating that a negative test is a strong indicator

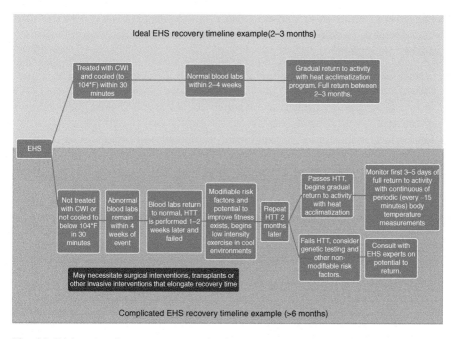

Fig. 4.9 Dichotomy of two common exertional heat stroke recovery scenarios based on initial treatment provided. *Top line* represents ideal or optimal return scenario; *bottom line* represents a complicated recovery scenario. *HTT* heat tolerance testing, *CWI* cold water immersion

for successful return to the military without further EHS incidents. Currently, insufficient data are available to support the HTT as a diagnostic test, but it does serve as a functional test to assess a person's responses within that moment. We believe a successful HTT should be a tool that is incorporated into a larger decision-making process that considers other factors impacting an individual's ability to return to a pre-EHS lifestyle. Although the HTT has been determined to be a functional test of heat tolerance, it does not account for modifiable factors such as aerobic capacity, training, acclimatization status, or body fat, which have all been demonstrated as significant predictors of HTT outcomes [59, 60]. Therefore, the status of each of these items must be assessed at the time of the HTT to determine if further improvement may be possible via these modifiable factors.

In addition to the return criteria and progression outlined above, particular considerations need to be included for the activity that the individual will be returning to, specifically if the individual is headed back to the military, sport, or labor industry. As noted, a return to military duty represents the most stringent criteria for return. This is because a military member may be sent back to duty or assignment in an area where his/her duties may not be regulated or monitored, placing that individual at risk for a subsequent EHS. Additionally, many military missions may rely upon a group dynamic, where if one member of the team is incapacitated or unable to perform their duty, the entire group would be placed at risk. These types of high-stakes scenarios are what lead military return to duty decisions regarding EHS patients to lean on the conservative end. Within the Israel Defense Forces protocol, the HTT is performed about 6 weeks following the EHS and is not performed before complete clinical recovery [56, 57]. The following criteria are followed for the Israel Defense Forces HTT:

- Individual core temperature must be below 37.5 °C (99.5 °F) at the time of testing.
- Walks on treadmill for 120 minutes at 5 km/h with 2% incline.
- Environment is controlled to maintain 40 °C (104 °F) and 40% relative humidity.
- Individuals are instructed to avoid tobacco, alcohol, and caffeine prior (24 h) to the test.
- Individuals are instructed to sleep at least 7 hours the night before and drink 0.5 L of water the hour before the test.
- Heat intolerance is determined when core body temperature elevates above 38.5 °C, heart rate elevates above 150 bpm, or when either does not plateau [57]. Core temperature plateau is defined as an increase not more than 0.45 °C during the second hour of the test [61].
- If response is abnormal, soldier is scheduled for a second test 1–3 months later.
- If the second test is abnormal, the soldier is defined as heat intolerant and cannot continue combat military service but may serve in other capacities.

Certainly one of the points that should be emphasized is that this test has been performed for over 40 years with very good success. However these results are specific to relatively young and fit individuals, and these testing parameters may not be applicable or practical for other populations such as athletes or laborers. Within the

US military, the HTT is used as a discretionary test for service members whose duty assignment or training may demand objective data to the ability of that service member's ability to return to duty. This decision is typically left to the clinician who must consider the clinical picture, the HTT results, and the specific duty demands that will be asked of the individual [62].

When applying the HTT to an athletic population, it has been criticized for not being sport specific or reflective of the demands of a specific sport [63–65]. It is generally accepted that the HTT is a good initial screening tool for advancement and progression towards a full return to activity as a failed test is a strong indicator that the individual is not prepared to progress at that point in time. While there have been some attempts to create a sport-specific protocol, no standardized or validated protocol has been established for athletes or a specific sport. A study by Mee et al. [64] is most promising, as it examined athletes within the same environmental conditions as the Israel Defense Forces HTT but asked that they run at 9 km/h for 30 minutes at 2% incline (passing criteria was met if rectal temperature remained below 39.7 °C). While this study was performed on healthy individuals, it did demonstrate good agreement and low variability within the results, which may be a step in the right direction to identify a higher intensity HTT that may be a better predictor for success within athletes following an EHS. Therefore, while there is not a sport-specific HTT, the standard HTT still provides a good starting point within the athletic population for early identification of individuals who undoubtedly should not return to sport if they are unable to pass the HTT. These individuals should also be assessed for modifiable risk factors (fitness, acclimatization status, and body fat) to determine if there is room for improvement via one of these factors. If so, a second test may be deemed appropriate in ~2–3 months after the athlete has had time to address these modifiable risk factors. While there is no guarantee for athletes who pass the HTT, they should continue their progression forward with close monitoring by the medical staff until they are able to demonstrate appropriate physiological responses to the demands of their sport. As noted above, athletes should be monitored during the initial weeks of returning to activity and demonstrate a successful full return to normal practices before tapering active medical monitoring.

The HTT is used even less so within the laborer population. The authors are unable to find or provide any literature that demonstrates the use or validity of the HTT within the laborer population. This is likely because the EHS recovery process for a laborer is likely to be handled by a primary care physician who may not be versed in treatment for EHS nor have access to facilities that would house the equipment necessary to conduct a HTT. The laborer industry is likely to suffer from the same limitations as the sporting world where there may be a wide variety of demands, individuals, ages, and fitness levels, which would all impact their results and interpretation of their results for the traditional HTT. Much more research is required to determine the need and validity of the HTT within the laborer population.

When determining an individual's ability to return to duty, sport, or work, it is important to consider the modifiable factors contributing to the body's heat tolerance that include the individual's body size (waist circumference, body fat), exercise intensity, hydration status, clothing/equipment/load, fitness status, dietary supplements, drugs, sleep deprivation, and fatigue [59–61, 66–70]. These will all be important when determining the cause and prognosis of an individual who has had an EHS. While at this point, it is not clear which particular biological markers can be used to identify recovery or future risk for EHS, the same holds true with regard to the diagnostic feasibility of the HTT. Current best practices combine the use of blood biomarkers, overall clinical picture, results of a HTT, and ability to successfully complete a progressive return to activity protocol to determine if an athlete, soldier, or laborer should return to their given field. Future research is needed to identify the utility and validity of the HTT within athletes and laborers.

Summary

EHS is a medical emergency requiring prompt recognition, assessment, management, and care to optimize survivability. It is the responsibility of all medical providers that may be involved with EHS care (i.e., athletic trainers, EMS, emergency department physicians, sports medicine physicians) to be educated and trained in current evidence-based best practices for managing this condition. While not 100% preventable, 100% survival is possible when proper steps are taken to assess (i.e., determination of CNS dysfunction and body temperature using rectal thermometry) and treat (i.e., whole-body CWI) EHS.

References

1. Casa DJ, DeMartini JK, Bergeron MF, Csillan D, Eichner ER, Lopez RM, et al. National Athletic Trainers' Association position statement: exertional heat illnesses. J Athl Train. 2015;50(9):986–1000.
2. Lopez RM, Jardine JF. Exertional heat illnesses. In: Casa DJ, editor. Sport and physical activity in the heat: maximizing performance and safety. Cham: Springer; 2018. p. 313–30.
3. Rav-Acha M, Hadad E, Epstein Y, Heled Y, Moran DS. Fatal exertional heat stroke: a case series. Am J Med Sci. 2004;328(2):84–7.
4. Kerr ZY, Register-Mihalik JK, Pryor RR, Pierpoint LA, Scarneo SE, Adams WM, et al. The association between mandated preseason heat acclimatization guidelines and exertional heat illness during preseason high school American football practices. Environ Health Perspect. 2019;127(4):47003.
5. Bouchama A, Knochel JP. Heat stroke. N Engl J Med. 2002;346(25):1978–88.
6. Epstein Y, Roberts WO. The pathophysiology of heat stroke: an integrative view of the final common pathway. Scand J Med Sci Sports. 2011;21(6):742–8.
7. Pedersen BK, Hoffman-Goetz L. Exercise and the immune system: regulation, integration, and adaptation. Physiol Rev. 2000;80(3):1055–81.
8. Cannon JG. Inflammatory cytokines in nonpathological states. News Physiol Sci. 2000;15:298–303.
9. Hietala J, Nurmi T, Uhari M, Pakarinen A, Kouvalainen K. Acute phase proteins, humoral and cell mediated immunity in environmentally-induced hyperthermia in man. Eur J Appl Physiol. 1982;49(2):271–6.

10. Hammami MM, Bouchama A, Shail E, Aboul-Enein HY, Al-Sedairy S. Lymphocyte subsets and adhesion molecules expression in heatstroke and heat stress. J Appl Physiol Bethesda (1985). 1998;84(5):1615–21.

11. Leon LR. Heat stroke and cytokines. Prog Brain Res. 2007;162:481–524.

12. Leon LR, Bouchama A. Heat stroke. Compr Physiol. 2015;5(2):611–47.

13. Yan Y-E, Zhao Y-Q, Wang H, Fan M. Pathophysiological factors underlying heatstroke. Med Hypotheses. 2006;67(3):609–17.

14. Lin MT. Pathogenesis of an experimental heatstroke model. Clin Exp Pharmacol Physiol. 1999;26(10):826–7.

15. Epstein Y, Hadad E, Shapiro Y. Pathological factors underlying hyperthermia. J Therm Biol. 2004;29(7–8):487–94.

16. Lambert GP. Role of gastrointestinal permeability in exertional heatstroke. Exerc Sport Sci Rev. 2004;32(4):185–90.

17. Vandermark LW, Adams WM, Asplund C, Hosokawa Y, Casa DJ. Heat stroke. In: Chopra JS, Sawhney IMS, editors. Neurology in tropics. 2nd ed. New Delhi: Reed Elsevier India; 2015. p. 896–908.

18. Lambert GP. Intestinal barrier dysfunction, endotoxemia, and gastrointestinal symptoms: the 'canary in the coal mine' during exercise-heat stress? Med Sport Sci. 2008;53:61–73.

19. Leon LR, Helwig BG. Heat stroke: role of the systemic inflammatory response. J Appl Physiol (1985). 2010;109(6):1980–8.

20. Belval LN, Casa DJ, Adams WM, Chiampas GT, Holschen JC, Hosokawa Y, et al. Consensus statement- prehospital care of exertional heat stroke. Prehosp Emerg Care. 2018;22(3):392–7.

21. Casa DJ, Pagnotta KD, Pinkus DP, Mazerolle SM. Should coaches be in charge of care for medical emergencies in high school sports? Athl Train Sports Health Care. 2009;1(4):144–6.

22. Casa DJ, Becker SM, Ganio MS, Brown CM, Yeargin SW, Roti MW, et al. Validity of devices that assess body temperature during outdoor exercise in the heat. J Athl Train. 2007;42(3):333–42.

23. Ganio MS, Brown CM, Casa DJ, Becker SM, Yeargin SW, McDermott BP, et al. Validity and reliability of devices that assess body temperature during indoor exercise in the heat. J Athl Train. 2009;44(2):124–35.

24. Miller KC, Hughes LE, Long BC, Adams WM, Casa DJ. Validity of core temperature measurements at 3 rectal depths during rest, exercise, cold-water immersion, and recovery. J Athl Train. 2017;52(4):332–8.

25. Huggins R, Glaviano N, Negishi N, Casa DJ, Hertel J. Comparison of rectal and aural core body temperature thermometry in hyperthermic, exercising individuals: a meta-analysis. J Athl Train. 2012;47(3):329–38.

26. Lee SM, Williams WJ, Fortney Schneider SM. Core temperature measurement during supine exercise: esophageal, rectal, and intestinal temperatures. Aviat Space Environ Med. 2000;71(9):939–45.

27. Gagnon D, Lemire BB, Jay O, Kenny GP. Aural canal, esophageal, and rectal temperatures during exertional heat stress and the subsequent recovery period. J Athl Train. 2010;45(2):157–63.

28. Casa DJ, Guskiewicz KM, Anderson SA, Courson RW, Heck JF, Jimenez CC, et al. National athletic trainers' association position statement: preventing sudden death in sports. J Athl Train. 2012;47(1):96–118.

29. Armstrong LE, Casa DJ, Millard-Stafford M, Moran DS, Pyne SW, Roberts WO. American College of Sports Medicine position stand. Exertional heat illness during training and competition. Med Sci Sports Exerc. 2007;39(3):556–72.

30. Binkley HM, Beckett J, Casa DJ, Kleiner DM, Plummer PE. National Athletic Trainers' Association position statement: exertional heat illnesses. J Athl Train. 2002;37(3):329–43.

31. Casa DJ, Almquist J, Anderson SA, Baker L, Bergeron MF, Biagioli B, et al. The inter-association task force for preventing sudden death in secondary school athletics programs: best-practices recommendations. J Athl Train. 2013;48(4):546–53.

32. National Athletic Trainers' Association. Inter-association taskforce on exertional heat illnesses consensus statement [Internet]. 2003. https://www.nata.org/sites/default/files/inter-association-task-force-exertional-heat-illness.pdf.

33. Mazerolle SM, Scruggs IC, Casa DJ, Burton LJ, McDermott BP, Armstrong LE, et al. Current knowledge, attitudes, and practices of certified athletic trainers regarding recognition and treatment of exertional heat stroke. J Athl Train. 2010;45(2):170–80.

34. Nedimyer AK, Chandran A, Hirschorn RM, Adams WM, Pryor RR, Casa DJ, et al. Exertional heat stroke management strategies: a comparison of practice and intentions between athletic trainers who did and did not treat cases during high school football preseason (abstract). J Athl Train. 2019;54(6 Suppl):S-69.

35. Casa DJ, Kenny GP, Taylor NAS. Immersion treatment for exertional hyperthermia: cold or temperate water? Med Sci Sports Exerc. 2010;42(7):1246–52.

36. DeMartini JK, Casa DJ, Stearns R, Belval L, Crago A, Davis R, Jardine J. Effectiveness of cold water immersion in the treatment of exertional heat stroke at the Falmouth Road Race. Med Sci Sports Exerc. 2014;47(2):240–5.

37. Adams WM, Hosokawa Y, Casa DJ. The timing of exertional heat stroke survival starts prior to collapse. Curr Sports Med Rep. 2015;14(4):273–4.

38. Adams WM. Exertional heat stroke within secondary school athletics. Curr Sports Med Rep. 2019;18(4):149–53.

39. McDermott BP, Casa DJ, Ganio MS, Lopez RM, Yeargin SW, Armstrong LE, et al. Acute whole-body cooling for exercise-induced hyperthermia: a systematic review. J Athl Train. 2009;44(1):84–93.

40. Casa DJ, McDermott BP, Lee EC, Yeargin SW, Armstrong LE, Maresh CM. Cold water immersion: the gold standard for exertional heatstroke treatment. Exerc Sport Sci Rev. 2007;35(3):141–9.

41. Proulx CI, Ducharme MB, Kenny GP. Effect of water temperature on cooling efficiency during hyperthermia in humans. J Appl Physiol Bethesda Md (1985). 2003;94(4):1317–23.

42. Miller KC, Truxton T, Long B. Temperate-water immersion as a treatment for hyperthermic humans wearing American football uniforms. J Athl Train. 2017;52(8):747–52.

43. Friesen BJ, Carter MR, Poirier MP, Kenny GP. Water immersion in the treatment of exertional hyperthermia: physical determinants. Med Sci Sports Exerc. 2014;46(9):1727–35.

44. Sloan RE, Keatinge WR. Cooling rates of young people swimming in cold water. J Appl Physiol. 1973;35(3):371–5.

45. Lemire BB, Gagnon D, Jay O, Kenny GP. Differences between sexes in rectal cooling rates after exercise-induced hyperthermia. Med Sci Sports Exerc. 2009;41(8):1633–9.

46. Lemire B, Gagnon D, Jay O, Dorman L, DuCharme MB, Kenny GP. Influence of adiposity on cooling efficiency in hyperthermic individuals. Eur J Appl Physiol. 2008;104(1):67–74.

47. Miller KC, Long BC, Edwards J. Necessity of removing American football uniforms from humans with hyperthermia before cold-water immersion. J Athl Train. 2015;50(12):1240–6.

48. Miller KC, Swartz EE, Long BC. Cold-water immersion for hyperthermic humans wearing American football uniforms. J Athl Train. 2015;50(8):792–9.

49. Hosokawa Y, Adams WM, Belval LN, Vandermark LW, Casa DJ. Tarp-assisted cooling as a method of whole-body cooling in hyperthermic individuals. Ann Emerg Med. 2017;69(3):347–52.

50. Luhring KE, Butts CL, Smith CR, Bonacci JA, Ylanan RC, Ganio MS, et al. Cooling effectiveness of a modified cold-water immersion method after exercise-induced hyperthermia. J Athl Train. 2016;51(11):946–51.

51. Adams WM. An alternative method for treating exertional heat stroke: tarp-assisted cooling. Athl Train Sports Health Care. 2019;11(3):101–2.

52. Goddard CJ, Warnes TW. Raised liver enzymes in asymptomatic patients: investigation and outcome. Dig Dis Basel Switz. 1992;10(4):218–26.

53. American College of Sports Medicine, Armstrong LE, Casa DJ, Millard-Stafford M, Moran DS, Pyne SW, et al. American College of Sports Medicine position stand. Exertional heat illness during training and competition. Med Sci Sports Exerc. 2007;39(3):556–72.

54. Poussel M, Guerci P, Kaminsky P, Heymonet M, Roux-Buisson N, Faure J, et al. Exertional heat stroke and susceptibility to malignant hyperthermia in an athlete: evidence for a link? J Athl Train. 2015;50(11):1212–4.
55. Sagui E, Montigon C, Abriat A, Jouvion A, Duron-Martinaud S, Canini F, et al. Is there a link between exertional heat stroke and susceptibility to malignant hyperthermia? PLoS One. 2015;10(8):e0135496.
56. Epstein Y. Heat intolerance: predisposing factor or residual injury? Med Sci Sports Exerc. 1990;22(1):29–35.
57. Moran DS, Erlich T, Epstein Y. The heat tolerance test: an efficient screening tool for evaluating susceptibility to heat. J Sport Rehabil. 2007;16(3):215–21.
58. Schermann H, Heled Y, Fleischmann C, Ketko I, Schiffmann N, Epstein Y, et al. The validity of the heat tolerance test in prediction of recurrent exertional heat illness events. J Sci Med Sport. 2018;21(6):549–52.
59. Druyan A, Amit D, Makranz C, Moran D, Yanovich R, Epstein Y, et al. Heat tolerance in women—reconsidering the criteria. Aviat Space Environ Med. 2012;83(1):58–60.
60. Lisman P, Kazman JB, O'Connor FG, Heled Y, Deuster PA. Heat tolerance testing: association between heat intolerance and anthropometric and fitness measurements. Mil Med. 2014;179(11):1339–46.
61. Druyan A, Ketko I, Yanovich R, Epstein Y, Heled Y. Refining the distinction between heat tolerant and intolerant individuals during a heat tolerance test. J Therm Biol. 2013;38(8):539–42.
62. Casa DJ, editor. Sport and physical activity in the heat: maximizing performance and safety. Cham: Springer; 2018.
63. Johnson EC, Kolkhorst FW, Richburg A, Schmitz A, Martinez J, Armstrong LE. Specific exercise heat stress protocol for a triathlete's return from exertional heat stroke. Curr Sports Med Rep. 2013;12(2):106–9.
64. Mee JA, Doust J, Maxwell NS. Repeatability of a running heat tolerance test. J Therm Biol. 2015;49–50:91–7.
65. Roberts WO, Dorman JC, Bergeron MF. Recurrent heat stroke in a runner: race simulation testing for return to activity. Med Sci Sports Exerc. 2016;48(5):785–9.
66. Hursel R, Westerterp-Plantenga MS. Thermogenic ingredients and body weight regulation. Int J Obes. 2010;34(4):659–69.
67. Lyons J, Allsopp A, Bilzon J. Influences of body composition upon the relative metabolic and cardiovascular demands of load-carriage. Occup Med (Lond). 2005;55(5):380–4.
68. Ricciardi R, Deuster PA, Talbot LA. Metabolic demands of body armor on physical performance in simulated conditions. Mil Med. 2008;173(9):817–24.
69. Vaughan RA, Conn CA, Mermier CM. Effects of commercially available dietary supplements on resting energy expenditure: a brief report. ISRN Nutr. 2014;2014:650264.
70. Adams WM, Belval LN. Return-to-activity following exertional heat stroke. Athl Train Sports Health Care. 2018;10(1):5–6.

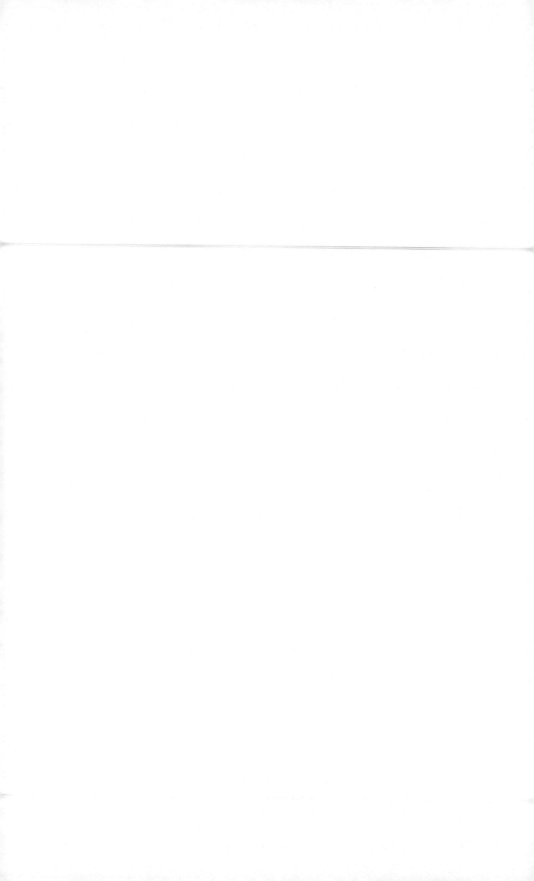

Chapter 5
Heat Exhaustion

Lawrence E. Armstrong

Introduction

Athletes, recreational enthusiasts, laborers, and soldiers occasionally experience a common failure during their activities: inability to continue exercise in a hot environment. Known as exertional heat exhaustion (H_{EX}), this illness is categorized with heat cramps, heat syncope, and the medical emergency heat stroke in the International Classification of Diseases [1]. It represents the most common illness encountered during summer sports, military activities, and year-round indoor industrial heat exposures [2–4], yet it proves to be enigmatic for clinicians and physiologists for two reasons. First, the duration and intensity of exercise, the degree of stress placed on the heart and blood vessels, rate of water and salt loss in sweat, as well as the amount of heat stored in skeletal muscle and internal organs affect the type and extent of physiological responses that act to restore homeostasis. These responses or abnormal responses may be observed as signs and symptoms involving the nervous, cardiovascular, muscular, excretory, and gastrointestinal systems of the body; they also are influenced by multiple, interacting, inherent, and environment factors. Second, anyone (e.g., even healthy, highly-trained world class endurance athletes) can experience H_{EX} if he/she exercises or labors beyond personal physiological limits, in a hot environment, for a prolonged period of time.

During the mid-1960s, this complex clinical situation prompted extended collaboration between the Medical Research Council, the Climatic Physiology Committee (United Kingdom), and the National Academy of Sciences-National Research Council Subcommittee on Thermal Factors in the Environment (United States). These groups acted to update the heat illness categories published in the

L. E. Armstrong (✉)
Hydration & Nutrition, LLC, Newport News, VA, USA

Department of Kinesiology (Professor Emeritus), University of Connecticut, Storrs, CT, USA
e-mail: lawrence.armstrong@uconn.edu

© Springer Nature Switzerland AG 2020
W. M. Adams, J. F. Jardine (eds.), *Exertional Heat Illness*,
https://doi.org/10.1007/978-3-030-27805-2_5

World Health Organization's 1957 *Manual of the International Classification of Diseases, seventh revision* [5]. In an editorial summary of recommendations, Minard [6] described three categories of H_{EX}: salt and/or water depletion, anhidrotic, and unqualified. To that date, these categories best explained the complicated clinical picture of H_{EX} by classifying diseases according to cause, with environmental heat as the unifying etiologic factor. In 2019, the International Classification of Diseases Tenth Revision contains ten codes specific to "effects of heat and light" [1]. Three different codes for H_{EX} are specified: anhydrotic (T67.3), due to salt depletion (T67.4), and unspecified (T67.5).

The aforementioned complexity and difficulty of classifying H_{EX} has been acknowledged in various research and clinical publications. For example, DeGroot et al. [7] conducted a retrospective chart review of exertional heat illness casualties admitted to Martin Army Community Hospital, Fort Benning, GA from 2009 to 2012. All cases with a primary ICD-9 diagnostic code for heat illness from April 1 to October 31 of each year were included. Medical record analyses indicated the following number of cases for each category of H_{EX}: anhidrotic, 3; salt depletion, 1; and unspecified, 107. DeGroot et al. [7] stated that textbooks generally agree on the definition of heat exhaustion as well as diagnostic criteria. However, his analysis suggested that there is considerable variability in how clinicians interpret and apply these criteria with respect to ICD-9 coding. In addition, Armstrong and Lopez [8] noted that severe cases of exertional heat exhaustion in athletes are difficult to distinguish in the field from cases of exertional heat stroke because these illnesses share common signs and symptoms. Both conditions involve a deep internal temperature of 39–40 °C (i.e., which is widely accepted as the threshold for the onset of exertional heat stroke) that may or may not be evaluated in a field setting. Similarly, when evaluating exertional heat illnesses at a large summer road race, DeMartini et al. [9] acknowledged that the term heat exhaustion has been scrutinized because of its lack of distinguishing diagnostic criteria and uncertain pathophysiology.

Table 5.1 [6, 10–19] illustrates the evolution of selected paradigms and clinical features of H_{EX}, from 1935 to 2015. Considering the variety and complexity in Table 5.1, it is reasonable to pose two questions, "How can we reconcile the diverse observations and reports regarding H_{EX}?" and "Are the pathophysiology and signs/symptoms of H_{EX} similar in all sport, military, and industrial settings?"

Etiology

In September of 1912, Naval Surgeon Charles N. Fiske presented a report to the attendees of the International Congress on Health & Hygiene in Washington, D.C. [20]. His accounts of heat casualties aboard more than 20 US seagoing vessels (1861–1911) demonstrated that the term "heat prostration" was used sparingly through the year 1877, in reference to both heat exhaustion and heat stroke, without standardized diagnostic criteria. From 1885 forward, the term heat exhaustion was used extensively. Due to the coal-fired boilers that propelled ships during that

Table 5.1 Exertional heat exhaustion descriptions and classifications spanning 80 years

Etiology	Pathophysiology	Signs and symptoms of heat exhaustion	Treatment/management	Authors/purpose
Observations of humans living in tropical climates, working in industrial settings, and exercising in artificial laboratory environments distinguish two clusters of relevant physiological responses: (1) circulatory insufficiency and (2) electrolyte imbalance. These disorders have multiple common etiological factors	(1) Circulatory insufficiency occurs when the combined stresses of exercise and ambient heat exceed the cardiac capacity to maintain normal functions. Aggravated by fluid-electrolyte losses (2) Electrolyte imbalance is defined as a low serum chloride (Cl⁻) conc. of ≤100 mEq/L (sodium [Na⁺] conc. ≤139 mEq/L), primarily due to replacement of water loss in sweat without replacement of electrolytes	(1) Vertigo, fainting, collapse, nausea, headache, vomiting, respiratory disturbance, fatigue, and exhaustion are present in varying proportions. (2) Reduced serum Na⁺ and Cl⁻ conc. Loss of body weight. Tingling leading to muscle cramps. Vomiting and diarrhea. Normal rectal temperature Heat exhaustion and heat cramps often are observed with overlapping symptoms. Hyperpyrexia (i.e., heat stroke) and life-threatening loss of body water (20–25% of body mass) are classified as distinct disorders	Both (1) and (2) respond rapidly to intravenous (i.v.) saline administration	Lee, report to the Royal Society of Tropical Medicine and Hygiene, UK [10]

(continued)

Table 5.1 (continued)

Etiology	Pathophysiology	Signs and symptoms of heat exhaustion	Treatment/management	Authors/purpose
Industrial labor, mining and military activities. Exercise-induced sweating that leads to dehydration and large salt losses in sweat. Elevated internal body temperature or skeletal muscle cramps may or may not be involved. Long duration of heat exposure each day	Classified four types of heat exhaustion: *anhydrotic*: sweating deficiency usually preceded by severe prickly heat (miliaria rubra): *salt deficiency*: inadequate replacement of salt loss due to sweat and urine losses, leading to dehydration and reduced blood volume; *water deficiency*: lack of drinking water or low volume intake; and *exercise-induced* (e.g., marching or digging)	*Anhydrotic*: General physical and mental loss of energy and initiative, irritability, loss of appetite, difficulty sleeping and working. While under heat stress, intense warmth, dyspnea, tachycardia and distress. Eventual collapse with possible loss of consciousness. Skin is dry except on the face, palms, soles of the feet, and axillae. *Salt deficiency (Type I)*: collapse with pallor, sweating, vomiting, and sometimes muscle cramps. Hemoconcentration. Urine is concentrated with small volume and low sodium concentration. *Water deficiency (Type II)*: thirst, vague discomfort, anorexia, impatience, sleepiness, weariness, dizziness. Tingling, dyspnea, cyanosis in advanced cases. Walking pace cannot be maintained, inability to stand, incoordination, hysteria, or delirium. *Exercise-induced*: exertion is halted voluntarily due to exhaustion or collapse. Syncope may occur if upright posture is sustained after exercise	Heat exhaustion treatment options are not described	Weiner and Horne, UK Medical Research Council, Climatic Physiology Committee report [11]

As part of updated nomenclature and classification of heat illnesses, three types of heat exhaustion are recognized: (a) salt and/or water depletion, (b) anhidrotic, and (c) unqualified	The pathophysiologies of heat disorders are not described	In this one-page document, specific signs and symptoms of heat disorders are not described. General descriptions include (a) salt and/or water depletion is used as a compromise term in the field, where physicians rely on clinical observations and judgment without the aid of laboratory tools; (b) extensive obstruction of sweat-gland ducts leads to impaired evaporative cooling, with loss of heat tolerance; and (c) diagnosis by exclusion Distinct from heat exhaustion, transient heat fatigue is presented as a new heat illness classification, to designate the deterioration of skilled performance occasionally observed in an otherwise normal adult during short exposures to extreme heat. Recovery is prompt upon return to a cool environment	Heat exhaustion treatment options are not described	Minard summary of UK and US government medical and research committee joint efforts [6]

(continued)

Table 5.1 (continued)

Etiology	Pathophysiology	Signs and symptoms of heat exhaustion	Treatment/management	Authors/purpose
Soldiers working or marching in hot or hot-wet environments. Heavy sweating with inadequate water and salt replacement. Excessive cardiovascular demand and water-electrolyte depletion exist in all cases. Two forms of heat exhaustion are distinguished: water depletion and salt depletion	Heat exhaustion is due to the combination of excessive cardiovascular demand (i.e., reduced "effective" organs), reduced "effective" plasma volume, reduced venous return to the heart (due to vasodilation in skin and active muscle), and sweat-induced depletion of water and salt. A single episode of heat exhaustion does not imply predisposition to heat injury	The symptoms of heat exhaustion are non-specific. No combination of presenting symptoms and signs is characteristic of this illness. Each patient requires careful clinical evaluation addressed to the presenting complaints, including thirst, syncope, profound physical fatigue, nausea, vomiting, hyperventilation with carpopedal spasm, dyspnea, muscle cramps, confusion, anxiety and agitation, mood change, orthostatic dizziness, ataxia, hyperthermia, and frontal headache. Water depletion and salt depletion heat exhaustion exhibit subtly different signs and symptoms. This is a functional illness and is not associated with evidence of organ damage	Removal of gear or clothing and rest in a shaded-ventilated area encourages spontaneous cooling. Pouring cool water over the skin encourages skin vasoconstriction and venous return to the heart. Extracellular volume is replenished rapidly by i.v. fluid. Patients with tachycardia at rest or orthostatic signs should initially receive normal saline in i.v. boluses of 200–250 cc to restore circulatory function. More than 2 L of normal saline should not be administered without laboratory surveillance	USARIEM Heat Illness Guide for Medical Officers [12]

Endurance running in a hot environment, including training and competition. The most susceptible individuals are those who exercise at or near their maximal capacity, are dehydrated, are not physically fit, and are not heat acclimatized	Failure of the cardiovascular responses to strenuous workload, high ambient temperature, and dehydration. Such dehydration reduces exercise capacity due to decreased circulating blood volume, blood pressure, sweat rate, and skin blood flow	Heat exhaustion has no known harmful, chronic effects. Symptoms may include headache, extreme weakness, dizziness, vertigo, heat cramps in skeletal muscles, sensation of heat on the head or neck, vomiting, nausea, irritability, and goose flesh. Depending on the severity of signs and symptoms, agitation, hyperventilation, muscle incoordination, impaired judgment, and confusion may be seen. Fainting may or may not accompany heat exhaustion. During the early stage, the patient may appear ashen-gray, the blood pressure may be low, and the pulse rate may be elevated	Oral rehydration is preferred for patients who are conscious, coherent, and without vomiting. Intravenous fluids facilitate rapid recovery; 5% dextrose sugar in either 0.45% saline (NaCl) or 0.9% saline is most commonly administered	ACSM Exertional Heat Illness Position Stand [13]

(continued)

Table 5.1 (continued)

Etiology	Pathophysiology	Signs and symptoms of heat exhaustion	Treatment/management	Authors/purpose
During exercise, repetitive muscle pumping action assists venous return to the heart. On cessation of exercise, this muscle assistance to blood flow ceases, and venous blood return may diminish rapidly enough to produce nausea, collapse, or syncope. Although this form of syncope may occur in the absence of EHI, clinical evaluation is warranted because the symptoms may be due to hypovolemia	Exertional heat exhaustion is a reversible, non-life-threatening multisystem disorder reflecting the inability of the circulatory system to meet the demands of thermoregulatory, muscular, cutaneous, and visceral blood flow. It represents primarily a syndrome of dehydration without serious metabolic complications. This is a reversible system dysfunction without evidence of organ damage or severe metabolic consequences	This illness usually involves minor elevations of internal temperature (<40 °C), but it can be associated with a very high rectal temperature in cases of severe heat exhaustion. If hyperthermia greater than 104 °F (40 °C) is measured rectally, rapid cooling to a body temperature of less than 102 °F (38.99 °C), rest, and rehydration are essential to prevent progression to heat stroke. Levels of progressive orthostatic signs and symptoms are proposed. *Mild*: faintness, dizziness, wobbly legs, stumbling gait, blurred or tunnel vision, blackout. *Exertional heat syncope*: collapse with brief (>3 min) loss of consciousness. *Severe*: evaluated via tilt tests. Shock or cardiovascular collapse are possible.	*Mild*: symptoms are rapidly improved by water and salt replacement, a cool environment, and rest. *Moderate-to-Severe*: patients with orthostatic hypotension are better treated with 1–2 liters of i.v. normal or half-normal saline, starting at a rate of 250–500 ml/h, and their responses are monitored. A history or evaluation that suggests hyponatremia (i.e., drinking large volume of water) or severe salt and water deficits indicates laboratory monitoring	Gardner and Kark, heat illness diagnosis, management, surveillance[a] [14]

	NATA Exertional Heat Illness Position Statement [15]
Exercise (heat) exhaustion is the inability to continue exercise and is associated with any combination of heavy sweating, dehydration, sodium loss, and energy depletion. It occurs most frequently in hot, humid environments	
Athletes with exercise (heat) exhaustion may exhibit these signs and symptoms: dehydration, dizziness, lightheadedness, syncope, headache, nausea, anorexia, diarrhea, decreased urine output, persistent muscle cramps, pallor, profuse sweating, chills, cool/ clammy skin, weakness, intestinal cramps, hyperventilation, and a rectal temperature that ranges between 36 °C (97 °F) and 40 °C (104 °F). Severe heat exhaustion is difficult to distinguish from exertional heat stroke without measuring rectal temperature. Cognitive changes are usually minimal, but bizarre behavior, hallucinations, altered mental status, confusion, disorientation, and coma suggest more serious conditions	The goal of athlete safety is addressed through the recognition of heat illness and a well-developed plan to evaluate and treat affected athletes. This includes knowledge of the common early signs and symptoms, a rectal thermometer to measure deep body temperature, a cooling zone (shaded, fans, air conditioned), a plan for emergency evacuation if needed, and a mobile phone to communicate with emergency personnel
In athletes, cumulative dehydration develops insidiously over several days and is typically observed during the first few days of a season or in tournament competition Cumulative dehydration can be detected by measuring daily prepractice and postpractice weights. The cumulative effects of a 1% fluid loss per day occurring over several days create an increased risk for heat illness and decreased exercise performance	

(continued)

Table 5.1 (continued)

Etiology	Pathophysiology	Signs and symptoms of heat exhaustion	Treatment/management	Authors/purpose
Selected intrinsic etiological factors: inadequate heat acclimatization, low physical fitness status, high percent body fat, dehydration, gastrointestinal illness, salt deficiency, medications (e.g., antihistamines, diuretics), dietary supplements (e.g., ephedra), motivation to push oneself to extreme limits. Selected extrinsic factors: Intense or prolonged exercise with few rest breaks; high ambient temperature, humidity, and sun exposure; minimal access to fluids before and during practice and rest periods; inappropriate work/rest ratios based on intensity and wet bulb globe temperature (WBGT); insulative clothing and equipment; lack of education and awareness of early warning signs among coaches, athletes, and medical staff; no emergency plan	Heat exhaustion is a moderate illness characterized by the inability to sustain adequate cardiac output, resulting from strenuous physical exercise and environmental heat stress. Inherent needs to maintain blood pressure and essential organ function, combined with a loss of fluid due to acute dehydration, create a challenge the body cannot meet, especially if intense exercise continues unabated	Most important criteria are (a) obvious difficulty continuing intense exercise in the heat, (b) lack of severe hyperthermia (usually <40 °C) although mild hyperthermia may be seen at the time of the incident (100°–103 °F, 37.7°–39.4 °C) and (c) lack of severe CNS dysfunction. Other salient findings may include physical fatigue, dehydration, electrolyte depletion, ataxia or coordination problems, syncope, dizziness, profuse sweating, pallor, headache, nausea, vomiting, diarrhea, stomach/intestinal cramps, persistent muscle cramps, and rapid recovery with treatment	The following procedures are recommended if heat exhaustion is suspected: move the athlete from activity to a shaded or air-conditioned area. Remove excess clothing and equipment. If hyperthermic, cool the athlete until rectal temperature is ~ 101 °F (38.3 °C). Lie the athlete supine with legs propped above heart level. If the athlete is not nauseated, vomiting, or experiencing CNS dysfunction, rehydrate orally with chilled water or sports drink. Alternatively, implement i.v. normal saline therapy. Monitor heart rate, blood pressure, respiratory rate, rectal temperature, and CNS status. Transport to an emergency facility if improvement is not rapid	Inter-Association Task Force Statement [16]

Military training or operations in high ambient temperature, humidity, and solar radiation with low air movement. Exercise in a hot environment produces metabolic heat, increased internal body temperature, body water loss as sweat, reduced blood volume, peripheral blood pooling in dilated and compliant skin, loss of splanchnic vasoconstriction, and reduced venous return to the heart	Heat exhaustion is not associated with evidence of organ damage. It occurs when the body cannot sustain cardiac output at a level that is necessary to meet the combined demands of skin blood flow for thermoregulation and blood flow to exercising skeletal muscle	The signs and symptoms include generalized weakness, fatigue, ataxia, dizziness, headache, nausea, vomiting, malaise, hypotension, tachycardia, muscle cramps, hyperventilation and transient alteration of mental status. Sweating may be profuse	Treatment and management details are similar to the above technical report (USARIEM 91–3, 1991). Although patients with heat exhaustion experience rapid clinical recovery, they need at least 24 h of rest and rehydration under medical supervision. Determine the reason for heat exhaustion (e.g., ratio of work-to-rest, water intake, coincident illness, or medication) and develop a plan to avoid similar episodes in the future	Department of the Army Technical Report, heat stress control, heat casualty management [17]

(continued)

Table 5.1 (continued)

Etiology	Pathophysiology	Signs and symptoms of heat exhaustion	Treatment/management	Authors/purpose
Several lines of evidence suggest that heat exhaustion Results from peripheral vascular dilation resulting in hypotension and cardiovascular insufficiency. If the air humidity is high, evaporative cooling is impaired, signaling the body to increase skin blood flow that aids nonevaporative heat loss. This explains why heat exhaustion commonly occurs on humid days	Exercise exhaustion may be triggered by some combination of reduced peripheral and central muscle activation, dehydration, depletion of energy stores, or electrolyte imbalance. In hot environments, post-exercise collapse may be due to postural hypotension	It is clinically difficult to distinguish athletes with exhaustion in cool conditions from those who collapse in hot conditions. The signs and symptoms of heat exhaustion are neither specific nor sensitive. During the acute stage, blood pressure is low, the pulse and respiratory rates are elevated, and the patient appears sweaty, pale and ashen. Muscle cramps may or may not exist. In the field, rectal temperature measurement may discriminate between severe heat exhaustion (<40 °C, <104 °F) and heat stroke (>40 °C)	The athlete should be moved to a cool-shaded area, helped to remove excess clothing, placed in a supine position with legs elevated, and monitored (heart rate, blood pressure, rectal temperature, respiratory rate, and central nervous system status). If rectal temperature cannot be measured promptly, empiric cooling therapy should be considered, especially if central nervous symptoms exist. The majority of athletes will resolve collapse within 30 min with leg elevation, oral fluids, and rest. An athlete who does not improve should be transported to an emergency facility. Oral fluids are preferred for rehydration in athletes who are conscious, able to swallow well, and not losing fluids via vomiting or diarrhea. If blood pressure, pulse, and rectal temperature indicate, i.v. fluids facilitate rapid recovery. The primary goal of i.v. therapy is intravascular volume expansion with saline, to protect organ function and improve blood pressure when signs of shock are observed. The most commonly recommended i.v. fluids are normal saline or 5% dextrose in normal saline. The 5% dextrose provides glucose for cell energy	ACSM Exertional Heat Illness Position Stand [18]

			NATA Exertional Heat Illness Position Statement [19]
Heat exhaustion is defined as the inability to effectively exercise in the heat, secondary to a combination of cardiovascular insufficiency, hypotension, energy depletion, and central fatigue. This condition manifests with an elevated internal body temperature (usually <40.5 °C) with a high rate or volume of skin blood flow, heavy sweating, and dehydration. This illness most often affects non-acclimatized or dehydrated individuals with a body mass index >27 kg/m²	Heat exhaustion results from a combination of cardiovascular insufficiency, energy depletion, and central fatigue	Heat exhaustion may be present if the patient demonstrates excessive fatigue, faints, collapses, or presents with minor cognitive changes (e.g., headache, dizziness, confusion) while performing physical activity. Other signs and symptoms of exertional heat exhaustion may include fatigue, weakness, dizziness, headache, lightheadedness, vomiting, nausea, low blood pressure, and impaired muscle coordination. The NATA strongly recommends that rectal temperature be measured because in cases of heat exhaustion it is usually less than 40.5 °C (105 °F), a characteristic that differentiates it from exertional heat stroke	Cease exercise, move the athlete to a cool-shaded area, remove excess clothing and equipment, elevate legs to promote venous return to the heart, monitor vital signs, and provide fluids. If intravenous fluids are needed or if recovery is eventful and not rapid (≤ 30 min), i.v. fluid should be administered under the care of a physician. If the condition worsens during or after treatment, emergency medical treatment should be activated

Note: The above statements are synopses written by the present author. They are not verbatim quotations from original publications

a This document classifies numerous exertion-related heat illness syndromes as *exertional heat illness* (EHI). These syndromes form a continuum of multisystem illnesses, which are divided into three levels on the basis of severity: (1) *mild EHI*, which includes heat exhaustion, mild dehydration, and heat cramps; (2) *intermediate EHI*, which includes exertional heat injury and mild rhabdomyolysis, renal insufficiency, orthostatic hypotension, heat-related syncope, and reversible electrolyte and metabolic disturbances; and (3) *severe EHI*, which includes heat stroke, severe rhabdomyolysis, liver necrosis, acute renal failure, cardiovascular collapse, and marked electrolyte or metabolic disturbances

b This document introduced the illness classification named *exertional heat injury*, defined as a moderate-to-severe heat illness characterized by organ (e.g., liver, renal) and tissue (e.g., gut, muscle) injury associated with sustained high body temperature resulting from strenuous exercise and environmental heat exposure. Body temperature is usually but not always greater than 40.5 °C (105 °F). Exertional heat injury is distinguished from exertional heat exhaustion and exertional heat stroke (i.e., a medical emergency) involving central nervous system dysfunction manifested as collapse, aggressiveness, irritability, confusion, seizures, and altered consciousness period, the most common etiology of heat exhaustion involved heavy labor in or near the engine room, high humidity, and extreme temperatures reaching 140–210 °F. In recognition of this remarkably stressful working environment, the US Navy began to modify the below-deck working environment, wall insulation, and air ventilation systems around 1909; also, newly installed oil-burning engines no longer required moving coal by hand, and the work load of sailors was reduced considerably. From 1909 to 1911, the annual rate of heat exhaustion casualties in the US Navy fell by 43%.

Physical exhaustion is vaguely defined as the inability to continue exercise and occurs with strenuous effort in all environments, from cool to hot. As ambient temperature rises above 20 °C (68 °F) and heat stress increases, the time to reach exhaustion decreases [21]. Although the exact mechanism of physical exhaustion has not been discovered, termination of exercise due to exhaustion may result from brain fatigue (i.e., decreased central activation) and subsequently reduced skeletal muscle force output that is influenced by either a whole-body fluid-electrolyte imbalance or depleted energy stores. The H_{EX} that occurs in hot environments may or may not involve the same mechanism as physical exhaustion, but it clearly is more pronounced [18].

Collapse at or near the finish line of an endurance or ultra-endurance event is a common reason for athletes to receive treatment at the medical tent. This benign condition (i.e., a form of exercise-associated collapse) is defined as inability to stand or walk unaided as a result of lightheadedness, dizziness, faintness, or syncope and is confirmed after endurance running by a drop of systolic blood pressure greater than 20 mmHg when moving from a lying to an erect posture [22]. Such exercise-associated collapse occurs in 1.1% of race starters at the finish of cool or mild weather marathons (41–68 °F, 5–20 °C) [23]; in ultramarathon events that involve hours of strenuous upright exercise, the prevalence is considerably greater [23, 24]. The pathophysiology of this exercise-associated collapse (EAC) is believed to involve postural hypotension when a runner finishes [24, 25], due to inactivation of the calf muscle pump, blood pooling in the compliant veins of the lower extremities, reduced atrial filling pressure, and subsequent syncope. Unfortunately, some authorities have interpreted these observations to mean that H_{EX} does not exist as a distinct entity, that the word "heat" is not necessary to describe this condition and extrapolate their observations to mean that the pathophysiology of H_{EX} simply involves postural hypotension [24, 25]. This is unfortunate because (a) the existence of one disorder (i.e., postural hypotension) does not disprove the existence of another; (b) the exertional heat illnesses were not named or classified as heat illnesses because patients were hyperthermic, rather the word heat referred to the environment as a stressor (e.g., heat cramps do not involve a high rectal temperature); and (c) numerous investigators have observed H_{EX} in a variety of scenarios and concluded that H_{EX} is more complex than postural hypotension per se (Table 5.2) [25–35]. In the paragraphs below, published reports of H_{EX} cases (see section titled Signs & Symptoms) demonstrate that dizziness, orthostatic rise of heart rate, syncope, and collapse are not universally observed.

Table 5.2 Characteristics of exertional heat exhaustion in diverse scenarios

Etiology	Pathophysiology	Signs and symptoms of heat exhaustion	Treatment/management	Authors/purpose
Heat exhaustion that developed across multiple days as a result of large water-electrolyte losses and inadequate replacement				
Below-deck strenuous labor aboard US naval ships with inadequate ventilation, often humid conditions. Long duration work shifts	Not stated, likely because the pathophysiology apparently was not clearly understood	This publication provided the original description of heat exhaustion, distinct from heat stroke (pg. 584) but not distinguished from heat cramps. The symptoms of heat exhaustion included "slight fever" or the subnormal skin temperature of shock, pallor, dull blue or gray-blue skin color, drenching perspiration, weakness of voluntary and involuntary muscles, and embarrassment of circulation and respiration. Skeletal muscle fiber twitching and violent painful cramps of the abdomen, arms, and legs were prominent in some cases	Valid treatment options, from the perspective of today's knowledge, are not described	Fiske 1913. A 35-year report of sailor heat illnesses that led to casualties and deaths [26]
Hard labor performed by US Navy sailors shoveling in 100 °F and 100% relative humidity. Some engine rooms reported air temperatures exceeding 54 °C (130 °F). Long duration work shifts	The author acknowledged little understanding of the pathophysiology underlying heat exhaustion (i.e., why some men have heat cramps but others do not.	Heat exhaustion patients were prostrated when admitted with cold moist skin, rapid pulse, and no cramps. When the hot ambient conditions of Hawaii were encountered on consecutive days, the conditions below deck were extremely stressful, even for young experienced sailors. The crew felt physically "washed out"	Valid treatment options, from the perspective of today's knowledge, are not described	Phelps, a summary of heat exhaustion aboard US Navy ships in 1924–1925 [27]

(continued)

Table 5.2 (continued)

Etiology	Pathophysiology	Signs and symptoms of heat exhaustion	Treatment/ management	Authors/purpose
Military activities of UK armed forces in Iraq. The average daily shade temperature for the month of August 1930 was 115 °F (46 °C) with 122 °F (50 °C) maximum, often with low relative humidity. Long duration work shifts each day. No deaths occurred	Environmental heat stress. Metabolic acidosis is presented as a theoretical pathological factor, but little evidence supports this theory	A 1–3 day prodromal period of malaise, weakness of the legs, headache, constipation and small urine volume often is observed in residents, which may not involve direct exposure to the sun. Severe cases involve collapse and circulatory shock; in some, this occurred at night and involved no exercise. The patient is pale, bathed in cold-clammy perspiration, mentally apprehensive, and may be in acute discomfort due to violent cramps of the abdominal and leg muscles. If untreated for hours or days, mild rectal hyperthermia of 101 °F (38.3 °C) can progress to 108 °F (42.2 °C), and coma or convulsions may occur	Preliminary treatment for shock. The effect of i.v. infusion is dramatic in that vomiting and muscle cramps cease. Patients are nearly convalescent within 48 h	Morton, 1932. Military medical report regarding troop activities [28]

In underground mines, the environmental conditions are: 86–96 °F (30–35 °C), a very high relative humidity of 90–96%, and air velocities of 100–250 ft./min (30.5–76.2 m/min). Internal heat production is maintained during 8-h shifts. High relative humidity and temperature discourage sweat evaporation. Miners wear only a pair of shorts and boots. Once on the surface, heat stress is removed. Usually the worker who is engaged in sustained shoveling, although at half his working capacity, suffers heat illness. Older miners are rarely employed underground after the age of 45 years, due to increased incidence of heat illness	The authors include salt-deficiency heat exhaustion, heat cramps, and mixed water-electrolyte depletions in the category named "heat exhaustion" because their etiologies all involve inadequate salt or water replacement after losses (acute or chronic), incurred during labor. Proportionately, the salt imbalance is greater when only water is replaced, and the basic pathology involves extracellular dehydration. No deaths occurred	This publication presented a very comprehensive clinical description of advanced/severe heat exhaustion. Pure water depletion is not seen in this setting because both water and salt are lost in sweat. The signs and symptoms represent salt depletion heat exhaustion and mixed fluid-electrolyte depletions The average patient body fluid loss was 12% of body weight. Skin turgor and elasticity were markedly decreased and eyeballs were sunken. Skin was cool or cold, often clammy, but at times dry. Nearly all patients confirmed that they had sweat profusely and felt very hot. Collapse during labor was common. Systolic blood pressure was low (80–90 mmHg) and peripheral pulse could not be palpated. In mild or moderate cases, the pulse increased markedly upon standing and the patient fainted. Nausea, vomiting, and weakness were common Laboratory findings included a low serum Cl⁻ conc. (group mean of 86 mEq/L) with normal-to-low Na⁺ and normal potassium (K⁺) conc. Hematocrit was elevated. Urine Cl⁻ conc. was low in all cases	Electrolyte loss is indisputable. Therapy is designed to provide accurate water and electrolyte replacement, in consideration of the patient's daily water and salt turnover, relief of muscle cramps, and correction of osmotic imbalance. Extracellular osmolality is reduced, thus i.v. saline is the fastest and best treatment. Normal saline is used for the initial 2 liters of fluid replacement; thereafter, half-normal saline in 5% dextrose is dispensed. Oral fluids may exacerbate vomiting	King and Barry, 1962. Description of workers in deep underground mines of South Africa [29]

Table 5.2 (continued)

Etiology	Pathophysiology	Signs and symptoms of heat exhaustion	Treatment/management	Authors/purpose
A 110.5 kg man performed intermittent high-intensity treadmill running during a research study; 56 min of exercise (57–66% of VO_{2max}) was accomplished during each 100 min heat exposure (days 1–7), except day 8. Although physiological adaptations progressed normally through day 5, heat exhaustion occurred on the eighth day of exercise-heat exposure	Increased cardiovascular strain was evidenced by greater heart rate change (day 1, +71 beats·min^{-1} and day 8, +96 beats·min^{-1}) and greater plasma volume change (day 1, −10.7% and day 8, −16.2%) post-exercise. Pre-exercise body mass decreased by 3.6 kg from day 1 to day 8 of heat acclimation. Calculations indicated a mild 8-day whole-body Na$^+$ deficit of 3.8 g (166 mEq/8d) and an extracellular volume contraction of 0.72 L	This individual reported no signs or symptoms of heat exhaustion during exercise on days 1–7. Exercise was terminated prematurely only on day 8 and the following symptoms of salt depletion heat exhaustion were observed: vomiting, muscular weakness, fatigue, and abdominal muscle cramps. Heat exhaustion on day 8 was fore-warned by loss of body weight (− 5.4 kg during the 72 h preceding the episode), increased heart rate (days 5–8), and increased rectal temperature (days 7–8) during exercise. Plasma cortisol (i.e., a marker of general body stress) and beta-endorphin (i.e., a sensitive index of heat stress) were elevated on day 8 (twofold and six–ninefold, respectively, above days 1 and 4)	On day 8, investigators moved the participant from the hot laboratory environment to an air-conditioned room. A physician managed his recovery for 48 h post-exercise, including encouragement to increase dietary water and salt intake as tolerated	Armstrong et al., 1988. A case report of monitored heat exhaustion [30]
Religious pilgrims walk across the desert in ambient temperatures that often exceed (113 °F) 45 °C, 50% relative humidity. Hundreds of people, many elderly, succumb to heat illness and are treated at field medical sites along the course	Heat exhaustion patients exhibit hypovolemia and intact mental function with rectal temperature <40 °C. Their hemodynamic changes reflect a hyperdynamic circulation with tachycardia and high cardiac output	Heat exhaustion patients ($n = 29$) and a control group ($n = 31$) with no clinical symptoms were assessed via non-invasive echocardiography. Patients demonstrated peripheral vasodilatation. There were no cardiac signs of major hypovolemia in heat exhaustion patients, with a left ventricular size that was only mildly smaller than that of controls, and with no marked collapse of the inferior vena cava. Signs of arterial vasodilatation were reflected in the descending aortic flow, with a higher cardiac output maintained by increased heart rate	Specific treatment options are not described.	Shahid et al., 1999. Heat exhaustion during religious pilgrimage [31]

Heat exhaustion that developed within a single day or event as a result of water-electrolyte loss and reduced peripheral vascular resistance

Controlled observations of male laborers involved shoveling gravel for 1 h in either a hot environment (dry bulb, 96–98 °F, 35.6–36.7 °C; wet bulb, 94–95 °F, 34.4–35 °C) or a mild environment, then standing upright with arms hanging freely. Pulse rate, respiratory rate, and systolic–diastolic blood pressures were measured	Standing in the mild environment after exercise resulted in no participant collapse. Thus, the observed collapses were truly heat-induced. The most noteworthy differences between these groups were changes in the circulatory system as indicated by pulse rate and blood pressure. The six men who collapsed while standing in the heat exhibited a feeble and slow pulse, a fall in systolic (and often but not invariably diastolic) pressure, and a decrease in pulse pressure (i.e., the difference of systolic minus diastolic). This was a vasovagal form of collapse that likely involved pooling of blood in the extremities and visceral organs. Those men who did not collapse exhibited a high pulse rate, steady blood pressures, and a large pulse pressure, indicative of appropriate physiological responses to upright posture	Of the 36 test participants, only six experienced great distress and collapse. Their syncope was transient and recovery was rapid, once they were removed to a mild environment. The 30 unaffected men stood in the heat without signs or symptoms for 60 min post-exercise. The first signs of syncope were forward bending of the head, closing of the eyes, sighing, absence of body tone, body restlessness, and a verbal request to lean or sit down. At this stage, fainting was imminent. Participants reported weakness, lassitude, nausea, giddiness, and a period of blackness. This is one of the few published studies in which experimental test participants experienced syncope and collapse. This likely occurred because of the requirement to stand for 1 h in the heat	Air movement across the skin is an effective measure to counteract syncope and collapse	Weiner, 1938. Heat collapse research study [32]

(continued)

Table 5.2 (continued)

Etiology	Pathophysiology	Signs and symptoms of heat exhaustion	Treatment/management	Authors/purpose
Strenuous labor in a deep Australian underground mine (1800 m maximum depth) in hot ambient conditions. Cases of heat exhaustion were reported by telephone; miners were retrieved and transported to a medical center. The heat exhaustion incidence rose in a dose-response manner when ambient conditions reached >33 °C, 91.4 °F dry bulb, >28 °C, 82.4 °F web bulb globe temperature, and <1.5 m/sec air velocity	Heat exhaustion is caused by the inability of the circulatory system to simultaneously supply sufficient blood flow to the skin to achieve heat loss and to supply the vital organs and exercising skeletal muscle. This illness usually is due to hypovolemia resulting from varying degrees of water and salt loss. The urine specific gravity at presentation was strongly correlated with the incidence of heat exhaustion; see Fig 6.1.	A total of 106 miners were included in this study, which spanned 12 months. The incidence of heat exhaustion therefore was 94.2/1000 workers/year. The most commonly observed symptoms were nausea, fatigue, headache, cramps, dizziness and vomiting. Symptom details appear in Table 5.5, which may be compared to Table 5.2. People with heat exhaustion rarely experienced confusion, ataxia, convulsions, or prolonged unconsciousness; the authors noted that these strongly suggest exertional heat stroke	Treatment consisted of either oral fluids or i.v. normal saline, given in an air-conditioned treatment room of the medical center	Donoghue et al., 2000. Heat exhaustion in miners [33]
This brief review paper proposes that heat exhaustion in marathons actually is post-exercise collapse when athletes are fully conscious with no other serious medical conditions, have postural hypotension (blood pressure <100 mm Hg), and low heart rates (<100 beats·min^{-1}). This paper suggests that dehydration is not an important etiological factor in heat exhaustion	Low peripheral vascular resistance is present in patients with heat illness. When high air temperature increases skin temperature, peripheral resistance in blood vessels decreases and cutaneous blood flow increases. Because peripheral resistance provides compensation for upright posture, reduced arterial blood pressure becomes the critical event. Theoretically, this may be accompanied by a vasodilation response in skeletal muscle	Low peripheral vascular resistance may result in postural hypotension, faintness, blacking out, collapse, and weakness with or without vomiting	Lying supine with feet above the level of the head relieves hypotension	Noakes et al. 2007. Marathon runner collapse [25]

			Specific treatment options are not described	
This brief review paper considers the causes of marathon collapse related to physical exhaustion, heat exhaustion, and dehydration	During severe exercise-heat stress (i.e., high skin and internal temperatures), cardiac output can decrease below levels observed during exercise in temperate environments. In combination with vasodilated skin and muscle, dehydration accentuates cardiovascular strain. Other factors that may contribute to post-race collapse include reduced skeletal muscle pump activity and an altered cerebrovascular response to orthostatic challenge	Athletes who finish a marathon and collapse are typically fully conscious but are unable to stand without support		Kenefick and Sawka, 2007. Marathon runner collapse [34]
Ten healthy men participated in controlled laboratory experiments that evaluated the effects of control (C), partial (P), and full (F) American football uniforms on cardiovascular and thermal responses during mixed mode exercise in a hot, humid environment (33 °C, 91.4 °F; 49% rh). During 19 of 30 trials, participants halted exercise as a result of volitional exhaustion	Seven participants in group C completed the entire 80-min protocol (box lifting and treadmill walking), 3 in P, and 1 in F. Exhaustion occurred during the F and P trials at the same mean internal temperature (39.3 °C, 102.7 °F). Hypotension influenced exhaustion during exercise. Skin temperatures, measured at two sites, were greater during both P and F; this likely reduced peripheral resistance and increased skin blood flow	Systolic blood pressure decreased during box-lifting exercise in the heat. Also, both systolic and diastolic pressures decreased at the end of treadmill walking Diastolic pressures suggested that cardiac filling decreased as a result of lower pressure during diastole and stroke volume decreased. To maintain cardiac output, the mean final heart rates (C, 164; P, 178; F, 180 beats·min^{-1}) were necessarily high in experiments P and F, indicating great cardiovascular strain at the time of exhaustion. The mean internal temperatures at the end of exercise ranged from 38.7–39.2 °C, 101.7–102.3 °F		Armstrong et al., 2010. Exhaustion during uniformed exercise [35]

Note: The above statements are synopses written by the present author. They are not verbatim quotations from original publications

Clinical and controlled laboratory research studies refine the above field observations of runners and clarify the nature of H_{EX}. For example, Sawka et al. [36] observed healthy men during two experiments (i.e., one euhydrated and one dehydrated to −8% of total body water) involving treadmill exercise (180 min heat exposure, 50 min walking per hour) in a hot-dry (49 °C) environment. Exhaustion in this harsh environment ended 27 of 34 experiments and always occurred before a rectal temperature of 40 °C was achieved, across a wide range (37.6–39.7 °C). The large body water loss reduced the internal temperature that could be tolerated. Other research studies have shown that (a) exercise performed in a cool environment does not induce H_{EX}; (b) mild exercise (40–50% VO_{2max}) in hot environments (34–39 °C, 93–102 °F) does not induce H_{EX} unless significant fluid-electrolyte loss and cardiovascular strain exist; and (c) cumulative dehydration across 3 days can result in H_{EX} [30, 36]. Thus, both dehydration and a high ambient temperature influence the prevalence of H_{EX}. Interesting support for the previous sentence appears in the clinical observations of laborers who worked in a deep metalliferous mine [33] at dry bulb temperatures ranging from 31.0 to 43.0 °C and experienced H_{EX}. When the urine specific gravities of these laborers at presentation were plotted against the cumulative percentage of H_{EX} ($n = 87$), the authors discovered the relationship shown in Fig. 5.1. Urine specific gravity is a widely recognized biomarker of hydration status; a value of 1.020 is often viewed as the threshold for the onset of dehydration, and values ≥1.030 represent frank dehydration. Eighty-five percent of H_{EX} patients (see Fig. 5.1) presented at the infirmary with a urine specific gravity of 1.020–1.040, indicating that their dehydration ranged from mild to severe. Further, virtually no H_{EX} cases (<5%) occurred at wet bulb globe temperatures <28.0 °C or dry bulb temperatures <33.0 °C.

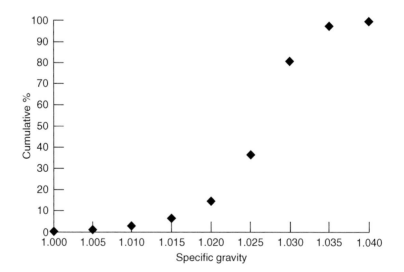

Fig. 5.1 Cumulative incidence of heat exhaustion events, categorized on the basis of each patient's urine specific gravity upon arrival at the medical infirmary. Data represent 87 laborers who worked in a hot-humid, deep metal ore mine. (From Donoghue et al. [33] with permission)

Table 5.3 Water and salt (NaCl) losses during prolonged military and industrial activities in hot environments

Measurements	Duration of effort	
	1 day of desert living[a]	1 work shift (8 h)[b]
Total volume of sweat lost	5–14 L/24 h[a]	5–11 L/8 h[b]
Total NaCl lost in sweat	4–28 g NaCl/24 h[c]	15–20 g NaCl/8 h[b]
Sweat rate	0.7–1.1 L/h[a,d]	0.6–1.4 L/h[d,e]

[a]Data represent soldiers living, marching and working in the desert [41]
[b]Data represent South African laborers working in a deep underground mine [29]
[c]Calculated recognizing that 1 L of sweat typically contains 0.8–2.0 g NaCl in heat acclimatized individuals
[d]A sweat rate of 3.5 L/h can be maintained for several hours by some individuals [41]
[e]Calculated on the basis of one 8-h work shift

Documented cases of H_{EX} (see Table 5.1) indicate that the following are important etiological characteristics in athletic, industrial, and military settings [37]: high ambient temperature/humidity/solar radiation with slow air movement, strenuous or prolonged exercise, large sweat loss, whole-body electrolyte imbalance, circulatory insufficiency for the task at hand, and lack of heat acclimatization. Table 5.3 [29, 38], for example, provides quantitative examples of documented water and sodium chloride losses of soldiers and laborers. Clearly, such 24-h deficits greatly exceed the water and salt consumed in an ordinary Western diet that provides 2000 Kcal/day. It is relevant that 8–10 days of exercise-heat acclimatization reduces NaCl losses in sweat and urine, improves orthostatic intolerance, enhances cardiovascular stability, and expands plasma (extracellular) volume [39–41].

Pathophysiology

The pathophysiology of H_{EX} involves perturbations of total body water, whole-body sodium balance, plasma volume, plasma concentration, and cardiovascular stability. When deficits of water and sodium are large, numerous systems of the body are negatively affected. This dysfunction ultimately arises from the patient's fluid-electrolyte losses in sweat and urine, exercise duration and intensity, cumulative dehydration across days, environmental heat stress, cardiovascular physical fitness, heat acclimatization status, and dietary intake of salt and water.

Figure 5.2 depicts whole-body sodium and water balance in two dimensions. The vertical axis represents the continuum of extracellular exchangeable sodium, from excess to deficit. The horizontal axis represents the continuum of total body water from deficit (hypohydration) to fluid overload. Three forms of H_{EX} are depicted in Fig. 5.2: predominant water depletion (WD), mixed salt and water depletion, and predominant salt depletion (SD). Their names are self-explanatory. Because urine and sweat both contain water and electrolytes, pure WD and pure SD are seldom observed. Complicating recognition and treatment, the mixed salt and water depletion heat exhaustion in Fig. 5.2 may result in signs and symptoms of both WD and SD.

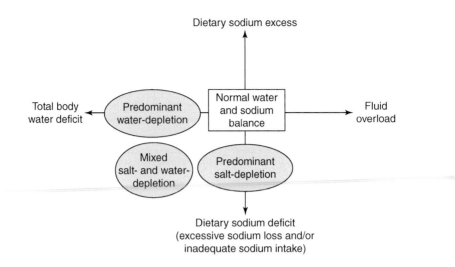

Fig. 5.2 Sodium and water imbalances as etiologic factors in the development of three types of heat exhaustion: predominant water depletion, predominant salt depletion, and mixed water depletion plus salt depletion

Table 5.4 presents a compilation of signs and symptoms that inform the pathophysiology associated with WD and SD (see text above and Fig. 5.2), as reported by multiple authors [38, 42–44]. It is firstly important to note the usual time of development for these fluid-electrolyte disorders. WD can occur during a single day or event, within a few hours if replacement is minimal. SD, however, usually requires 3–5 days to develop, as a result of consistent NaCl losses in sweat. Indeed, Tables 5.2 and 5.4 are organized into two subsections that reflect these distinct rates of illness development. In a few rare individuals, a perfect storm of personal characteristics occurs when a very high sweat rate (e.g., 2.5–3.0 L/h) and a very high sweat sodium concentration (e.g., 40–80 mEq Na^+/L; 2.3–4.6 g NaCl/L) are inherited hereditary traits; these persons develop signs and symptoms faster than most people (i.e., may be the first to seek medical care). Thus, an adult potentially could lose 5.8–13.8 g NaCl/h during strenuous exercise-heat exposure. When compared to the average daily dietary intake of adults in the USA (3.4 g NaCl/d and 3.3 L water/d [45, 46]), these losses clearly indicate that this adult would require supplemental water and salt replacement and could benefit from dietary counseling. It is worth noting that anyone who lives or works in hot surroundings on a low salt diet is vulnerable to salt depletion if dietary intake is further reduced by nausea or heat-induced anorexia or if electrolytes are lost via vomiting or diarrhea [47].

The pathophysiology of WD and SD is different, in that predominant WD (i.e., by virtue of increased extracellular-plasma osmolality) induces water to leave the intracellular space and dehydrates cells [47]. As WD progresses, reabsorption of sodium from the renal tubules is augmented in an attempt to maintain extracellular volume at the expense of intracellular fluid; a small 24-h urine vol-

Table 5.4 Signs and symptoms of salt depletion and water depletion heat exhaustion [41–44]

Signs and symptoms	Predominant salt depletion heat exhaustion	Predominant water depletion heat exhaustion
Time to develop	3–5 days	Within 1 day or 1 event
Nausea	Yes	Yes
Anorexia	Yes	Yes
Fatigue, weakness	Yes	Yes
Loss of skin turgor	Yes	Yes
Mental dullness, apathy	Yes	Yes
Tachycardia at rest	Yes	Yes
Dry mucous membranes	Yes	Yes
Muscle cramps	Present in most cases[a]	No
Vomiting	Present in most cases[a]	No
Plasma volume	Decreased	Normal until advanced
Hemoconcentration	Yes	Slight when advanced
Orthostatic rise of heart rate	Yes[a]	Absent until advanced
Plasma Na+/Cl− concentration	Diminished	Average or slightly increased
Urine Na+/Cl− concentration	Negligible	Normal
24-h urine volume	Normal until advanced[a]	Scant
Thirst	Mild or absent[a]	Prominent
Increased rectal temperature	Yes	Present in most cases

[a]These signs and symptoms may distinguish salt depletion from water depletion heat exhaustion in field settings

ume is excreted from the outset. When WD becomes severe, the brain does not maintain blood volume despite profound cellular dehydration; both resting pulse rate and internal body temperature rise. In contrast, predominant SD (i.e., due to decreased extracellular tonicity) osmotically induces water to leave the extracellular space (i.e., slightly expanding intracellular volume) and stimulates diuresis because less sodium is available for reabsorption by the kidneys [48]. The extracellular fluid (e.g., plasma) contains most of the metabolically available sodium in the body and therefore is affected most by salt depletion, in the form of a considerably reduced extracellular fluid volume [47]. Thus, the reduced blood volume, stroke volume, and cardiac output observed in SD patients influence muscular weakness, fatigue, and orthostatic rise of heart rate during exercise in a hot environment (Tables 5.4 and 5.5). SD and heat cramps often appear concurrently, due to the expanded intracellular volume and decreased extracellular sodium (see the section below titled Recognition, para. 1 and 2; also see Chap. 6 in this book) [48].

Clinical and scientific publications since 1935 present a variety of pathophysiological explanations for H_{EX}. In addition to the preceding three paragraphs, Table 5.1 illustrates this point by summarizing 11 documents that were written by respected physicians and physiologists, professional organizations, and government agencies.

Table 5.5 Signs and symptoms of heat exhaustion observed in laborers working in a deep underground mine[a] [33]

Signs and symptoms[b,c]	Number of patients who reported[b,d]	Percent of 106 patients who reported each sign or symptom
Nausea	86	81
Fatigue	83	78
Headache	71	67
Muscle cramps	69	65
Dizziness	60	57
Vomiting	50	47
Diarrhea	10	9.4
Transient loss of consciousness	2	1.9
Confusion	1	0.9
Convulsions	0	0

[a]This metalliferous mine in tropical, arid Australia (1800 m maximum depth; mean ambient dry bulb temperature was 37.4 °C/99.3 °F and mean wet bulb globe temperature was 31.5 °C/88.7 °F) employed 1252 workers whereas the above data refer to 106 patients treated at the medical clinic
[b]A total of 118 miners were treated for heat exhaustion across 1 year (incidence of 94.2/1000 workers/y), of which 106 were included in the above data base
[c]Compare to Tables 5.4 and 5.6
[d]Although the mean dry bulb temperature was 37.4 °C and the mean wet bulb globe temperature was 31.5 °C, few or no H_{EX} cases occurred below a dry bulb temperature of 33 °C or a wet bulb globe temperature of 28 °C

Specifically, column 2 of Table 5.1 presents the following diverse pathophysiological paradigms: postural hypotension, excessive cardiovascular demand (e.g., circulatory insufficiency), electrolyte imbalance, sweating deficiency, high-intensity exercise, central fatigue, and depletion of energy stores. It is highly unlikely that *all* of these states of perturbed homeostasis exist in any single patient at one point in time. But, assuming that the observations in Table 5.1 are accurate, all of these pathophysiologies exist in some patients, at different points in time and in different scenarios. This suggests that our present paradigm and classification of H_{EX} [3, 5, 7] may be too simplistic to explain a complex illness, involving the responses and dysfunction of multiple organ systems. This also may explain why the "unspecified" category of H_{EX} was selected by military physicians to classify 96% of soldiers with H_{EX} [7], and why H_{EX} often is diagnosed by exclusion.

Table 5.1 contains two examples of heat illness classifications that differ from ICD classes. The first, published by Gardner and Kark [14], categorizes numerous heat-related syndromes (i.e., dehydration, heat cramps, H_{EX}, heat stroke, heat syncope, rhabdomyolysis, renal insufficiency) as mild, intermediate, and severe exertional heat illness, on the basis of severity of symptoms and physiological dysfunction. The second example, published by the National Athletic Trainers' Association [19], proposes a class of illnesses named exertional heat injury that was distinct from heat stroke and H_{EX}. This class was defined as moderate-to-severe heat illness characterized by organ and tissue injury, associated with sustained high body temperature and resulting from strenuous exercise-heat stress. The US Armed Forces Health Surveillance Center [49] utilizes a similar illness classification named heat injury and defines this class as heat exhaustion with evidence of organ (liver, renal, stomach) and/or muscle (rhabdomyolysis) damage, but without the neurological signs and symptoms of heat stroke.

Recognition

Virtually all physiological functions rely on homeostasis of total body water and electrolytes. Thus, when deficits or water and sodium are large, numerous systems of the body are affected negatively. Because each patient's work environment, activity level, fluid-electrolyte losses, physical fitness, and heat acclimatization status are different, the signs and symptoms of H_{EX} vary from person to person. Yet, Table 5.4 suggests that SD and WD may be distinguished in field settings by evaluating the presence of muscle cramps, vomiting, orthostatic rise of heart rate, 24-h urine volume, and thirst. This has not been tested in a field clinical trial, but Dinman and Horvath [50] reported that SD and WD could *not* be distinguished by physicians who treated laborers in the aluminum industry; however, this may have been due to the absence of laboratory tests (e.g., plasma and urinary sodium) in their infirmary.

Several forms of skeletal muscle cramps and spasms have been documented and have varying etiologies (e.g., nocturnal, writer's, injury-induced), but exertional heat cramps have been recognized as unique because they develop when a whole-body sodium deficiency exists (see Fig. 5.2), subsequent to prolonged exercise-heat stress and a large sweat loss [51]. Thus, SD and muscle cramps often occur concurrently, as described in Tables 5.4 and 5.5. In fact, the majority of publications summarized in Tables 5.1 and 5.2 describe muscle cramps and SD in the same patients. Exertional heat cramps are described in detail in Chap. 6 of this book; however one publication is noteworthy from the perspective of SD. W.S.S. Ladell, a noted physiologist during the mid-twentieth century, learned during repeated trials in his laboratory that he was susceptible to heat cramps. His classic paper [52], titled Heat Cramps, described the results of experiments in which he self-induced a negative salt balance in himself on 20 occasions (out of 26 trials) by exercising in a 37.8 °C (100 °F) environment. His mean negative balance was 21.3 g (range, 11–34 g) of NaCl (i.e., equivalent to 364 mEq NaCl and 143 mEq Na$^+$), and his total sweat loss per experiment ranged from 1.0–8.0 L. Ladell concluded that both intracellular overhydration (i.e., expansion) and an extracellular chloride (i.e., sodium) concentration decrease were required for heat cramps to occur. Ladell's descriptions of water movements between fluid compartments were strikingly similar to other descriptions of SD [38, 42–44].

Table 5.6 presents complaints that were reported by 13 young men during self-paced running in a 41.2 °C (106.2 °F) environment [30, 53]. Although these data do not describe H_{EX} patients, they provide a picture of the early warning symptoms that runners might experience during exercise-heat exposure. These complaints involved the central nervous, integumentary, gastrointestinal, cardiovascular, and muscular systems of the body. The most commonly reported complaints appear in the top rows of the table. The two bottom rows of Table 5.6 illustrate the beneficial effects of heat acclimation, in that both the number of complaints and the number of premature exercise terminations (see footnote g) on days 1–4 were three times greater than the number reported on days 5–8. This statistic demonstrates that the ill effects of strenuous exercise-heat stress are modifiable, not immutable, and show systematic heat acclimatization to be a fundamental aspect of H_{EX} prevention.

Table 5.5 summarizes observations made on 106 miners (1252 total employees) who worked in a deep underground mine and who presented with H_{EX} [33]. Five observations are especially relevant to this chapter. First, the most commonly reported signs and symptoms (i.e., nausea, fatigue, headache, muscle cramps, dizziness, vomiting) can serve as guiding indicators during the recognition of H_{EX}. Second, hematocrit, hemoglobin, and osmolality values were elevated, indicating that H_{EX} patients were dehydrated. Third, intravenous fluids (1–4 L) were administered to 47% of these patients, usually resulting in rapid improvement; patients who preferred oral rehydration usually had longer recovery periods. Fourth, laboratory tests indicated metabolic acidosis in 63% of H_{EX} cases; this may have resulted from increased anaerobic metabolism (i.e., due to mild hyperthermia) or a compensatory response to metabolic alkalosis induced by hyperventilation [33]. Finally, few or no heat exhaustion cases (<5%) occurred below psychrometric wet bulb globe temperatures of 28 °C or dry bulb temperatures of 33 °C.

Comparing the signs and symptoms in Tables 5.4, 5.5, and 5.6 is informative because each table represents a different aspect of H_{EX} and exercise-heat stress. The former compares the body's responses to two distinct fluid-electrolyte depletion states (also see Fig. 5.2). Table 5.6 delineates the premonitory clues and signs/symptoms of illness that occurred during 100 min of strenuous, intermittent running in a hot environment. The latter table represents a summary of patient visits to a medical center in a deep Australian mine. Considered in toto, these three tables illustrate that (a) because the time to develop signs and symptoms varies, depending on the predominant form of H_{EX} involved (i.e., WD, within 1 day or event; SD, 3–5 days; Tables 5.3 and 5.4), the patient history can inform clinical decisions; and (b) signs and symptoms of H_{EX} vary across situations and activities. Further, Tables 5.4, 5.5, and 5.6 have three symptoms in common: nausea, muscular weakness, and fatigue. Not only does this suggest that runners, athletes, and laborers should be alert for these symptoms but also that physicians and nurses can value these symptoms as useful diagnostic indicators of H_{EX}, especially when all three are observed concurrently.

Regarding post-exercise hypotensive collapse (as described above in the section titled Etiology), Tables 5.4, 5.5, and 5.6 indicate that dizziness and orthostatic rise of heart rate were rare occurrences in these clinical and physiological publications. Similarly, neither collapse nor frank syncope occurred.

Among the significant illnesses that occur in field settings, shared signs and symptoms complicate the recognition of H_{EX} [54]. For example, mental status

Table 5.6 Complaints reported during 8 days of self-paced running in a 41.2 °C (106.2 °F) environment[a,b]

Complaints[c,d,e]	Experimental days								
	1	2	3	4[e]	5[e]	6	7	8	8-day incidence
"Heat sensations" with flushed skin on head and torso	1	1	2	2		1			7
Chills	1	2	1	1	1	1			7
Abdominal cramps		2						2	4
Piloerection (goose flesh)	2	2							4
Resting tachycardia (>160 beats·min^{-1} for 5 min)	1	1	1	1					4
Extreme muscular weakness				1					1
Vomiting and nausea								1	1
Dizziness				1					1
Hyperirritability							1		1
Daily complaint totals	5	8	4	6	1	2	1	3	30
Premature exercise termination[g]	6	5	2	3	2	1	2	0	21

[a]13 healthy, well-nourished young men participated in 8 days of intermittent treadmill running as part of a heat acclimation research study [53] with a total heat exposure of 100 min/d
[b]Exercise involved nine self-paced running periods (5–10 min each) that were alternated with nine rest periods (2–10 min each)
[c]All were transient and reversible
[d]Complaints do not include those of a single participant who developed salt depletion on day 8 (see Table 5.2 for details) [30]
[e]Compare to Tables 5.4 and 5.5
[f]This research protocol involved 2 days of rest without exercise-heat exposure between days 4 and 5 (weekend)
[g]Exercise was terminated if heart rate exceeded 180 beats·min^{-1}, if heart rate did not fall below 160 beats·min^{-1} during any 5 min period of rest, if rectal temperature exceeded 39.5 °C, or if signs and symptoms of heat stress warranted premature termination of trials in the opinion of the physician medical monitor

changes (i.e., clouded sensorium) are observed in cases of exertional heat stroke, hyponatremia, and H_{EX}, but not syncope. Elevated rectal temperature, an invariable symptom of heat stroke (>39–40 °C, 102.2–104.0 °F), is mildly present in H_{EX} (39.5–40.5 °C, 103.1–104.9 °F), and is unlikely in heat syncope and hyponatremia. Thus, the assessment of a potentially heat-injured athlete centers around two clinical criteria: mental status and rectal temperature. Frequently, H_{EX} will cause mild confusion, irritability, incoordination, and fatigue. In a field setting, if a patient exhibits significant mental status change, the medical staff should assume that he/she has heat stroke or hyponatremia. Heat stroke can be verified by taking rectal temperature. Symptomatic hyponatremia arises from fluid overload and is most often encountered when exercise lasts longer than 3–4 h; this fluid-electrolyte disorder is verified by analyzing serum sodium (<130–135 mEq/L). Today, a handheld sodium analyzer (e.g., i-STAT, Abbott, Princeton, NJ) has become a standard instrument in the medical tents of mass participation endurance events.

Treatment and Management

Treatment begins with recognition of H_{EX} signs and symptoms (above). After exercise stops, move the athlete to a cool-shaded area, remove excess clothing, and elevate legs in a supine position to promote venous return to the heart [19]. Monitor heart rate, blood pressure, respiratory rate, and central nervous system status. Measure rectal temperature with a thermometer that has a maximum reading ≥ 106 °F, 41.1 °C. If hyperthermia (>104 °F, 40 °C) is detected, cool the athlete until rectal temperature decreases to ~ 102 °F (38.9 °C). Although full body, cold water immersion is the most effective method to lower internal temperature, and the resulting peripheral vasoconstriction supports central blood volume, this therapy typically is not necessary if heat stroke has been ruled out [18, 19].

If the patient is not vomiting, nauseated or experiencing central nervous system dysfunction, rehydrate orally. A history that suggests hyponatremia (i.e., a large water intake) or severe salt and water deficits (i.e., a small water intake) indicates laboratory monitoring [14]. An athlete who does not improve within 30 min of initiating therapy should be transported to an emergency facility [18].

Treatment of exertional heat cramps (e.g., via oral rehydration, i.v. fluid, or eating sodium-rich foods such as canned soup) has the same goal as SD therapy: counteracting a whole-body NaCl deficit (see Fig. 5.2) secondary to prolonged exercise and large sweat loss in a hot environment [51]. Saline administration brings rapid resolution of exertional heat cramps [52]. Additional details appear in Chap. 6 of this book.

Although mild orthostatic hypotension with no other symptoms may be treated with rest and leg elevation, exertional H_{EX} cases that involve large fluid losses and tachycardia at rest should be treated by the judicious administration of i.v. fluid. Patients should initially receive intravenous boluses of 200–250 cc, and their responses should be monitored. More than 2 L of normal saline should not be given without laboratory surveillance. Solutions of 5% dextrose sugar in either 0.45% saline (NaCl) or 0.9% saline are most commonly prescribed [13]. Fluid loss can be estimated as 1.5 L (1.6 qt) of water and 2 g of NaCl per hour of continuous moderate-to-heavy exertion.

Severe Heat Exhaustion

During exercise in a hot environment, cardiac output increases up to four times the resting rate, and as much as 20% of cardiac output may be directed to the skin and peripheral circulation [55]. Dehydration and intercompartmental fluid shifts further reduce effective central blood volume, and compensation must occur to maintain cardiac output during exercise in the heat. After maximal stroke volume is reached, compensation is accomplished by increased heart rate until exhaustion occurs. If it were not for intense vasoconstriction of the splanchnic circulation, kidneys, and inactive muscle, a serious deficit of arterial volume would result [56]. Loss of splanchnic vasoconstriction or blood pooling in the skin and extremities (i.e., loss of peripheral resistance) signals that (a) cardiovascular compensations (i.e., peripheral resistance, calf muscles pumping venous return to the heart) are insufficient, (b) serious hypotension exists (e.g., systolic blood pressure <90 mmHg), (c) circulatory shock is possible, and (d) exhaustion and collapse are imminent [54, 57].

When collapse or altered mental status is observed, severe H_{EX} should be suspected because maximal cardiovascular compensation has been reached and hyperthermia accentuates this cardiovascular insufficiency [8, 36]. Although hyperthermia makes severe H_{EX} difficult to distinguish from exertional heat stroke, H_{EX} can be verified in most cases by three characteristics: a rectal temperature below 40 °C, normal serum enzyme levels, and consciousness [36]. Figure 5.3 illustrates the relationships between H_{EX}, severe H_{EX}, and exertional heat stroke. If rectal temperature cannot be measured promptly and laboratory tests are not available, cooling should be initiated, especially if central nervous symptoms are present.

Signs and symptoms of severe H_{EX} should be treated immediately [17]. These may include high internal body temperature, confusion/disorientation, vomiting, involuntary bowel movement, convulsions, a weak or rapid pulse, agitation, unresponsiveness or coma, and shock.

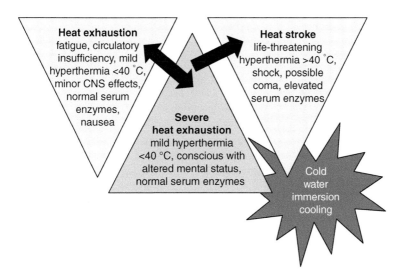

Fig. 5.3 Relationship of heat exhaustion to heat stroke. If exercise-heat stress is excessive, or if heat exhaustion is not recognized and managed, the patient may progress to severe heat exhaustion. Heat exhaustion and heat stroke may occur independently of the other, with few or no common signs or symptoms. However, severe heat exhaustion may progress to heat stroke (e.g., life-threatening hyperthermia >40 °C; may involve cardiovascular shock and coma) if cardiovascular compensation is maximal and hyperthermia adds additional stress to an existing cardiovascular insufficiency

Return to Daily Activities

Prognosis is best when mental acuity was not altered and serum enzymes (e.g., alanine aminotransferase, aspartate aminotransferase, lactate dehydrogenase, and creatine phosphokinase) remained within normal limits on the day of the H_{EX} episode. If known, rule out the underlying condition or illness that predisposed the athlete.

Same-day return to activity is not recommended [19]. Rectal temperature and hydration status should be normal. A simple check of urine volume (i.e., >1 L/24 h) and urine color (i.e., pale yellow or straw color) will allow the patient to self-assess hydration status [18]. Individuals who experienced mild H_{EX} and possess a high level of fitness may return to exercise within 24–48 h, under medical supervision. They should gradually increase the intensity and duration of training across several days.

Because 8–10 consecutive days of exercise-heat stress (i.e., heat acclimatization) improve orthostatic intolerance markedly [39, 40], prognosis and effective management involve guided outdoor exercise-heat exposures. Heat acclimatization produces beneficial physiological adaptations, including increased blood volume, decreased heart rate, enhanced ability to tolerate exercise in a hot environment, earlier onset of sweating, and decreased internal body temperature [41].

Determining the reasons for the initial H_{EX} event (e.g., ratio of work-to-rest, water intake, coincident illness, or medication) will help the patient avoid similar episodes in the future [17]. Avoiding cumulative dehydration across consecutive days [15] and eating a balanced diet (i.e., avoiding a low salt diet) represent healthy fluid-electrolyte habits. Although time consuming, straightforward methods exist to measure sweat rate, sweat electrolyte contents, dietary intake of salt, and a whole-body sodium deficit [58].

Finally, the attending physician should consider the following questions, which emphasize pertinent predisposing factors for H_{EX} [8]. Is the patient unfit or overweight with a body mass index >27 $kg·m^{-2}$? How many previous exercise-heat exposures did the patient have (e.g., to induce heat acclimatization)? Does the patient have both a high sweat rate and concentrated sweat (i.e., high NaCl content), which represent a perfect storm of personal inherited characteristics? Chapter 3 in this book considers predisposing factors in greater detail.

Summary

The Introduction section above posed two questions, "How can we reconcile the diverse observations and reports regarding H_{EX}?" and "Are the pathophysiology and signs/symptoms of H_{EX} similar in all sport, military, and industrial settings?" Regarding the former question, the pathophysiology of H_{EX} involves loss of total body water, reduced whole-body exchangeable sodium, inadequate water and salt consumption, reduced plasma volume, and increased plasma concentration. The signs and symptoms of H_{EX} differ, depending on the extent of salt and water derangements (see Fig. 5.2), as well as the sufficiency of regulatory responses that maintain cardiac output, blood pressure, total body water, and fluid osmolality. For example, the reduced blood volume, stroke volume, and cardiac output observed in SD patients influence muscular weakness, fatigue, nausea, and orthostatic rise of heart rate during exercise in a hot environment (Tables 5.4 and 5.5). Regarding the latter question, athletic, industrial, and military situations pose a variety of thermal, fluid regulatory, and cardiovascular challenges. The resulting signs and symptoms may differ, depending on whether water or salt depletion predominates and the extent of hyperthermia. Specifically, SD usually requires 3–5 days to develop, whereas WD may develop within 1 day or event. Recognition and therapy are optimized when clinicians and emergency responders know the H_{EX} signs and symptoms that reflect fluid-electrolyte imbalance and cardiovascular insufficiency: nausea, muscular weakness, fatigue, ashen skin, hypotension, and mild rectal temperature elevation.

References

1. World Health Organization. ICD-10 : international statistical classification of diseases and related health problems: tenth revision. 2nd ed. Geneva: World Health Organization; 2004. http://www.who.int/iris/handle/10665/42980. Accessed 17 Sept 2019.
2. Carter R III, Cheuvront SN, Williams JO, Kolka MA, Stephenson LA, Sawka MN, et al. Epidemiology of hospitalizations and deaths from heat illness in soldiers. Med Sci Sports Exerc. 2005;37(8):1338–44.
3. Harduar Morano L, Watkins S. Evaluation of diagnostic codes in morbidity and mortality data sources for heat-related illness surveillance. Public Health Rep. 2017;132(3):326–35.
4. Coris EE, Ramirez AM, Van Durme DJ. Heat illness in athletes: the dangerous combination of heat, humidity and exercise. Sports Med. 2004;34(1):9–16.
5. World Health Organization. Manual of the international statistical classification of diseases, injuries, and causes of death: based on the recommendations of the seventh revision conference, 1955, and adopted by the ninth World Health Assembly under the WHO nomenclature regulations, vol. 2. Geneva: WHO; 1957.
6. Minard D. Nomenclature and classification of heat disorders. JAMA. 1965;191:854.
7. DeGroot DW, Mok G, Hathaway NE. International classification of disease coding of exertional heat illness in US Army soldiers. Mil Med. 2017;182(9):e1946–50.
8. Armstrong LE, Lopez RM. Return to exercise training after heat exhaustion. J Sport Rehabil. 2007;16:182–90.
9. DeMartini JK, Casa DJ, Belval LN, Crago A, Davis RJ, Jardine JJ, Stearns RL. Environmental conditions and the occurrence of exertional heat illnesses and exertional heat stroke at the Falmouth Road Race. J Athl Train. 2014;49(4):478–85.
10. Lee DHK. The human organism and hot environments. Trans R Soc Trop Med Hyg. 1935;29:7–30.
11. Weiner JS, Horne GO. A classification of heat illness. Brit Med J. 1958;28:1533–5.
12. Department of the Army and Air Force. Heat illness: a handbook for medical officers. Technical note 91–3. Natick: U.S. Army Research Institute of Environmental Medicine; 1991.
13. Armstrong LE, Epstein Y, Greenleaf JE, Haymes EM, Hubbard RW, Roberts WO, Thompson PD. American College of Sports Medicine position stand: heat and cold illnesses during distance running. Med Sci Sports Exerc. 1996;28(12):i–x.

14. Gardner JW, Kark JA. Clinical diagnosis, management, and surveillance of exertional heat illness. In: Pandolf KB, Burr RE, editors. Textbook of military medicine. Medical aspects of harsh environments. Washington, DC: Office of the Surgeon General; 2001. p. 231–79.

15. Binkley HM, Beckett J, Casa DJ, Kleiner DM, Plummer PE. National Athletic Trainers' Association position statement: exertional heat illnesses. J Athl Train. 2002;37(3):329–43.

16. Casa DJ, Almquist J, Anderson S. Inter-association task force on exertional heat illnesses consensus statement. NATA News. 2003;6:24–9.

17. Department of the Army and Air Force. Heat stress control and heat casualty management. In: Technical bulletin medical 507. Natick: U.S. Army Research Institute of Environmental Medicine; 2003.

18. American College of Sports Medicine, Armstrong LE, Casa DJ, Millard-Stafford M, Moran DS, Pyne SW, Roberts WO. American College of Sports Medicine position stand. Exertional heat illness during training and competition. Med Sci Sports Exerc. 2007;39(3):556–72.

19. Casa DJ, DeMartini JK, Bergeron MF, Csillan D, Eichner ER, Lopez RM, et al. National Athletic Trainers' Association position statement: exertional heat illnesses. J Athl Train. 2015;50(9):986–1000.

20. Fiske CN. The effects of exposure to intense heat on the working organism. In: Transactions of the fifteenth international congress on hygiene and demography, Washington D.C., September 23–28, 1912. Ann Arbor: University of Michigan Library; 1913.

21. Galloway SD, Maughan RJ. Effects of ambient temperature on the capacity to perform prolonged cycle exercise in man. Med Sci Sports Exerc. 1997;29(9):1240–9.

22. Holtzhausen LM, Noakes TD. The prevalence and significance of post-exercise (postural) hypotension in ultramarathon runners. Med Sci Sports Exerc. 1995;27(12):1595–601.

23. Roberts WO. A 12-yr profile of medical injury and illness for the Twin Cities Marathon. Med Sci Sports Exerc. 2000;32(9):1549–55.

24. Speedy DB, Noakes TB, Holtzhausen LM. Exercise-associated collapse: postural hypotension, or something deadlier? Phys Sportsmed. 2003;31(3):23–9.

25. Noakes TD. Reduced peripheral resistance and other factors in marathon collapse. Sports Med. 2007;37(4–5):382–5.

26. Fiske CN. The effects of exposure to intense heat on the working organism. Am J Med Sci. 1913;145:565–85.

27. Phelps JR. Heat cramps and heat exhaustion on board ships of the navy in recent months. US Navy Bull. 1926;24:145–54.

28. Morton TS. The etiology and treatment of heat exhaustion and heat hyperpyrexia, with special reference to experiences in Iraq. J R Army Med Corps. 1932;59:200–11.

29. King BA, Barry ME. The physiological adaptations to heat-stress with a classification of heat illness and a description of the features of heat exhaustion. S Afr Med J. 1962;36:451–5.

30. Armstrong LE, Hubbard RW, Szlyk PC, Sils IV, Kraemer WJ. Heat intolerance, heat exhaustion monitored: a case report. Aviat Space Environ Med. 1988;59(3):262–6.

31. Shahid MS, Hatle L, Mansour H, Mimish L. Echocardiographic and Doppler study of patients with heatstroke and heat exhaustion. Int J Card Imaging. 1999;15(4):279–85.

32. Weiner JS. An experimental study of heat collapse. J Ind Hyg Toxicol. 1938;20:389–400.

33. Donoghue AM, Sinclair MJ, Bates GP. Heat exhaustion in a deep underground metalliferous mine. Occup Environ Med. 2000;57(3):165–74.

34. Kenefick RW, Sawka MN. Heat exhaustion and dehydration as causes of marathon collapse. Sports Med. 2007;37(4–5):378–81.

35. Armstrong LE, Johnson EC, Casa DJ, Ganio MS, McDermott BP, Yamamoto LM, et al. The American football uniform: uncompensable heat stress and hyperthermic exhaustion. J Athl Train. 2010;45(2):117–27.

36. Sawka MN, Young AJ, Latzka WA, Neufer PD, Quigley MD, Pandolf KB. Human tolerance to heat strain during exercise: influence of hydration. J Appl Physiol (1985). 1992;73(1):368–75.

37. Stearns RL, Casa DJ, O'Connor FG, Kenny GP. Exertional heat stroke. In: Casa DJ, Stearns R, editors. Preventing sudden death in sport and physical activity. Burlington: Jones & Bartlett; 2017. p. 71–92.

38. Adolph EF. Physiology of man in the desert. New York: Interscience; 1947.
39. Bean WB, Eichna LW. Performance in relation to environmental temperature. Reactions of normal young men to simulated desert environment. Fed Proc. 1943;2:144–58.
40. Poh P, Armstrong LE, Casa DJ, Pescatello LS, McDermott BP, Emmanuel H, et al. Orthostatic hypotension after 10 days of exercise-heat acclimation and 28 hours of sleep loss. Aviat Space Environ Med. 2012;83(4):403–11.
41. Armstrong LE, Maresh CM. The induction and decay of heat acclimatisation in trained athletes. Sports Med. 1991;12(5):302–12.
42. Vaamonde CA. Sodium depletion. In: Papper S, editor. Sodium: its biological significance. Boca Raton: CRC Press; 1980. p. 208–34.
43. Marriott HL. Water and salt depletion. Springfield: Charles C. Thomas; 1950. p. 12–73.
44. McCance RA. Medical problems in mineral metabolism. Lancet. 1936;227:704–10.
45. Drewnowski A, Rehm CD, Constant F. Water and beverage consumption among adults in the United States: cross-sectional study using data from NHANES 2005–2010. BMC Public Health. 2013;13:1068. https://doi.org/10.1186/1471-2458-13-1068.
46. U.S. Department of Health and Human Services and U.S. Department of Agriculture. Dietary guidelines for Americans. 8th ed. Washington, D.C: Office of Disease Prevention and Health Promotion; 2015–2020. http://health.gov/dietaryguidelines/2015/guidelines/. Accessed 17 Sept 2019.
47. Leithead CS, Lind AR. Heat stress and heat disorders. Philadelphia: F.A. Davis; 1964. p. 143–69.
48. Ladell WS. The changes in water and chloride distribution during heavy sweating. J Physiol. 1949;108:440–50.
49. Armed Forces Health Surveillance Center: Armed Forces Reportable Medical Events Guidelines and Case Definitions. 2017. https://health.mil/Military-Health-Topics/Combat-Support/Armed-Forces-Health-Surveillance-Branch. Accessed 17 Sept 2019.
50. Dinman BD, Horvath SM. Heat disorders in industry. A reevaluation of diagnostic criteria. J Occup Med. 1984;26:489–95.
51. Bergeron MF. Exertional heat cramps. In: Armstrong LE, editor. Exertional heat illnesses. Champaign: Human Kinetics; 2003. p. 91–102.
52. Ladell WS. Heat cramps. Lancet. 1949;254:836–9.
53. Armstrong LE, Hubbard RW, Kraemer WJ, DeLuca JP, Christensen EL. Signs and symptoms of heat exhaustion during strenuous exercise. Ann Sports Med. 1987;3:182–9.
54. Armstrong LE, Anderson JM. Heat exhaustion, exercise-associated collapse, and heat syncope. In: Armstrong LE, editor. Exertional heat illnesses. Champaign: Human Kinetics; 2003. p. 57–90.
55. Åstrand PO, Rodahl K. A textbook of work physiology: physiological bases of exercise. 2nd ed. New York: McGraw-Hill; 1977.
56. Hubbard RW. The role of exercise in the etiology of exertional heatstroke. Med Sci Sports Exerc. 1990;22(1):2–5.
57. Hubbard RW, Armstrong LE. The heat illnesses: biochemical, ultrastructural and fluid-electrolyte considerations. In: Pandolf KB, Sawka MN, Gonzalez RR, editors. Human performance physiology and environmental medicine at terrestrial extremes. Indianapolis: Benchmark Press; 1988. p. 305–59.
58. Armstrong LE, Casa DJ. Methods to evaluate electrolyte and water turnover of athletes. Ath Train Sports Health Care. 2009;1:169–79.

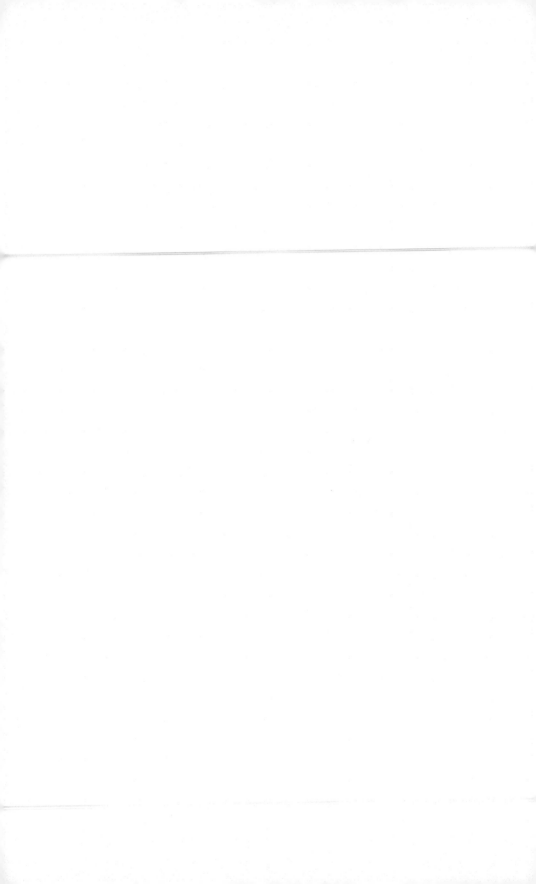

Chapter 6
Exercise-Associated Muscle Cramps

Kevin C. Miller

Introduction

The year is 2014. The Miami Heat are in the National Basketball Association (NBA) Finals for the fourth consecutive year. They are attempting to become the first basketball team since 2002 to win three consecutive NBA championships. Headlining the matchup was one of the greatest, and highest paid, professional basketball players of all time—LeBron James. At the time, James won the NBA's coveted most valuable player award four times in the preceding 6 years. The matchup was set. The Heat would be playing the San Antonio Spurs.

Game 1 of the NBA Finals occurred on a Friday night in San Antonio, Texas. Oddly, the air conditioning was broken in AT&T stadium, and the on-court temperature exceeded 90 °F (32.2 °C). With a little over 7 minutes remaining in the game, James was forced to exit the biggest game of his season because of exercise-associated muscle cramps (EAMC) in his legs. The medical staff admirably treated James' EAMC as best, and as fast, as they could. James struggled but was able to return to the court. In the end, the medical staff's efforts would be unsuccessful.

With 4:16 remaining in the game, the Heat faced a 4-point deficit. James got the ball, stared down his opponent, made a hard jab step left, crossed the ball over to his right, drove to the basket, and laid the ball in the hoop for 2 points! There was just one problem. When James landed from his jump, he just stood there. He could not move or get back down the court to play defense. James called to his medical staff and told them his legs were cramping again. Ever so slowly, James cautiously walked off the court. Eventually, his pain and cramping became too much, and he needed his teammates to carry him to the bench.

K. C. Miller (✉)
School of Rehabilitation and Medical Sciences, Central Michigan University,
Mount Pleasant, MI, USA
e-mail: mille5k@cmich.edu

© Springer Nature Switzerland AG 2020   117
W. M. Adams, J. F. Jardine (eds.), *Exertional Heat Illness*,
https://doi.org/10.1007/978-3-030-27805-2_6

James never returned to Game 1 after that. With the best player out of the game, the Spurs went on to win the game with a final score of 110–95. When all was said and done, the Miami Heat's best player played just 5 of 12 minutes in the fourth quarter of Game 1. In his post-game remarks, James remarked:

> It's something [*talking about EAMC*] you try to prevent, you try to control. I mean, I got all the fluids I need to get. I do my normal routine I've done. It was inevitable for me tonight, throughout the conditions, you know, out there on the floor. I lost all the fluids I was putting in the last couple of days. It sucks not being out there for your team, especially at this point in the season.

He continued:

> Drank a lot at halftime, even, changed my uniform, just tried to get the sweat up off of you. Our training staff tried to do the best they could by giving us ice bags and cold towels on timeouts, keep us dry.

When we evaluate this game, several questions come to mind. Were James' EAMC truly inevitable? Were the EAMC caused by the fluids he lost while playing in those hot conditions, and, if so, why was James the only player to get debilitating EAMC during that game? Were the fluids, ice bags, and cold towels the best treatments for his EAMC? Was there anything James or the medical staff could have done to prevent the EAMC from occurring in the first place?

Athletes, laborers, soldiers, and other physically active persons may experience painful, involuntary contractions of skeletal muscle during the course of their exertional activity. These exercise-associated muscle cramps (EAMC) are especially common injuries though estimates of their prevalence are wide-ranging. In athletes, EAMC incidence ranges from 40% to 70% [1]. In a large 4-year prospective cohort study of over 26,000 ultra-distance marathoners, EAMC occurred in 1.9 of every 1000 runners [2]. In American football players, EAMC prevalence was 3.07 per 1000 athlete exposures [3]. Some authors [4] even estimated 95% of physically active individuals have experienced at least one EAMC in their lifetimes.

Despite affecting so many people, significant confusion exists around the cause, prevention, and treatment of EAMC. Part of this confusion stems from inappropriate terminology to describe EAMC and the association of muscle cramping with general medical conditions (e.g., hypothyroidism, kidney dysfunction) or their treatments (e.g., dialysis). While muscle cramping can occur as a side effect of medications, underlying disease, or medical treatment, EAMC are a unique injury in that they occur in otherwise healthy individuals. For example, they are not the muscle cramps experienced by athletes during an exertional sickling episode. Unlike EAMC, sickling cramps tend to be less painful, have no preliminary "twitching" preceding full cramping, occur alongside general muscle weakness, and are due to oxygen starvation in the muscle [5].

Confusion also exists because of inappropriate terminology. Terms like "spasms," "tics," "twinges," and "contractures" are inappropriate because, unlike EAMC, these conditions are usually painless or electrically silent on electromyogram [6]. "Heat cramps" and "exertional heat cramps" are also inappropriate terms because EAMC occur in cool and temperature-controlled climates [7], are not associated with elevated body core temperatures [8], do not occur concurrently with the onset of severe heat-related illnesses like exertional heat stroke, and are not relieved by cooling. Moreover, if EAMC were due to "heat," the best treatment for EAMC (i.e., stretching) would be ineffective. While a number of inappropriate terms, beliefs, and treatments for EAMC still exist today, great strides have been made in the last 50 years toward better understanding their pathophysiology.

Pathophysiology of Exercise-Associated Muscle Cramping

The pathophysiology of EAMC is controversial, though two main theories have emerged over the last 100 years [9–11]. The earliest attempts to understand EAMC began in the early twentieth century and associated EAMC with strenuous work in the heat, excessive fluid consumption, and losses of blood chloride [12, 13]. Then, in the late 1940s, Ladell [14] performed a series of experiments and made two primary observations: EAMC rarely occurred without salt deficiencies and intravenous fluid replacement appeared to relieve EAMC. It was from these early works that the "dehydration/electrolyte imbalance" theory emerged.

The Dehydration/Electrolyte Imbalance Theory

Water and electrolytes are essential for maintaining normal body functioning. The human body is 50–70% water, and our body's fluids are divided between two main areas known as the intracellular (i.e., inside the cells) and extracellular compartments (i.e., outside the cells). Quite simply, water is essential for maintaining cellular integrity and function, and death occurs in a matter of days if water is prohibited. Similarly, electrolytes like sodium, potassium, and chloride play important roles in body fluid balance, nerve conduction, and muscle contraction to name a few. Since fluid and electrolytes are the main components in sweat, their loss during exercise is often associated with EAMC genesis [1]. In fact, the dehydration/electrolyte imbalance theory is the most widely believed theory for EAMC genesis. Eighty-eight percent of collegiate athletes [15] and 92% of medical professionals [16] believe dehydration or electrolyte imbalance cause EAMC.

Proponents of the dehydration/electrolyte imbalance theory posit losses in sodium and chloride from exercise-induced sweating causes a large deficit in whole-body exchangeable sodium. Consequently, fluid shifts out of the interstitium (i.e., the space surrounding muscle cells) and into the blood vessels. The interstitium then contracts until there is mechanical deformation of peripheral nerve endings and an increase in the concentration of excitatory neurotransmitters (e.g., acetylcholine), metabolites, and electrolytes [9]. Then, select motor nerve terminals become hyperexcitable, spontaneously discharge, and result in EAMC.

Support for the Dehydration/Electrolyte Imbalance Theory

Advocates [9, 17] for the dehydration/electrolyte imbalance theory primarily cite three lines of evidence for support. First, early observational studies of occupational workers (e.g., miners) showed EAMC were relieved by ingesting salt and fluids [12, 13]. Second, research shows fluid does shift from the interstitium to the vasculature during exercise [18]. Costill et al. [18] demonstrated that 40–60% of total body water loss during exercise came from the interstitium as subjects exercised to a body mass deficit of ~6%. Finally, case reports [19, 20] and field studies [21, 22] demonstrated some athletes with a history of EAMC had higher sweat rates and sweat sodium concentrations than athletes without a history of EAMC. Of note was the field study known as the "Sweaty Sooners Study." Stofan et al. [21] compared sweat rates, sweat sodium concentrations, and sweat potassium concentrations of five American football players with a history of EAMC (i.e., cramp-prone) to five athletes without a history of EAMC (i.e., non-crampers). The primary results were the cramp-prone athletes lost about 500 mL more sweat and had higher sweat sodium concentrations (55 mmol/L vs. 25 mmol/L) than the non-crampers. The term "salty sweaters" originated after this study and is still used today to describe individuals with EAMC [17].

Limitations of the Dehydration/Electrolyte Imbalance Theory

The dehydration/electrolyte imbalance theory suffers from numerous physiological inconsistencies and limitations:

1. There is no evidence of athletes with acute EAMC having higher interstitial excitatory neurochemicals or mechanical deformation of nerve terminals than athletes not experiencing EAMC.
2. Proponents of this theory [9] cite the work by Costill et al. [18] to support the claim that large volumes of fluid move from the interstitium to the vasculature during exercise. However, there is often no mention that Costill et al. [18] also measured intracellular and extracellular electrolyte concentrations so they could calculate resting muscle membrane potential. Simply put, resting membrane potential provides an indication of how easy a muscle cell is to depolarize and contract. Normally, a muscle's resting membrane potential is around −85 mV. The muscle cell will not contract unless the membrane depolarizes (i.e., becomes more positive). Once the muscle cell receives enough excitatory stimuli from a nerve to reach its threshold potential (normally around −50 mV), it contracts. Interestingly, Costill et al. [18] noted resting membrane potential remained fairly constant and even *decreased* slightly (i.e., became more negative) after subjects became severely hypohydrated. If the dehydration/electrolyte imbalance theory were true, resting membrane potential should have

increased, thereby making the muscle membrane more easily depolarized and more likely to develop spontaneous contractions. Yet, this did not occur.

3. Numerous cohort studies demonstrated plasma electrolyte concentrations [8, 23, 24] plasma volume [8, 24], blood volume [8, 24], and body weight losses [22–25] were within normal limits and not different between athletes who did and did not experience EAMC during exercise. Consequently, the volume and concentration of the fluid bathing the muscles and corresponding fluid pressures that drive fluid between compartments were comparable between crampers and non-crampers.

4. There are no data in humans to support the idea that interstitium pressure is higher in individuals with EAMC. This may be due to the technically daunting nature and difficulty of taking this measurement in humans. However, in an animal model, interstitial compartment pressure was actually lower when animals were dehydrated than hydrated [26]. This is contradictory to what the dehydration/electrolyte imbalance theory proposes.

5. In some instances [20, 21], athletes with a history of EAMC lost up to 10 grams of sodium (more than four times the recommended sodium intake per day) via exercise-induced sweating. However, not one subject in every observational study showing "crampers" lost large quantities of sweat, and electrolytes actually developed EAMC during or after exercise [19–22].

6. The studies comparing sweat characteristics in athletes with and without a history of EAMC did not control for numerous factors affecting sweat electrolyte concentrations (e.g., diet, acclimatization status, and exercise intensity) [27]. Thus, it is impossible to determine whether the higher sweat electrolyte concentrations were due to the athletes having a history of EAMC or some other confounding variable. Moreover, the observational research design these studies [19–22] employed prohibits cause and effect inferences.

7. The studies [21, 22] showing high sweat electrolyte concentrations in cramp-prone athletes had very small sample sizes ($n < 6$ cramp-prone and $n < 8$ non-crampers). This is problematic because sweat electrolyte concentrations vary considerably [27]. Sweat sodium concentration in athletes can vary between 15 mmol/L and 100 mmol/L. Baker et al. [28] determined that the average sweat sodium concentration in over 500 male and female athletes from a variety of skill and endurance sports was 44 ± 18 mmol/L. In 2018, Miller et al. [29] completed the largest cohort study to date comparing male and female Division 1 collegiate athletes with and without a self-reported lifetime occurrence of EAMC (245 athletes with EAMC history, 95 athletes without EAMC history). They observed sweat sodium concentration of cramp-prone athletes varied from 25 ± 3 mmol/L to 51 ± 12 mmol/L, whereas non-crampers varied from 21 ± 4 mmol/L to 50 ± 11 mmol/L [29]. Receiver operating characteristic area under the curve (AUC) analysis further indicated sweat rate, sweat sodium concentration and content, sweat potassium concentration and content, and sweat chloride concentration and content were not predictive (i.e., values ranged from 0.46 to 0.57) of EAMC in nine of ten sports. However, sweat rate, sweat sodium content, sweat potassium content, and sweat chloride content were predictive of

EAMC history in American football players (AUC values ranged from 0.65 to 0.72). Discrepancies between our data and others [21, 22] are likely due to how authors defined "crampers." We used self-reported lifetime history of EAMC to define crampers, whereas other scientists [21, 22] required medical documentation of EAMC occurrence, intravenous fluid replacement, or inability to continue participation to define crampers. Admittedly, our [29] definition was prone to recall bias. However, the latter definition was overly restrictive since many EAMC go unreported to medical professionals and few EAMC require IV fluids to treat [24] or cause athletes to discontinue exercise [30]. Thus, the athletes in the "salty sweater" studies [20–22] were well within normal limits for sweat electrolyte concentrations in athletes.

8. Muscle cramp susceptibility was unaffected when muscle cramps were induced in a rested, unexercised muscle of mildly (3% body mass reduction) and severely (up to 5% body mass reduction) hypohydrated subjects [31, 32]. Unlike the prospective cohort studies which also demonstrated similar body mass reductions in athletes with and without EAMC [8, 23–25], these two laboratory studies [31, 32] isolated the effects of fatigue from dehydration. By doing so, the authors [31, 32] demonstrated that mild and severe levels of hypohydration and up to 4 grams of sodium loss did not alter muscle cramp risk.

9. When subjects ingested sports drinks at a similar rate as their sweat losses during a calf-fatiguing protocol, EAMC still occurred 70% of the time [33].

10. There is a disconnect between the known treatment for EAMC (i.e., stretching) and purported cause of EAMC if the dehydration/electrolyte imbalance theory was true. Gentle static stretching alleviates EAMC but does not add any electrolytes or fluid to the body. If dehydration or electrolyte imbalance elicited EAMC, then stretching should not alleviate them.

11. Cramp-prone athletes consume similar volumes of fluid during exercise as non-crampers [21, 22]. Thus, EAMC do not seem to be caused by some athletes failing to drink enough during exercise.

For these reasons, several prominent professional organizations, including the National Athletic Trainers Association [34] and American College of Sports Medicine [35], noted that the level of evidence supporting the dehydration/electrolyte imbalance theory was weak.

The Altered Neuromuscular Control Theory

As an alternative to the dehydration/electrolyte imbalance theory, Schwellnus et al. [36] proposed the altered neuromuscular control theory in 1996. Originally, they [36] proposed exercise-induced fatigue causes an increase in excitatory activity from muscle spindles along with a concomitant decrease in inhibitory activity from Golgi tendon organs. Consequently, the exercising muscle's alpha motor neuron pool becomes increasingly excitable and elicits EAMC. Schwellnus [10] later revised this theory in 2009 to include other potential EAMC risk factors (e.g., muscle injury) which could result in overexcitation of the alpha motor nerve. Most recently, other authors [37, 38] have amended the altered neuromuscular control theory by emphasizing the likelihood that the pathophysiology of EAMC is multi-factorial and, potentially, unique within and between individuals. Thus, a greater emphasis was put on how risk factors interact to alter neuromuscular control and elicit EAMC (Fig. 6.1). Furthermore, there is a strong likelihood that once an EAMC occurs, a positive feedback loop is created which contributes to the recurrence and sustainability of EAMC (Fig. 6.2).

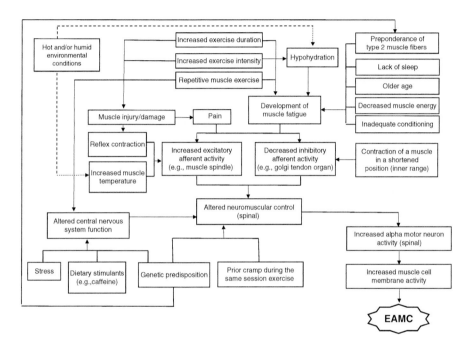

Fig. 6.1 Altered neuromuscular control theory for the pathogenesis of exercise-associated muscle cramps (*dashed arrow used for the sole purpose of improving clarity of the "hot and/or humid environmental conditions" pathway*). (Adapted from Schwellnus [10], with permission)

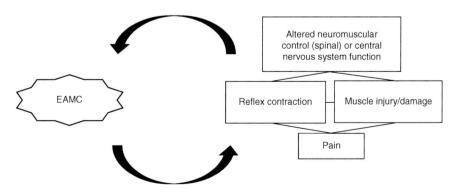

Fig. 6.2 Positive feedback loop demonstrating risk factors which may precipitate maintenance or increased susceptibility to future exercise associated muscle cramping

Support for the Altered Neuromuscular Control Theory

At its core, the altered neuromuscular control theory emphasizes the influence of risk factors on muscle afferents (e.g., muscle spindles and Golgi tendon organs) and neuromuscular control. Several observations from the literature indicate muscle afferents are essential for normal neuromuscular control and may contribute to EAMC development:

1. EAMC most commonly affect muscles that span two joints. The most common muscles to develop EAMC in distance runners were the hamstrings (48%), quadriceps (38%), and calves (14%) [24]. When muscles contract in shortened positions, the alpha motor neuron pool receives less inhibition from Golgi tendon organs [39].
2. Cramps can be alleviated by electrically stimulating Golgi tendon organs [40].
3. Electromyograms from cramping muscles and voluntary contractions demonstrate similar timing and amounts of inhibition. This suggests similar spinal pathways are utilized during normal muscle contractions and cramping [40].
4. Non-crampers produced significantly stronger amounts of inhibition than individuals who developed cramps [40].
5. Cramp duration was shorter, and cramp intensity was less severe when authors induced muscle cramps following a peripheral nerve block [41]. This suggests spinal involvement was necessary for cramp induction and maintenance.
6. Elevations in muscle temperature affect muscle afferent activity, especially muscle spindles [42]. In animal models, muscle spindle discharge frequency was 2–4 times higher when a warm muscle (35 °C) changed length than a cold muscle (25 °C) [43, 44]. By extension, alpha motor neuron excitability would also increase as muscle temperature increased. Since body core temperature and muscle temperatures increase faster under uncompensable conditions, this may explain why EAMC occur more frequently under hot and humid conditions [3].
7. The altered neuromuscular control theory better explains how static stretching relieves EAMC (see Treatment of EAMC section). Since muscle afferents contribute to the pathophysiology of EAMC, it is necessary to discuss the primary risk factors that affect muscle afferent activity and neuromuscular control.

Fatigue may affect neuromuscular control and play a role in the pathophysiology of EAMC. EAMC tend to occur near the end of competitions or exercise sessions when fatigue is the highest. In distance runners, EAMC did not occur until after 24–28 km (14.9–17.4 miles) [8, 24]. Maughan [8] noted 33% of the marathon runners with EAMC developed them in the last 1.5 km (0.9 mile) of the race. EAMC also tend to occur when athletes exercise at intensities higher than anticipated, when exercise intensity is increased, and when specific muscles are targeted [25, 33, 44]. Altering exercise in these ways would tend to induce fatigue faster. In fact, Jung et al. [33] induced EAMC in as little as 15 minutes when a calf-fatiguing protocol was used.

These observations are also consistent with the neurophysiology literature on muscle cramping. Electrically induced fatigue increased resting muscle spindle discharge frequency and firing rate [45] while also decreasing Golgi tendon organ activity [46]. Moreover, the following factors may also influence the onset of fatigue: having a preponderance of less fatigue-resistant muscle fibers (e.g., type II fibers), dehydration, lack of or diminished quality of sleep, exhausted muscle energy stores, age, and lack of conditioning [1, 2, 47]. Consequently, athletes who fail to prepare themselves against the onset of fatigue from any of these sources may be increasing their susceptibility to EAMC via fatigue-induced changes in the neuromuscular system.

Pain and/or psychological stress may also be risk factors for EAMC by influencing neuromuscular control [48, 49]. In three different cohort studies examining risk factors for EAMC, muscle injury, pre-race muscle damage, and pain were predisposing factors to EAMC [50–52]. In one study, pre-race creatine kinase (i.e., an indicator of muscle damage) levels were 35% higher in athletes who developed EAMC during an ultramarathon than non-cramping athletes [51]. Summers et al. [52] noted that low back pain that resulted in rugby players missing playing time was a risk factor for calf EAMC. From the neurophysiology literature, the presence of painful illnesses and conditions increased action potential activity in muscles suggesting pain increased muscle activity [53]. Moreover, Golgi tendon organ activity decreased followed experimentally induced muscle pain [54]. Interestingly, when pain was induced by injecting glutamate into a muscle's latent trigger point, Ge et al. [49] elicited an increase in muscle action potential activity and even elicited muscle cramps. Moreover, when hypertonic saline was injected into a muscle to increase nociceptor activity, scientists could induce cramping with fewer electrical stimulations than when isotonic saline was injected [48]. Similarly, psychological stress may also influence neurological control. Ironman athletes with EAMC predicted they would finish a race approximately 40 minutes faster than their actually time [25]. This may have resulted in higher stress which may have increased central nervous system and/or muscle activity [55]. These observations suggest pain and stress may alter neurological activity and predispose athletes to EAMC.

A history of EAMC is one of the best predictors of future EAMC and is consistent with the altered neuromuscular control theory. Miller et al. [56] observed cramp-prone individuals required fewer electrical stimulations to induce cramping than individuals without a history of cramping. Moreover, almost 90% of their [56] subjects with a history of cramping also had a familial history of cramping. Thus, there may be a genetic predisposition to EAMC. Prior EAMC also appear to predict EAMC recurrence; 71% of distance runners reported having more than three EAMC despite attempts by clinicians or athletes at treatment [24]. Recent laboratory studies confirm this observation; cramp susceptibility was higher for up to 60 minutes following a volitionally induced cramp in rested, unexercised subjects [57]. This increased susceptibility may be due to cramping causing nervous system excitation [58]. Overall, the altered neuromuscular control theory is more consistent with the muscle cramping literature and does not suffer from as many limitations as the dehydration/electrolyte imbalance theory.

Limitations of the Altered Neuromuscular Control Theory

The altered neuromuscular control theory is not without limitations, and several questions remain unanswered. First, it is unclear how fatigue alters muscle spindle or Golgi tendon organ activity. Second, it is unknown to what extent individuals must become fatigued to develop EAMC and whether this fatigue level can be modulated (positively or negatively) by other factors. Numerous highly trained and well-conditioned athletes develop EAMC, and their history of training is often not predictive of EAMC [51, 59]. Third, it is unclear whether central or peripheral fatigue or any other singular factor is more important than another to the pathophysiology of EAMC. Fourth, many of the prospective cohort studies examining athletes with and without EAMC rely on question-naires for information about past EAMC [23, 25, 51, 52, 59]. Thus, there may be some recall bias in the responses. Finally, while neurophysiology studies on muscle cramping have greatly improved our understanding of how other factors unrelated to fatigue can alter neuromuscular control, uncertainty exists regard-ing the application of their results to EAMC. Further research is needed to clarify whether exercise induces similar changes in muscle afferents and neuro-muscular control.

Recognition of Exercise-Associated Muscle Cramping

Clinically, EAMC are easily recognized. During an acute EAMC, individuals will be in noticeable pain with all, or sections of, their skeletal muscle firm, pulsing, and/or bulging involuntarily. Concomitantly, there may be alterations in joint position due to the sustained involuntary contraction. For example, the ankle and toes may point downward (i.e., plantarflexed) if the calf is actively cramping. Typically, EAMC last a few seconds or minutes and affect the skeletal muscles which cross two joints (e.g., quadriceps, hamstrings, calves) [24]. Moreover, some individuals are able to sense EAMC are imminent or articulate they "feel like they will cramp" [19]. This "cramp-prone state" usually precedes the onset of full EAMC and is often an indicator an individual needs to modify or cease their activity level or EAMC will occur.

Though easily recognized, EAMC severity varies considerably. In most cases, EAMC are mild and do not impair athletic performance [8, 23, 24]. However, some athletes may be unable to complete athletic events because of EAMC. Hoffman and Fogard [30] reported 5% of ultramarathoners were unable to finish a competition because of EAMC. While rare, reports of hospitalization due to EAMC have been reported [60] though advanced diagnostic testing and blood work are often unre-markable in individuals with EAMC [23, 24, 61].

Treatment of Exercise-Associated Muscle Cramping

The immediate treatment for individuals experiencing an acute EAMC is slow, gentle static stretching of the muscle until the EAMC subsides. Static stretching is the most utilized treatment by clinicians to relieve EAMC [16] and is also a common self-treatment used by athletes if they experience EAMC during competitions [24]. Static stretching may alleviate EAMC via two mechanisms. The simplest explanation is static stretching elongates the muscle, thereby physically separating the contractile proteins and prevents the muscle from contracting. When muscles are unable to contract, they cannot cramp [62]. Alternatively, static stretching may increase tension in muscle tendons, thereby increasing inhibitory signals from Golgi tendon organs and lowering the excitability of the alpha motor neuron pool [36, 39].

Once the EAMC has dissipated and the athlete is no longer in pain, clinicians should rule out other potentially dangerous conditions (e.g., low blood glucose, high body temperatures). If athletes do not present with signs or symptoms of other dangerous general medical conditions, clinicians can focus on identifying the potential underlying factors which preceded the EAMC. Since the cause of EAMC is likely multifactorial, clinicians must thoroughly question athletes to determine the underlying cause of EAMC (Table 6.1) and then target those factors with appropriate interventions.

Many individuals use food, drinks, and other home remedies to treat EAMC. Most of these ingestible remedies are associated with the belief that EAMC are due to electrolyte losses. For example, bananas and mustard are often advocated to cramp-prone athletes because of their electrolyte content. However, individuals must consume at least 2 servings of bananas (~3 bananas) and wait 30 minutes before a meaningful increase in blood potassium content occurs post-exercise [67]. Similarly, eating the equivalent of 30 mustard packets (141 grams) did not alter blood electrolytes up to 60 minutes post-ingestion in dehydrated subjects [68]. Thus, banana or mustard ingestion is too slow to relieve an acute EAMC.

Another popular EAMC remedy is ingestion of pickle juice. Pickle juice is sometimes recommended because of its high sodium content, and the assumption EAMC are caused by sodium losses [69]. Interestingly, ingesting small volumes (~80 mL) of pickle juice during an electrically induced muscle cramp relieved the cramps 37% faster than water and 45% faster than drinking nothing at all [70]. However, like mustard and bananas, the nutrients in pickle juice are not absorbed by the body quickly post-ingestion. Miller et al. [71] observed small volumes of pickle juice stayed in the stomach for at least 25 minutes. Moreover, several experimental studies showed blood electrolyte concentrations do not change significantly following ingestion of small volumes of pickle juice [68, 70, 72]. Consequently, Miller et al. [70] hypothesized pickle juice ingestion relieved cramping through an oropharyngeal reflex rather than electrolyte restoration. They further hypothesized it was the acetic acid (vinegar) in pickle juice that elicited the reaction. Further research is required to elucidate the ingredients that trigger this reflex as well as the pathway and receptors through which pickle juice relieves cramping.

Table 6.1 Questions to aid in the identification of EAMC risk factors

Question	Justification	Risk factor
1. Do you have any illnesses or medical conditions?	Muscle cramping may be associated with diseases [1]	Underlying illness
2. Did EAMC occur after a change in or start of medication or drug use?	Muscle cramping may be associated with medication use [1].	Medication side effect
3. How hard were you exercising before you developed EAMC?	EAMC occur in athletes with the fastest actual and predicted race times [2, 25, 59]	Fatigue
4. When did the EAMC occur during exercise (i.e., beginning, middle, end)?	EAMC tend to occur near the end of exercise or competitions [8, 24]	Fatigue
5. How much sleep did you get the night before your exercise session when EAMC occurred?	Sleep loss reduced muscle glycogen [63] and time to exhaustion and increased energy needs [64]	Premature fatigue
6. How hot and humid was it when you developed EAMC?	EAMC can occur under any environmental conditions though they do occur most frequently in summer months (e.g., August) [3]	Hypohydration, premature fatigue, unacclimatized to environment
7. Was the exercise session during which EAMC occurred novel in any way?	EAMC tended to occur more in untrained individuals [12] or during harder than anticipated events [65]	Overexertion and/or fatigue
8. What was your diet like in the days preceding the EAMC? Was it balanced and nutritious?	Diets low in carbohydrates may reduce muscle glycogen and the amount of work or exercise performed [66]	Premature fatigue
9. Did you consume stimulants (e.g., caffeine) before your exercise session?	Stimulants can increase excitability of the nervous system	Overexcitation of the nervous system
10. Were you recently injured?	Pain [48, 49, 52] and prior injury [51] are predictors of cramping	Overexcitation of the nervous system
11. What was your psychological state during the exercise session when EAMC developed?	Stress [55] or unrealistic expectations [25] may increase nervous system and/or excitability	Overexcitation of the nervous system
12. Did you consume enough fluids and/or electrolytes to replace your sweat losses?	Contribution of sweat losses to EAMC genesis is equivocal [21–24]. American football players with an EAMC history may benefit from fluid and electrolyte monitoring [29]	Hypohydration; premature fatigue

Table 6.1 (continued)

Question	Justification	Risk factor
13. Did the EAMC tend to stop once you stopped the activity?	Activity cessation and/or reduced pace can relieve EAMC [44]	Overexcitation of the nervous system
14. Do the EAMC tend to occur only in the muscles that were doing the most work?	EAMC tend to affect working muscles and may be mitigated with reeducation of synergistic muscles [44]	Overexcitation of the nervous system
15. Did EAMC occur during training or during competition?	EAMC tend to affect athletes more during competitions than training [25]	Overexcitation due to stress of competition; premature fatigue due to overexertion

EAMC exercise-associated muscle cramps. Questions appear in no particular order or level of importance after Questions 1 and 2

A popular and dangerous misconception is sports drinks can be consumed to treat EAMC because they contain electrolytes. Most commercially available sports drinks are hypotonic. This means they contain less sodium in them than the blood. Consequently, drinking sports drinks tends to reduce blood sodium concentration [73]. If hypotonic beverages, like sports drinks, are overconsumed, a rare but deadly condition known as exertional hyponatremia (i.e., low blood sodium) may occur [74]. Table 6.2 demonstrates the *dangerous* volume of a variety of popular sports drinks a person would need to ingest to fully replace ~5 grams of sodium and ~1 gram of potassium. While the volumes in Table 6.2 are already dangerous, even more concerning is that some authors [20, 21] report athletes with a history of EAMC can lose up to 10 grams of sodium during exercise! Sadly, athletes overconsuming dangerous volumes of fluid to prevent and treat EAMC are not hypothetical. In 2014, two otherwise healthy secondary school American football athletes died from exercise-associated hyponatremia. In both cases, the young men died because they were trying to treat and prevent EAMC by consuming sports drinks and/or water [75].

Unfortunately, once an EAMC occurs, the likelihood of recurrence is high. EAMC recurrence during exercise has been reported in several sports [19, 24]. Seventy-one percent (15 of 21) of distance runners with EAMC reported experiencing more than three EAMC during a 56-km road race [24]. Moreover, EAMC symptoms have been reported for hours after an initial EAMC [61]. Sulzer et al. [23] noted electromyography activity was 1–2 times higher in cramping muscles compared to control muscles within the same athletes for several minutes after EAMC cessation. Miller et al. [57] demonstrated cramp susceptibility was elevated up to 1 hour following a volitionally induced muscle cramp. Ross [58] noted the Hoffman reflex (an indicator of motor neuron excitability) was up to 9 times higher following a calf cramp. Miller et al. [76] confirmed and extended Ross's original observations [58] when it was noted the Hoffman reflex was 25%, 37%, and 44% higher than

Table 6.2 Volume of sports drink an athlete with EAMC would need to ingest to completely replace sodium and potassium losses

Sports drink	[Na+] of beverage, (g/L)	Volume needed to fully replace Na + lost, L (gal)	[K+] of beverage, (g/L)	Volume needed to fully replace K+ lost, L (gal)
A-Game	0.49	10.0 (2.7)	0.32	2.9 (0.8)
Accelerade[a]	0.62	7.9 (2.1)	0.25	3.8 (1.0)
All Sport	0.24	20.5 (5.4)	0.25	3.8 (1.0)
Body Armor SuperDrink	0.09	54.6 (14.4)	1.48	0.64 (0.2)
Gatorade, Original/ Fierce/G2/Organic/ Flow/Zero/Frost	0.46	10.7 (2.8)	0.13	7.23 (1.9)
Infuse Thirst Quencher	0.42	11.7 (3.1)	0.13	7.23 (1.9)
K+ Organic Sports Drink	0.25	19.6 (5.2)	0.15	6.3 (1.7)
Monster Energy Hydro Sports Drink	0.21	23.4 (6.2)	0.17	5.53 (1.5)
PowerAde, Original/ Zero	0.42	11.6 (3.1)	0.10	9.4 (2.5)
Propel Fitness Water	0.46	10.7 (2.8)	0.12	7.8 (2.1)
SoBe Water	0.13	37.8 (9.9)	0.15	6.3 (1.7)
Squincher	0.23	21.3 (5.6)	0.19	4.9 (1.3)
Staminade	0.38	12.9 (3.4)	0.19	4.9 (1.3)
Vitamin Water, Active Werk it	0.51	9.8 (2.6)	0.18	5.2 (1.4)

Estimates are based on the following assumptions and data from the literature on cramp-prone athletes: (1) an average sweat sodium concentration of 48.4 mmol/L (1.1 g/L) [19–22], (2) an average sweat potassium concentration of 5.4 mmol/L (0.21 g/L) [19, 22], (3) an average sweat rate of 2.23 L/h [19–22], and (4) a 2-hour, continuous exercise bout. Based on these assumptions, the athlete would need to replace 4.91 g of Na + and 0.94 g of K+

EAMC exercise-associated muscle cramp, [Na+] sodium concentration, [K+] potassium concentration
[a]Product sold as a powder and made per manufacturer instructions

baseline at 10, 30, and 60 minutes, respectively, following volitionally induced calf cramp. Since the subjects [57, 76] did not undergo exercise or any other intervention, muscle cramping, in and of itself, may precipitate future cramp episodes by increasing the excitability of the central nervous system. Therefore, it is imperative that clinicians and athletes continue to treat EAMC over time and not just immediately after EAMC cessation.

Return to Activity Following Exercise-Associated Muscle Cramping

EAMC usually cause temporary discomfort, and return to activity is self-regulated according to a person's tolerance. However, EAMC can prevent completion of athletic activity in rare cases [30]. Most athletes who develop EAMC are able to resume exercise following self-treatment (e.g., slowing pace or stretching) [24]. As mentioned previously, it is likely EAMC will recur if exercise continues since cramping, in and of itself, increases nervous system excitability [57, 76, 77]. If athletes suffer from persistent and recurrent EAMC despite several unsuccessful attempts at prevention, they should see a physician to undergo advanced medical screening to rule out predisposing medical conditions. Little is known about the long-term effects of EAMC on health and is an area ripe for further research.

Prevention of Exercise-Associated Muscle Cramping

The first step in preventing EAMC is to perform a thorough medical history to rule out predisposing illnesses or medications that could be triggering EAMC. Muscle cramps are often associated with diseases (e.g., diabetes, cirrhosis). Moreover, they may occur as side effects of certain medications or procedures (e.g., dialysis). Once these have been ruled out, clinicians may attempt targeted prophylactic strategies tailored toward an individual's unique risk factors. General, non-specific recommendations to prevent EAMC must be avoided (e.g., drink more fluids, consume more electrolytes). Instead, it is paramount to identify the possible triggers that precipitate the occurrence of EAMC since the pathophysiology of EAMC is likely unique within and between individuals.

Numerous EAMC risk factors have been proposed in the literature with varying degrees of support [1]. Several studies consistently show a prior history of EAMC, muscle damage/injury, and faster running times as significant EAMC risk factor [2, 25, 50–52, 56]. Conversely, stretching history, muscle flexibility, body mass index, weight, gender, dehydration, electrolyte losses, and age are less consistently identified as EAMC risk factors [23–25, 52, 59]. Because of the lack of consistency in risk factors and the likelihood of a multifactorial etiology, it is important to question athletes thoroughly, so their unique risk factors can be identified before starting an EAMC prevention program (see Table 6.1). Since the preponderance of evidence supports the altered neuromuscular control theory, the majority of these questions should revolve around the onset of fatigue or nervous system excitability. To aid in identifying an individual's risk factors, individuals can keep an "EAMC journal" in which they answer the questions posed in Table 6.1 and then look for patterns in the information when EAMC occur. Once an individual's unique risk factors are identified, risk factor-specific prevention strategies can be implemented.

For individuals with overexertion or fatigue as risk factors, several strategies can be utilized. However, these strategies must be implemented cautiously since data supporting the effectiveness of these strategies for EAMC is sparse and/or conflicting. Neuromuscular reeducation may help prevent EAMC. In a case report, persistent hamstring EAMC were eliminated when a triathlete incorporated gluteal exercises into his training regimen [44]. The authors [44] hypothesized that by utilizing his gluteal muscles more during exercise, the hamstrings muscles were less stressed and did not become as easily fatigued. Other strategies to prevent the premature onset of fatigue include utilizing training strategies which target the neurological system (e.g., plyometrics); training, as much as possible, at exercise intensities, durations, and with other stressors that mimic competition; acclimatizing to the environmental conditions before competition; and beginning exercise euhydrated.

Three EAMC prevention strategies deserve special attention given their popularity [16]: pre-event electrolyte supplementation, intravenous (IV) fluid use, and pre-event static stretching. Since many believe EAMC and electrolyte loss are associated, it is common for individuals to preload with electrolytes (e.g., sodium) prior to competition. However, pre-event sodium supplementation did not prevent EAMC occurrence in ultramarathoners [78]. Similarly, IV fluids are often given to prevent EAMC in professional sports. Seventy-eight percent of head athletic trainers in professional American football used pregame IVs (i.e., normal saline) to prevent EAMC [79]. While most of these medical professionals (59%) believed the IVs were very or extremely effective, there is not a single randomized, controlled study showing IVs prevent EAMC more effectively than oral fluids or nothing at all. Finally, many athletes and clinicians use pre-competition stretching to prevent EAMC [16]. Unfortunately, several prospective cohort studies and laboratory studies suggest stretching is not an effective prophylactic strategy for EAMC. Stretching frequency, total stretch duration, and timing of stretching were all non-predictors of EAMC in triathletes [25, 59], while gastrocnemius, hamstring, and hip flexor flexibility and range of motion did not predict EAMC in rugby players [52]. Several laboratory studies on stretching are consistent with these observations. Neither acute static stretching nor proprioceptive neuromuscular facilitation stretching techniques altered cramp susceptibility [80]. Similarly, Golgi tendon organ inhibition returned to normal within 1 minute of an acute bout of clinician-applied static stretching to the calf [81]. While a single bout of acute stretching may not affect EAMC genesis, there are no current data on long-term stretching's effect on EAMC. Given the low-cost and relative safety of stretching, more research is needed on this intervention before its use before competitions is completely disregarded.

Overall, preventing EAMC is difficult. Looming questions remain about the origin and predisposing factors of EAMC, and studying them is difficult because of their spontaneity and unpredictability. While scientists have made great attempts at rectifying this problem by inducing muscle cramps with maximum voluntary contractions and electrical stimulation, questions remain about these models' validity to EAMC. Moreover, there are no well-designed, blinded, randomized controlled studies comparing the effectiveness of various interventions on EAMC genesis, and some authors [82] estimate the placebo effect can explain 40–50% of effectiveness of cramp treatments. If EAMC are caused by a unique convergence of risk factors unique to individuals, many products or strategies may be at least partially effective. This may explain the numerous EAMC prevention methods utilized by clinicians as well as the perceived lack of effectiveness for many of these methods [16].

Summary

EAMC are common, painful injuries recognized by firmness and bulging of skeletal muscles. EAMC likely originate when a myriad of factors converge to increase nervous system excitability and alter neuromuscular control. Risk factors and their contribution to the pathophysiology of EAMC are still being identified. Gentle static stretching continues to be the most effective method of relieving acute EAMC followed by treatments specific to individual's risk factors. To prevent EAMC, it is necessary to first rule out any underlying medical conditions and then identify the intrinsic and extrinsic risk factors that precipitated EAMC. Once an individual's unique risk factors are identified, clinicians should attempt targeted strategies to prevent EAMC. Such strategies will likely be safer and more effective than generalized treatment advice (e.g., drink more fluids).

References

1. Schwellnus M, Drew N, Collins M. Muscle cramping in athletes—risk factors, clinical assessment, and management. Clin Sports Med. 2008;27(1):183–94.
2. Schwabe K, Schwellnus M, Derman W, Swanevelder S, Jordaan E. Less experience and running pace are potential risk factors for medical complications during a 56 km road running race: a prospective study in 26 354 race starters–SAFER Study II. Br J Sports Med. 2014;48(11):905–11.
3. Cooper E, Ferrara M, Broglio S. Exertional heat illness and environmental conditions during a single football season in the Southeast. J Athl Train. 2006;41(3):332–6.
4. Norris F, Gasteiger E, Chatfield P. An electromyographic study of induced and spontaneous muscle cramps. Electroencephalogr Clin Neurophysiol. 1956;9(1):139–47.
5. National Athletic Trainers'. Association consensus statement: sickle cell trait and the athlete. Dallas: National Athletic Trainer's Association; 2007. http://www.nata.org/statements/consensus/sicklecell.pdf. Accessed 25 Apr 2019.
6. Parisi L, Pierelli F, Amabile G, Valente G, Calandriello E, Fattapposta F, et al. Muscular cramps: proposals for a new classification. Acta Neurol Scand. 2003;107(3):176–86.
7. Jones BH, Rock PB, Smith LS, Teves MA, Case JK, Eddings K, et al. Medical complaints after a marathon run in cool weather. Phys Sportsmed. 1985;13(10):103–10.
8. Maughan R. Exercise induced muscle cramp: a prospective biochemical study in marathon runners. J Sports Sci. 1986;4(1):31–4.
9. Bergeron M. Muscle cramps during exercise—is it fatigue or electrolyte deficit? Curr Sports Med Rep. 2008;7(Suppl 4):S50–5.
10. Schwellnus M. Cause of exercise associated muscle cramps (EAMC)-Altered neuromuscular control, dehydration, or electrolyte depletion? Br J Sports Med. 2009;43(6):401–8.
11. Miller KC. Rethinking the cause of exercise-associated muscle cramping: moving beyond dehydration and electrolyte losses. Curr Sports Med Rep. 2015;14(5):353–4.
12. Moss K. Some effects of high air temperatures and muscular exertion upon colliers. Proc R Soc Lond B. 1923;95:181–200.
13. Talbott J. Heat cramps: a clinical and chemical study. J Clin Invest. 1933;12:533–49.
14. Ladell W. Heat cramps. Lancet. 1949;2:836–9.
15. Nichols PE, Jonnalagadda SS, Rosenbloom CA, Trinkaus M. Knowledge, attitudes, and behaviors regarding hydration and fluid replacement of collegiate athletes. Int J Sport Nutr Exerc Metab. 2005;15(5):515–27.

16. Stone MB, Edwards JE, Stemmans CL, Ingersoll CD, Palmieri RM, Krause BA. Certified athletic trainers' perceptions of exercise associated muscle cramps. J Sport Rehabil. 2003;12(4):333–42.
17. Eichner ER. The role of sodium in 'heat cramping'. Sports Med. 2007;37(4–5):368–70.
18. Costill DL, Coté R, Fink W. Muscle water and electrolytes following varied levels of dehydration in man. J Appl Physiol. 1976;40(1):6–11.
19. Bergeron MF. Heat cramps during tennis: a case report. Int J Sport Nutr. 1996;6(1):62–8.
20. Bergeron MF. Heat cramps: fluid and electrolyte challenges during tennis in the heat. J Sci Med Sport. 2003;6(1):19–27.
21. Stofan JR, Zachwieja JJ, Horswill CA, Murray R, Anderson SA, Eichner ER. Sweat and sodium losses in NCAA football players: a precursor to heat cramps? Int J Sport Nutr Exerc Metab. 2005;15(6):641–52.
22. Horswill CA, Stofan JR, Lacambra M, Toriscelli TA, Eichner ER, Murray R. Sodium balance during US football training in the heat: cramp-prone vs. reference players. Int J Sports Med. 2009;30(11):789–94.
23. Sulzer NU, Schwellnus MP, Noakes TD. Serum electrolytes in Ironman triathletes with exercise associated muscle cramping. Med Sci Sports Exerc. 2005;37(7):1081–5.
24. Schwellnus MP, Nicol J, Laubscher R, Noakes TD. Serum electrolyte concentrations and hydration status are not associated with exercise associated muscle cramping (EAMC) in distance runners. Br J Sports Med. 2004;38(4):488–92.
25. Schwellnus MP, Drew N, Collins M. Increased running speed and previous cramps rather than dehydration or serum sodium changes predict exercise associated muscle cramping: a prospective cohort study in 210 Ironman triathletes. Br J Sports Med. 2011;45(8):650–6.
26. Guyton AC. Interstitial fluid pressure: II. Pressure-volume curves of interstitial space. Circ Res. 1965;16:452–60.
27. Baker LB. Sweating rate and sweat sodium concentration in athletes: a review of methodology and intra/interindividual variability. Sports Med. 2017;47(Suppl 1):S111–28.
28. Baker LB, Barnes KA, Anderson ML, Passe DH, Stofan JR. Normative data for regional sweat sodium concentration and whole-body sweating rate in athletes. J Sports Sci. 2016;34(4):358–68.
29. Miller KC, Yeargin SW, McDermott BP. Sweat electrolyte concentrations and sweat rates of athletes with and without a history of muscle cramps. J Athl Train. 2018;52:S207–8.
30. Hoffman M, Fogard K. Factors related to successful completion of a 161-km ultramarathon. Int J Sports Physiol Perform. 2011;6(1):25–37.
31. Braulick KW, Miller KC, Albrecht JM, Tucker JME. Significant and serious dehydration does not affect skeletal muscle cramp threshold frequency. Br J Sports Med. 2012;47(11):710–4.
32. Miller KC, Mack GW, Knight KL, Hopkins JT, Draper DO, Fields PJ, Hunter I. Three percent hypohydration does not affect the threshold frequency of electrically induced muscle cramps. Med Sci Sports Exerc. 2010;42(11):2056–63.
33. Jung AP, Bishop PA, Al-Nawwas A, Dale RB. Influence of hydration and electrolyte supplementation on incidence and time to onset of exercise-associated muscle cramps. J Athl Train. 2005;40(2):71–5.
34. Casa DJ, DeMartini JK, Bergeron MF, Csillan D, Eichner ER, Lopez RM, et al. National Athletic Trainers' association position statement: exertional heat illnesses. J Athl Train. 2015;50(9):986–1000.
35. American College of Sports Medicine, Armstrong LE, Casa DJ, Millard-Stafford M, Moran DS, Pyne SW, Roberts WO. American College of Sports Medicine position stand: exertional heat illness during training and competition. Med Sci Sports Exerc. 2007;39(3):556–72.
36. Schwellnus M, Derman E, Noakes T. Aetiology of skeletal muscle 'cramps' during exercise: a novel hypothesis. J Sports Sci. 1997;15(3):277–85.
37. Miller KC. The evolution of exercise-associated muscle cramp research. ACSMs Health Fit J. 2018;22:6–8.
38. Qui J, Kang JK. Exercise associated muscle cramp—a current perspective. Sci Pages Sports Med. 2017;1:3–14.

39. Khan SI, Burne JA. Afferents contributing to autogenic inhibition of gastrocnemius following electrical stimulation of its tendon. Brain Res. 2009;1282:28–37.
40. Khan SI, Burne JA. Reflex inhibition of normal cramp following electrical stimulation of the muscle tendon. J Neurophysiol. 2007;98(3):1102–7.
41. Minetto MA, Holobar A, Botter A, Ravenni R, Farina D. Mechanisms of cramp contractions: peripheral or central generation. J Physiol. 2011;589(Pt 23):5759–73.
42. Mense S. Effects of temperature on the discharges of muscle spindles and tendon organs. Pflügers Arch. 1978;374(2):159–66.
43. Fischer M, Schäfer SS. Temperature effects on the discharge frequency of primary and secondary endings of isolated cat muscle spindles recorded under a ramp-and-hold stretch. Brain Res. 1999;840(1–2):1–15.
44. Wagner T, Behnia N, Ancheta W, Shen R, Farrokhi S, Powers CM. Strengthening and neuromuscular reeducation of the gluteus maximus in a triathlete with exercise associated cramping of the hamstrings. J Orthop Sports Phys Ther. 2010;40(2):112–9.
45. Nelson DL, Hutton RS. Dynamic and static stretch responses in muscle spindle receptors in fatigued muscle. Med Sci Sports Exerc. 1985;17(4):445–50.
46. Hutton RS, Nelson DL. Stretch sensitivity of Golgi tendon organs in fatigued gastrocnemius muscle. Med Sci Sports Exerc. 1986;18(1):69–74.
47. Telerman-Toppet N, Bacq M, Khoubesserian P, Coërs C. Type 2 fiber predominance in muscle cramp and exertional myalgia. Muscle Nerve. 1985;8(7):563–7.
48. Serrao M, Arendt-Nielsen L, Ge HY, Pierelli F, Sandrini G, Farina D. Experimental muscle pain decreases the frequency threshold of electrically elicited muscle cramps. Exp Brain Res. 2007;182(3):301–8.
49. Ge HY, Zhang Y, Boudreau S, Yue SW, Arendt-Nielsen L. Induction of muscle cramps by nociceptive stimulation of latent myofascial trigger points. Exp Brain Res. 2008;187(4):623–9.
50. Schwellnus MP, Swanevelder S, Jordaan E, Derman W, Van Rensburg DCJ. Underlying chronic disease, medication use, history of running injuries and being a more experienced runner are independent factors associated with exercise-associated muscle cramping: a cross-sectional study in 15778 distance runners. Clin J Sport Med. 2018;28(3):289–98.
51. Schwellnus MP, Allie S, Derman W, Collins M. Increased running speed and pre-race muscle damage as risk factors for exercise-associated muscle cramps in a 56 km ultra-marathon: a prospective cohort study. Br J Sports Med. 2011;45(14):650–6.
52. Summers KM, Snodgrass SJ, Callister R. Predictors of calf cramping in rugby league. J Strength Cond Res. 2014;28(3):774–83.
53. Hubbard DR, Berkoff GM. Myofascial trigger points show spontaneous needle EMG activity. Spine (Phila Pa 1976). 1993;18(13):1803–7.
54. Rossi A, Decchi B. Changes in Ib heteronymous inhibition to soleus motoneurones during cutaneous and muscle nociceptive stimulation in humans. Brain Res. 1997;774(1–2):55–61.
55. McNulty WH, Gevirtz RN, Hubbard DR, Berkoff GM. Needle electromyographic evaluation of a trigger point response to a psychological stressor. Psychophysiology. 1994;31(3):313–6.
56. Miller KC, Knight KL. Electrical stimulation cramp threshold frequency correlates well with the occurrence of skeletal muscle cramps. Muscle Nerve. 2009;39(3):364–8.
57. Miller KC, Long BC, Edwards JE. Muscle cramp susceptibility increases following a volitionally-induced muscle cramp. Muscle Nerve. 2017;56(6):E95–9.
58. Ross BH. Muscle cramp and the Hoffman reflex. XXth World Congress in Sports Medicine Handbook. Melbourne; 1974. p. 67–70.
59. Shang G, Collins M, Schwellnus MP. Factors associated with a self-reported history of exercise-associated muscle cramps in Ironman triathletes: a case-control study. Clin J Sport Med. 2011;21(3):204–10.
60. Edsall DL. Two cases of violent but transitory myokymia and myotonia apparently due to excessive hot weather. Am J Med Sci. 1904;155:1003.
61. Dickhuth HH, Röcker K, Niess A, Horstmann T, Mayer F, Striegel H. Exercise-induced, persistent and generalized muscle cramps. J Sports Med Phys Fitness. 2002;42(1):92–4.

62. Bertolasi L, De Grandis D, Bongiovanni L, Zanette G, Gasperini M. The influence of muscular lengthening on cramps. Ann Neurol. 1993;33:176–80.
63. Skein M, Duffield R, Edge J, Short MJ, Mündel T. Intermittent-sprint performance and muscle glycogen after 30 h of sleep deprivation. Med Sci Sports Exerc. 2011;43(7):1301–11.
64. Azboy O, Kaygisiz Z. Effects of sleep deprivation on cardiorespiratory functions of the runners and volleyball players during rest and exercise. Acta Physiol Hung. 2009;96(1):29–36.
65. Schwellnus MP. Muscle cramping in the marathon: aetiology and risk factors. Sports Med. 2007;37(4–5):364–7.
66. Balsom PD, Wood K, Olsson P, Ekblom B. Carbohydrate intake and multiple sprint sports: with special reference to football (soccer). Int J Sports Med. 1999;20(1):48–52.
67. Miller KC. Plasma potassium concentration and content changes after banana ingestion in exercised males. J Athl Train. 2012;47(6):648–54.
68. Miller KC. Electrolyte and plasma responses after pickle juice, mustard, and deionized water ingestion in dehydrated humans. J Athl Train. 2014;49(3):360–7.
69. Miller KC, Knight KL, Williams RB. Athletic trainers' perceptions of pickle juice's effects on exercise associated muscle cramps. Athl Ther Today. 2008;13:31–4.
70. Miller KC, Mack GW, Knight KL, Hopkins JT, Draper DO, Fields PJ, Hunter I. Reflex inhibition of electrically-induced muscle cramps in hypohydrated humans. Med Sci Sports Exerc. 2010;42(5):953–61.
71. Miller KC, Mack GW, Knight KL. Gastric emptying after pickle juice ingestion in rested, euhydrated humans. J Athl Train. 2010;45(6):601–8.
72. Allen ST, Miller KC, Albrecht JM, Garden-Robinson JA, Blodgett-Salafia EH. Ad libitum fluid intake and plasma responses after pickle juice, hypertonic saline and deionized water ingestion. J Athl Train. 2013;48(6):734–40.
73. Miller KC, Mack GW, Knight KL. Electrolyte and plasma changes after ingestion of pickle juice, water, and a common carbohydrate-electrolyte solution. J Athl Train. 2009;44(5):454–61.
74. Hew-Butler T, Rosner MH, Fowkes-Godek S, Dugas JP, Hoffman MD, Lewis DP, et al. Statement of the 3rd international exercise-associated hyponatremia consensus development conference, Carlsbad, California, 2015. Br J Sports Med. 2015;49(22):1432–46.
75. Stevens A. Update: Douglas county football player has died. Atlanta J Const. 11 Aug 2014. http://www.ajc.com/news/news/family-douglas-county-football-player-has-no-brain/ngy2X/. Accessed 25 Apr 2019.
76. Miller KC, Long BC, Edwards JE. Voluntarily-induced muscle cramp increases H-reflex amplitude (abstract). J Athl Train. 2016;51:S272.
77. Ross B, Thomas C. Human motor unit activity during induced muscle cramp. Brain. 1995;118(PT 4):983–93.
78. Hoffman MD, Stuempfle KJ, Valentino T. Sodium intake during an ultramarathon does not prevent muscle cramping, dehydration, hyponatremia, or nausea. Sports Med Open. 2015;1:39–45.
79. Fitzsimmons S, Tucker A, Martins D. Seventy-five percent of National Football League teams use pregame hyperhydration with intravenous fluid. Clin J Sport Med. 2011;21(3):192–9.
80. Miller KC, Harsen JD, Long BC. Prophylactic stretching does not reduce cramp susceptibility. Muscle Nerve. 2017;57(3):473–7.
81. Miller KC, Burne JA. Golgi tendon organ reflex inhibition following manually-applied acute static stretching. J Sports Sci. 2014;32(15):1491–7.
82. Miller T, Layzer RB. Muscle cramps. Muscle Nerve. 2005;32(4):431–42. Review.

Chapter 7
Minor Heat Illnesses

Gabrielle E. W. Giersch, Luke N. Belval, and Rebecca M. Lopez

Introduction

Exertional heat illnesses represent a large number of conditions and associated severities. Most commonly, those discussed (e.g., exertional heat stroke (EHS)) represent one end of the severity spectrum where the consequences of the condition affect mortality and morbidity. However, there are a host of minor conditions that occur subsequent to exercise in the heat that can impact an individual's health or ability to perform their best. These minor heat illnesses may increase the risk for developing more severe heat injuries, but are not required to develop in any particular order.

The goal of this chapter is to provide information on pathophysiology, recognition, treatment, and possible prevention of minor heat-related illnesses. Proper identification and management of these conditions is not only useful in efforts to maximize performance in the heat but also to distinguish relatively benign conditions from the symptoms of severe heat illnesses. This chapter will also focus on the status of the literature related to return to activity. This is an important factor for populations, including athletes, military personnel, and occupational workers, in order to gauge their readiness and health status for returning to their respective activities. This is impactful for all active populations who may be susceptible to heat illnesses in order to ensure enough time for recovery and reduce the risk of re-injury.

G. E. W. Giersch (✉) · L. N. Belval
Korey Stringer Institute, Department of Kinesiology, University of Connecticut, Storrs, CT, USA
e-mail: gabrielle.giersch@uconn.edu

R. M. Lopez
Athletic Training Post-Professional Program, Department of Orthopaedics & Sports Medicine, University of South Florida, Tampa, FL, USA

© Springer Nature Switzerland AG 2020
W. M. Adams, J. F. Jardine (eds.), *Exertional Heat Illness*,
https://doi.org/10.1007/978-3-030-27805-2_7

Heat Edema

Heat edema refers to the development of excess fluid when exposed to or when exercising in the heat [1]. Heat edema can present as swelling in joints or the extremities – especially the hands, ankles, and feet [1]. Heat edema is viewed as the mildest heat-related illness as there is minimal pain associated with the swelling [1, 2]. Heat edema does not directly contribute to increased risk of developing more severe heat-related illnesses but can inhibit movement and decrease comfort during physical activity. Furthermore, heat edema is more likely to occur in at-risk populations, such as those with poor circulation, and can generally prognosticate poor reactions to heat exposure.

Pathophysiology

It is believed that heat edema may be caused by the necessary increase in vasodilation during heat exposure, likely propagated by the increased need to send blood to the skin for purposes of heat dissipation. Vasodilation increases dry cooling capacity and is stimulated when performing physical activity in warm environments [3]. Vasodilation may also result in a pooling of interstitial fluid in the gravity-dependent extremities [2, 4]. Additional fluid compartment shifts occur as a result of the post-sweating increases in aldosterone and antidiuretic hormone that limit depletion of body sodium but results in fluid accumulation in joint spaces [5]. When the body is at a fluid deficit, these hormonal mechanisms increase in order to retain fluid and reduce the amount of fluid being lost to urine.

Recognition

Heat edema can be recognized by the distinct redness and swelling in the extremities. Heat edema is more likely to occur when individuals are unacclimatized [6] to the environmental conditions in which they are exposed. Heat edema will be uncomfortable for the individual affected and can hinder fine motor movements. It is important to distinguish heat edema from other more serious conditions (i.e., congestive heart failure, deep venous thrombosis, hyponatremia) which can also result in a buildup of interstitial fluid and lead to the development of edema. Heat edema largely results from an acute heat exposure, so differential diagnoses should take patient's activity and environmental exposure into account. Unlike acute injury, heat edema can present bilaterally and is typically more exaggerated in a distal fashion following prolonged standing or sitting. A thorough history and physical examination is likely to exclude systemic causes.

Treatment

Heat edema is typically a self-limiting condition. Heat edema can be behaviorally treated by cessation of exercise or heat exposure when possible, the elevation of extremities, or the use of compression garments in order to increase peripheral circulation [2]. From a treatment perspective, heat edema does usually resolve within a few days of heat acclimation/acclimatization, or with removal of heat exposure [4].

Return to Activity

An individual with heat edema should be removed from activity to properly evaluate the condition and rule out other more serious illnesses causing edema. Benign heat edema does not need to necessarily limit activity. Return to activity for heat edema is also relatively simple, whereby participants can return to activity as long as they can comfortably do so, and the edema is no longer present. Additionally, easing into heat exposure using appropriate heat acclimation/acclimatization strategies can enhance tolerance to physical activity in the heat and is the most potent tool to prevent exertional heat illnesses [7–9].

Transient Heat Fatigue

Pathophysiology

Transient heat fatigue is a mild heat illness that is thought to be caused by prolonged exposure to heat and refers to the physical discomfort and exhaustion that is associated with prolonged heat exposure. This broad definition typically applies to individuals who lack appropriate heat acclimation or acclimatization due to the overwhelming nature of heat when heat dissipation adaptations are not at their most effective. The greatest impact of transient heat fatigue is found in cognitive performance tasks, particularly those that require higher levels of concentration or higher-order thinking, which has been observed with prolonged heat exposure [10–12].

Recognition

Transient heat fatigue as a condition typically manifests as a syndrome of patient complaints that do not directly apply to other heat illnesses or lack sufficient severity. These complaints can include minor cognitive and mood disturbances and fatigue that is resolved by removal from heat exposure [10].

Treatment

The symptoms associated with transient heat fatigue are temporary and are usually rectified with the introduction of cool environmental temperatures (e.g., shade, indoors with air conditioning).The risk for developing transient heat fatigue and other minor heat illnesses is greater in a population that is unacclimatized/unacclimated or individuals who are at an increased risk for development of other heat illnesses [10].

Return to Activity

Return to activity from transient heat fatigue relies on the resolution of symptoms associated with transient heat fatigue, which usually occurs when activity is stopped and affected individuals are moved to a cool, shaded area to recover. Once removed from the hot environment and symptoms cease, the individual is able to return to activity. A consideration for this, particularly if individuals are unacclimatized, would be to gradually introduce heat exposures in order to ensure safety considerations.

Heat Rash (Prickly Heat)

Pathophysiology

Heat rash, also known as prickly heat or miliaria rubra, develops when sweat pores are clogged by fluid, skin, keratin, or dirt causing the sweat ducts to swell within the gland [13–15]. The ducts rupture producing superficial vesicles on the surface of the skin. These vesicles are raised and look similar to blisters on an erythematous base. With prolonged heat exposure, it may possibly lead to "tropical anhidrotic asthenia," a more severe case where sweating is inhibited on a larger level and is associated with heat exhaustion (see Chap. 5) [13–16].

Heat rash is more commonly reported during exercise in hot, humid environments on skin that has been covered in clothing [17]. While typically benign, miliaria rubra can lead to other more dangerous skin inflammation (miliaria profunda) or infections due to the trapping of bacteria on the skin surface [10].

Recognition

Heat rash is recognizable by small raised vesicles on the skin. These vesicles may be red in color themselves or surrounded by red skin [14]. Itching is the predominant clinical feature. While the condition's symptoms typically are related to the dermatologic reaction, an associated hypohidrosis can occur secondary to heat rash that impairs an individual's ability to exercise in the heat.

Treatment

Heat rash may be prevented by avoiding sweat-producing activities. When active in the heat, individuals should wear light, loose-fitting clothing. Heat rash can be treated by cessation of exercise or removal from heat exposure. Under those conditions, symptoms usually resolve within a few hours [13]. Hygiene may play a role in the prevention and management of the condition. After heat rash has presented, skin lesions should be treated with care. Itching is treated successfully with antihistamines.

Return to Activity

Return to activity is not affected by heat rash. While the symptoms of heat rash may alter perception surrounding performance and subsequent heat exposures, exercise performance would likely not be significantly affected by heat rash.

Sunburn

Pathophysiology

Sunburn is the heat-related condition that arises from radiant heat exposure that damages the epidermis. This damage can result in an inflammatory reaction of the dermis and proximal areas of the epidermis, similar to a first-degree burn. Sunburn impairs one's ability to sweat normally and impacts skin blood flow – disturbing the temperature gradient that is essential in dissipating stored body heat, thus increasing the risk for developing more severe heat illnesses when performing physical activity in the heat. Skin blood flow is an important factor for heat dissipation through dry and wet mechanisms. When this relationship is disturbed, e.g., sunburn, heat dissipation capacity is blunted (see Chap. 2 for further discussion on temperature regulation) [18].

Recognition

Swelling, redness, ulcerations, and pain are common symptoms associated with sunburn, and symptoms increase in magnitude with increasing severity of sunburn [1]. Symptom development usually occurs within 5 hours of an exposure incident but may not peak until up to 48 hours later [1].

Treatment

It has been commonly believed that when exposed to radiant heat, sunscreen, a protectant for sunburn, also inhibits heat dissipation through the sweat response. However, recent investigations have shown that some sweat-proof sunscreens did not impact sweating response to exercise in the heat; thus sunscreen can be utilized in order to prevent the development of sunburn when exposed to radiant heat [19]. With the inhibitory nature of sunburn, and the increased burden sunburn places on the thermoregulatory system, protection with increased clothing, or sunscreen protection, should be utilized to prevent the development of sunburn [1, 20].Treatment of sunburn depends on the severity of the condition. In milder cases, *Aloe vera* is a useful treatment to ease discomfort. In more severe cases, cold compresses and NSAIDs can be utilized to decrease discomfort and reduce any swelling associated with the burn.

Return to Activity

Sunburn does not prevent the participation in athletic or heat exposure events but should be treated prior to subsequent heat exposure in order to protect against further damage from solar radiation. Individuals with sunburn should avoid the sun until the inflammation resolves. For activities where exposure to the sun is unavoidable (e.g., sport, occupational work, military operations occurring outside), wearing clothing that covers the areas of the sunburn, but also are light, loosely woven and moisture wicking to optimize heat dissipation may provide added benefits.

As one of the primary methods of prevention of sunburn, sunscreen use is important to consider during exercise or physical activity in the heat. Though exercising with exposed skin introduces the risk of developing sunburn, sunscreen has previously been thought to decrease the capacity for heat dissipation mechanisms, by impairing the capacity to produce sweat onto the skin [19]. This relative ineffectiveness of sweating decreases the heat dissipation capacity through this primary mechanism during exercise [18]. This inability to dissipate heat to the fullest capacity increases the risk of developing more severe exertional heat illnesses due to the inability to decrease internal body temperature [1, 18]. Sweat-proof sunscreens may not affect the sweating response.

Heat Syncope

One of the least severe heat illnesses is heat syncope [21, 22]. Although heat syncope is considered to be of mild to moderate severity and non-life-threatening, this condition may have signs and symptoms similar to other more serious, potentially fatal conditions. Therefore, having a thorough understanding of the pathophysiology, recognition, and treatment following heat syncope can help ensure a safe return to activity.

Pathophysiology

Heat syncope is a fainting or syncopal episode that often results when an unacclimatized individual has either been standing for a prolonged amount of time or has a sudden change in posture [7]. Heat syncope can occur due to dehydration, lack of heat acclimatization, venous blood pooling in the extremities, hypotension, and reduced cardiac filling [7]. Heat syncope is often referred to as orthostatic dizziness, as changes in posture combined with heat stress can result in an attenuated baroreflex modulation and lead to orthostatic intolerance (Table 7.1) [23, 24]. It is known that heat stress can challenge the cardiovascular system during exercise; however, it is important to highlight the impact of heat stress on the cardiovascular system's ability to maintain blood pressure during prolonged standing or changes in posture in unacclimatized individuals (i.e., band members, military personnel, athletes standing on a sideline) [24–26]. Hypohydration can further exacerbate the effects of heat stress on orthostatic tolerance [27]. Blood pooling in the legs due to gravity can result in the need to attenuate a decrease in ventricular filling and stroke volume [24]. Prolonged standing results in increased skeletal muscle tension in the lower extremity, thereby, negatively affecting central blood volume and cerebral perfusion [27]. Orthostasis, or orthostatic hypotension, can lead to central hypovolemia, which requires changes within the cardiovascular system to counterbalance this condition [24]. The initial physiological adaptations that occur with heat acclimatization are cardiovascular in nature. Therefore, an individual who is not yet heat acclimatized, or who has heart disease and is standing in one place for a prolonged amount of time, will be more susceptible to heat syncope [7].

Recognition

Recognition of heat syncope and ruling out a more serious condition is critical for the healthcare provider. There are various causes of collapse in an exercising individual; therefore the clinician's primary goal is to rule out cardiac arrest or other life-threatening causes of collapse (i.e., exertional heat stroke, head injury, exertional sickling). Initial assessment of an athlete that has experienced syncope should include assessment of responsiveness, breathing, and heart rate [7]. Proper recognition of heat syncope consists of recognizing the symptoms, which may include dizziness, tunnel vision, a brief episode of fainting, and pale skin [7]. Once an acute cardiac etiology is ruled out, the clinician should ensure the patient is not experiencing exertional heat stroke. The key to ruling out exertional heat stroke is that with

Table 7.1 Ruling in heat syncope

Characteristics of condition	Differential diagnoses				
	Heat syncope	Cardiac arrest	Exertional heat stroke	Heat exhaustion	Exercise-associated collapse
Definition/pathophysiology	Orthostatic dizziness after standing in one place for prolonged time in the heat	Loss of cardiac function often due to cardiac dysrhythmias	Severe heat illness caused by increased metabolic heat production and/or inability to dissipate heat	Inability to continue exercise in the heat, often due to cardiac insufficiency and fluid and/or electrolyte depletion	Collapse in a conscious athlete that is unable to walk or stand [23] Occurs when the individual abruptly stops during intense exercise
Initial signs and symptoms	Fainting, hypotension	Unresponsive, lack of pulse, not breathing	Collapse and/or CNS dysfunction (acting out of sorts, combativeness, coma), rectal temperature >104 °F	Fatigue, pallor, weakness, headache, vomiting, dizziness	Inability to stand without assistance after cessation of exercise, dizziness, hypotension
Diagnostic criteria/ruling "in"	Syncope in unacclimatized individual that has been standing for a long time, rectal temperature <104 °F, rapid, weak pulse, initially hypotensive	Unresponsive, no pulse, not breathing, no signs of life	CNS dysfunction and rectal temperature >104 °F following exercise in the heat. Can be associated with organ-system dysfunction	Symptoms above in an individual that is not heat acclimatized and has been exercising in the heat. Rectal temperature <104 °F and minimal or no CNS dysfunction	Collapse and orthostatic intolerance in individual that has abruptly stopped exercising
Treatment	Elevate legs, monitor vital signs, move to cooler area and rehydrate	Activate EMS, CPR, AED	Aggressive cooling via cold water immersion until temperature reaches 102 °F	Move to cooler area, rehydrate if possible, cool the skin via ice towels, fanning, etc.	Elevate legs, monitor vital signs, move to cooler area, and rehydrate

CNS central nervous system, EMS emergency medical services, CPR cardiopulmonary resuscitation, AED automated external defibrillator heat syncope, core body temperature will typically remain below 40 °C (104 °F), whereas with exertional heat stroke (EHS), patients will have a dangerously elevated core body temperature, often greater than 104 °F. Those with EHS will also have an altered mental status. After a fainting episode, patients typically regain a normal mental status. The treatment for these conditions is vastly different; therefore, ruling out more serious conditions and confirming the diagnosis of heat syncope is extremely important.

Treatment

Treatment for heat syncope is similar to other syncopal episodes. Once more serious metabolic, cardiovascular, or neurologic disorders have been ruled out (i.e., primary survey), the patient should be placed in the Trendelenburg position, and vital signs should be monitored. If possible, the patient should be moved to a cooler area (air-conditioned or shaded area), and fluids should be given orally when the patient has regained consciousness and is coherent [7]. Attempts to cool via nonaggressive cooling methods (i.e., fanning, ice towels) may improve the patient's status; however, more aggressive cooling, such as cold water immersion, is not necessary since body temperature will not be dangerously elevated with heat syncope. Emphasis in treating a heat syncope patient should be placed on restoring cardiovascular function and ensuring signs and symptoms are no longer present.

Return to Activity

Return to exercise following heat syncope requires three important steps. Primarily, a more serious condition such as cardiac, EHS, or sickling should be ruled out. Secondly, healthcare providers should ensure all signs and symptoms from the syncopal episode have resolved. This would include normal vital signs, primarily blood pressure and heart rate, and restoration of normal hydration status. Lastly, the cause of the heat syncope should be determined and addressed prior to return to activity. If the patient lacked heat acclimatization prior to the syncopal episode, a gradual progression of heat exposure across 7–10 days should be introduced. The patient's hydration status should be measured via body mass changes or urinary field markers, such as urine color or specific gravity, to ensure the patient is euhydrated prior to being reintroduced to the warm environment. Additionally, it is imperative to educate the patient on maintaining a proper diet. If any of the signs or symptoms has not resolved or heat syncope should reoccur, the patient should be referred for a more extensive follow-up with a physician.

Conclusion

Understanding the development, pathophysiology, recognition, and treatment of minor heat illnesses is important for medical professionals. While minor heat illnesses lack the severity associated with exertional heat stroke and other medical emergencies, treating minor heat illnesses appropriately can enhance the acclimatization process and prevent the development of exertional heat illnesses.

References

1. Miners AL. The diagnosis and emergency care of heat related illness and sunburn in athletes: a retrospective case series. J Can Chiropr Assoc. 2010;54(2):107–17.
2. Lipman GS, Eifling KP, Ellis MA, Gaudio FG, Otten EM, Grissom CK, et al. Wilderness Medical Society practice guidelines for the prevention and treatment of heat-related illness. Wilderness Environ Med. 2013;24(4):351–61.
3. Charkoudian N. Skin blood flow in adult human thermoregulation: how it works, when it does not, and why. Mayo Clin Proc. 2003;78(5):603–12.
4. Yarbrough BE, Hubbard RW. Heat-related illnesses. In: Auerbach PS, Geehr EC, editors. Management of wilderness and environmental emergencies. St. Louis: Mosby; 1989. p. 119–43.
5. Horne GO, Mole RH. Mammillaria. Trans R Soc Trop Med Hyg. 1951;44(4):465–71.
6. Bailes BK, Reeve K. Prevention of heat-related illness. J Nurse Pract. 2007;3(3):161–8.
7. Casa DJ, DeMartini JK, Bergeron MF, Csillan D, Eichner ER, Lopez RM, et al. National athletic trainers' association position statement: exertional heat illnesses. J Athl Train. 2015;50(9):986–1000.
8. Pryor JL, Johnson EC, Roberts WO, Pryor RR. Application of evidence-based recommendations for heat acclimation: individual and team sport perspectives. Temperature. 2018;6(1):37–49.
9. Guy JH, Deakin GB, Edwards AM, Miller CM, Pyne DB. Adaptation to hot environmental conditions: an exploration of the performance basis, procedures and future directions to optimise opportunities for elite athletes. Sports Med. 2015;45(3):303–11.
10. Armstrong LE. Exertional heat illnesses. Champaign: Human Kinetics; 2003.
11. Piil JF, Mikkelsen CJ, Junge N, Morris NB, Nybo L. Heat acclimation does not protect trained males from hyperthermia-induced impairments in complex task performance. Int J Environ Res Public Health. 2019;16(5):716.
12. Piil JF, Lundbye-Jensen J, Trangmar SJ, Nybo L. Performance in complex motor tasks deteriorates in hyperthermic humans. Temperature (Austin). 2017;4(4):420–8.
13. Allen SD, O'Brien JP. Tropical anidrotic asthenia: a preliminary report. Med J Aust. 1944;2:335–6.
14. O'Brien JP. The etiology of poral closure; an experimental study of miliaria rubra, bullous impetigo and related diseases of the skin. I. an historical review of the causation of miliaria. J Invest Dermatol. 1950;15(2):95–101.
15. Shelley WB, Horvath PN. Experimental miliaria in man. J Invest Dermatol. 1950;14(3):193–203.
16. Bannister R. Acute anidrotic heat exhaustion. Lancet. 1959;2(7098):313–6.
17. Seto CK, Way D, O'Connor N. Environmental illness in athletes. Clin Sports Med. 2005;24(3):695–718. x

18. Coris EE, Ramirez AM, Durme DJ. Heat illness in athletes: the dangerous combination of heat, humidity and exercise. Sports Med. 2004;34(1):9–16.
19. Ou-Yang H, Meyer K, Houser T, Grove G. Sunscreen formulations do not interfere with sweat cooling during exercise. Int J Cosmet Sci. 2018;40(1):87–92.
20. Wells TD, Jessup GT, Langlotz KS. Effects of sunscreen use during exercise in the heat. Phys Sports Med. 1984;12(6):132–42.
21. Yamamoto T, Fujita M, Oda Y, Todani M, Hifumi T, Kondo Y, et al. Evaluation of a novel classification of heat-related illnesses: a multicentre observational study (Heat Stroke STUDY 2012). Int J Environ Res Public Health. 2018;15(9):1962.
22. Kenny GP, Wilson TE, Flouris AD, Fujii N. Heat exhaustion. Handb Clin Neurol. 2018;157:505–29.
23. Asplund CA, O'Connor FG, Noakes TD. Exercise-associated collapse: an evidence-based review and primer for clinicians. Br J Sports Med. 2011;45(14):1157–62.
24. Schlader ZJ, Wilson TE, Crandall CG. Mechanisms of orthostatic intolerance during heat stress. Auton Neurosci. 2016;196:37–46.
25. Crandall CG, Shibasaki M, Wilson TE. Insufficient cutaneous vasoconstriction leading up to and during syncopal symptoms in the heat stressed human. Am J Physiol Heart Circ Physiol. 2010;299(4):H1168–73.
26. Wilson TE, Cui J, Zhang R, Crandall CG. Heat stress reduces cerebral blood velocity and markedly impairs orthostatic tolerance in humans. Am J Physiol Regul Integr Comp Physiol. 2006;291(5):R1443–8.
27. Carter R 3rd, Cheuvront SN, Vernieuw CR, Sawka MN. Hypohydration and prior heat stress exacerbates decreases in cerebral blood flow velocity during standing. J Appl Physiol. 2006;101(6):1744–50.

Chapter 8
Molecular Aspects of Thermal Tolerance and Exertional Heat Illness Susceptibility

Elaine C. Lee, Jacob S. Bowie, Aidan P. Fiol, and Robert A. Huggins

Many questions about molecular mechanisms for both physiological adaptations to heat (i.e., acclimation and acclimatization) and increased susceptibility to exertional heat stroke remain unanswered. This chapter focuses on the few documented potential molecular and genetic factors in thermal tolerance and reduced or increased susceptibility to exertional heat stroke.

Molecular/Cellular Mechanisms of Thermal Tolerance and Exertional Heat Stroke Susceptibility

Immune Function Affects EHS Susceptibility and Pathophysiology

Exertional heat stroke (EHS) is clinically defined as a medical emergency defined by systemic hyperthermia (core body temperature ($T_c > 40$ °C with CNS dysfunction)) as per the National Athletic Trainers Association (NATA) position statement

E. C. Lee (✉) · J. S. Bowie · A. P. Fiol
Human Performance Laboratory, Department of Kinesiology, University of Connecticut, Storrs, CT, USA

Department of Kinesiology, University of Connecticut, Storrs, CT, USA
e-mail: elaine.c.lee@uconn.edu

R. A. Huggins
Human Performance Laboratory, Department of Kinesiology, University of Connecticut, Storrs, CT, USA

Department of Kinesiology, University of Connecticut, Storrs, CT, USA

Korey Stringer Institute, Department of Kinesiology, University of Connecticut, Storrs, CT, USA

© Springer Nature Switzerland AG 2020
W. M. Adams, J. F. Jardine (eds.), *Exertional Heat Illness*,
https://doi.org/10.1007/978-3-030-27805-2_8

(specifically, $T_c > 40.5$ °C) and other standards [1–3]. Historically, heat stroke (classical/undefined (HS) or EHS) has been thought to be caused by heat exposure or a combination of heat and exercise. However, heat stress alone does not fully capture the pathophysiology of heat stroke. In 2006, Lim proposed the dual pathway model (DPM) for heat stroke [4] which drew from observations made by Bouchama and Knochel [3]. In a 2018 review, Lim expands on this concept and proposed that HS is triggered by two independent pathways, whereby HS is triggered by heat sepsis at $Tc < 42$ °C and by heat toxicity at $Tc > 42$ °C [5]. Lim proposes that at different core temperatures, there are likely different mechanisms contributing to heat stroke. These models do not specifically address EHS separately. Asymptomatic (e.g., no CNS dysfunction) athletes with core temperatures up to 42 °C [6, 7] are documented in the literature, and research suggests that the critical thermal maximum, the lethal core temperature threshold, is between 41.6 °C and 42 °C [5]. Factors such as the duration of hyperthermia affect whether an athlete or laborer may develop EHS (see Chap. 4), and it appears from many examples in the literature that absolute core temperature is not a sole predictor of an individual's susceptibility for EHS. Pathophysiology of HS and EHS (and exertional heat illness (EHI)) includes multiple cellular mechanisms in addition to damage induced by thermal stress. Among the molecular/cellular mechanisms includes immune system-mediated pathophysiology primarily driven by endotoxemia and sepsis in select individuals.

A review of 12 years of military hospital records showed that >95% of heat stroke (HS/EHS) cases presented with mild fever, diarrhea, or an upper respiratory infection 2–3 days prior to the EHS event [8]. Febrile illness or other existing infection before commencing exercise in hot and humid conditions is known to be a predisposing risk factor for EHI/EHS [9–11]. For many different reasons, immune responses to infection may become extreme and cause tissue damage to the patient, resulting in an unchecked, exaggerated immune response called sepsis. Clinically, sepsis, septic shock, which can be part of the pathophysiology of EHS, can result in greater systemic effects through disseminated intravascular coagulation (DIC) [12], multi-organ dysfunction (MOD) [13], and CNS damage [1], which all feedback to stimulate the immune response further. The dysregulated immune response causes release of excess immune signaling molecules that serve as pyrogens, further raising T_c. This positive feedback loop causes further tissue damage, oxidative stress, and pyroptosis, a highly inflammatory form of programmed cell death. The immune system simultaneously releases anti-inflammatory cytokines to balance the inflammation which cause immunosuppression, but this negative feedback response may be inadequate. There is no singular causative factor in sepsis, septic shock, or HS/EHS-induced sepsis and subsequent DIC and MOD, but presence of endotoxins such as lipopolysaccharide (LPS) in the blood mediates the pathophysiological immune response in both sepsis and heat stroke. Exercise alone can result in elevated LPS which is exacerbated by environmental heat stress [14]. This has sparked interest in the role of sickness and other immune disturbances prior to exercise or heat stress as a predisposing factor (PDF) to HS (Table 8.1).

Endotoxemia is a damaging innate immune response caused by the presence of endotoxins such as LPS in the blood. LPS and other endogenous pyrogens are

Table 8.1 Comparison of the clinical symptoms of sepsis and septic shock to reported cases of heat stroke. Sepsis is defined as life-threatening organ dysfunction caused by a dysregulated host response to infection [15]. qSOFA: quick sequential organ failure assessment

Clinical symptoms (sepsis, septic shock)	Reports of EHS cases with clinical symptoms
qSOFA:	
Respiratory rate ≥22/min	[1, 3, 8, 13]
Altered mentation	[1, 3, 8, 13, 16]
Systolic blood pressure ≤100 mm hg	[8, 13, 16]
SOFA score >2 any of:	
Glasgow coma scale 10–12	[8, 13, 16]
Creatinine 2.0–3.4 mg/dL or greater	[8, 13, 16]
Urine output <500 mL/d	Dehydration [1]
Bilirubin 2.0–5.9 mg/dL or greater	[8, 13]
Septic shock symptoms:	
Hypotension requiring vasopressors to maintain MAP ≥65 mmHG	[13]
Serum lactate >2 mmol/L(18 mg/dL) despite adequate volume resuscitation	Normally elevated during exercise [16]
Disseminated intravascular coagulation	[13]

thought to raise the hypothalamic set point during exercise through the action of prostaglandin E_2 [17]. Endotoxemia/sepsis and systemic inflammation are likely major contributors to pathophysiology of EHS [18].

LPS is normally present in the protected environment of the intestine. The intestinal barrier consists of the biological barrier, the physical barrier, and the immune barrier. The biological barrier consists of a normal functional intestinal microbiota (IM), which helps to regulate pathogenic bacteria by competition [19]. The microbiota assists the host in breaking down molecules and providing essential vitamins. The physical barrier consists of the intestinal mucus layer, the epithelial cells, and the tight junctions which prevent translocation of pathogenic bacteria [20] into the circulation. The immune barrier consists of gut-associated lymphoid tissue (GALT) and tissue-specific lymphocytes which interact with the IM to maintain a healthy balance [21].

Intestinal barrier dysfunction during exercise-heat stress can be caused by reduced intestinal blood flow [17] which may result in tissue hypoxia and acidosis [22], oxidative and nitrosative stress [23], and the intestinal inflammatory response [14], all of which may result in increased LPS passage [24]. Nonsteroidal anti-inflammatory drugs (NSAIDS) which are frequently used by athletes have been shown to increase GI permeability [17, 25]. A review by Armstrong discussed the evidence showing that the IM of athletes can be modified by exercise and diet which a following review addressed specific nutritional recommendation [2, 26]. The chronic low-grade inflammation in obesity has been [18] associated in some cases with the presence of low levels of circulating LPS termed "metabolic endotoxemia" which supports the notion that diet and exercise induce beneficial adaptations in the gut [27]. Illness caused by infection with pathogenic bacteria has deleterious effects on intestinal epithelial barrier function not limited to diarrhea [28]. Chronic diseases such as inflammatory bowel disease are characterized by intestinal epithelial barrier dysfunction [29]. Given that the intestinal barrier is affected by so many factors related to metabolism, diet, and exercise, one could speculate that EHS patients may experience intestinal barrier damage due to diverse, individual factors.

Intestinal ischemia due to exercise and elevated T_c cause a breakdown of the gut barrier resulting in a "leaky gut" allowing toxins and bacteria to pass into the bloodstream. Exercise-induced hypoxia and other stress cause the breakdown of tight junctions and an inflammatory immune response [20]. The bulk of pathogens released into circulation are recognized and taken up by Kupffer cells in the healthy liver [2]. If the influx of pathogens overwhelms the filtering capacity of the liver, immune-activating substances such as LPS, lipoteichoic acid, lipopeptide, peptidoglycan, flagella, and bacterial DNA/RNA pass into the bloodstream [30] where they initiate a systemic innate immune response.

Once in systemic circulation, LPS, other pathogen-associated molecular patterns (PAMPs), or danger-associated molecular patterns (DAMPs) that may be increased by exercise [31, 32] are recognized by toll-like receptor 4 (TLR4) found on the surface of white blood cell membranes, specifically macrophages and monocytes [2, 33]. TLR4 binds LPS with the cooperation of LPS-binding protein (LBP), CD14, and myeloid differentiation protein-2 (MD-2) [30, 33]. After LPS binding, the TLR4/MD-2 complex stimulates two canonical pathways through TRIF and MyD88 that result in activation of transcription factors IRF3, NF-κB, and AP-1, which all increase production of inflammatory molecules including TNFα, IL-1β, and IL-18 [30]. The TRIF pathway specifically results in the release of type 1 interferons (IFN) which have a role in activating the cellular caspase recognition system and further redundant, inflammatory pathways [33].

In animal and cell culture models, administering agonists for multiple TLRs (enhancing TLR activity, including TLR2, −3, −4) during hyperthermia/fever (39.5 °C) increased pathogenesis of sepsis [34, 35]. More detailed mechanistic studies demonstrate that exposure to febrile-range temperatures of ~40 °C physically affects recruitment of LPS-induced transcription factors to different cytokines that are critical to inflammation (TNF-α and IL-1β) [36, 37]. Increasing TLR4 activity or LPS concentrations and inducing endotoxemia/sepsis appear to magnify the pathophysiological effects of exposure to febrile temperatures. This may be by modulation of inflammatory gene expression during hyperthermia/fever. The direct mechanistic links between endotoxemia and sepsis speak to the molecular and cellular impact that these pathways likely have in EHS if circulating LPS is increased during exercise in the heat and extremely so in some patients who develop EHS.

However, endotoxemia and sepsis do not entirely explain EHS susceptibility and pathophysiology; LPS-induced TLR4 signaling is only one partial aspect of the molecular mechanisms. This is demonstrated by experiments showing that a TLR4 blocker, eritoran, was not effective in clinical trials for sepsis treatment. These experiments resulted in the discovery of a noncanonical inflammasome pathway which may also be involved in LPS-induced inflammatory pathophysiology. In this pathway, cytosolic LPS recognition is mediated by direct binding to caspase-11 in mice and − 4/5 in humans [38, 39]. What immunologists understand and contribute to our understanding of immune system physiology in EHS is multifold (Fig. 8.1):

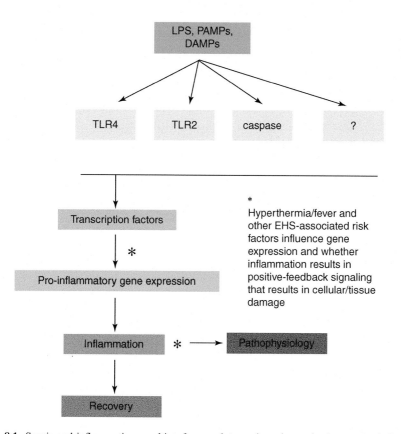

Fig. 8.1 Sepsis and inflammation resulting from endotoxemia and exercise-heat stress-induced signaling are likely highly complex. LPS (lipopolysaccharide) and specific LPS structural variants, pathogen-associated molecular patterns (PAMPs) from other bacterial components, danger-associated molecular patterns (DAMPs) that include endogenous heat shock proteins and lipoproteins, and other ligands directly bind TLR4 (toll-like receptor 4) during exercise, heat exposure, oxidative stress, and tissue damage to promote gene expression of multiple pro-inflammatory proteins. Other receptors such as TLR2, enzymes that can directly bind LPS, like caspase, and other potential noncanonical mechanisms funnel into multiple transcription factors to increase pro-inflammatory gene expression. The pro-inflammatory mediators themselves, including cytokines and heat shock proteins, may feedback positively to augment the entire signaling. Under normal, healthy conditions, an individual is able to recover from this acute systemic inflammation, but with a combination of other exacerbating factors, inflammation goes unchecked and resulting tissue damage and sepsis may contribute to EHS pathophysiology. Damage to specific organs like the brain and kidneys results in clinical manifestations associated with EHS above and beyond increases in core temperature

1. LPS is one of many ligands that directly bind to TLR4 to promote inflammation and sepsis inducing inflammatory pathways.
2. Other ligands that can stimulate TLR4 that are unstudied in EHS pathophysiology research include endogenous molecules that are important to exercise-heat stress responses.
3. Other bacterial components leaked from the gut during exercise-heat stress may stimulate TLR signaling.
4. TLR2 also contributes, by MyD88 signaling, to the production of inflammatory cytokines and is capable of binding ligands associated with cellular exercise-heat stress responses.
5. TLR4 signals by at least one noncanonical pro-inflammatory pathway that is yet unstudied in EHS animal models and patients.
6. Febrile temperatures.
7. Likely other context-dependent situations (e.g., sleep deprivation, endocrine dysfunction) affect the TLR4-dependent gene expression of specific cytokines. The signaling that links LPS in systemic circulation to pathophysiology associated with sepsis and perhaps heat stroke is likely complicated, involving multiple positive feedback mechanisms of inflammation and innate immune response that have yet been unstudied in EHS, specifically.

Cellular Heat Shock Response

In addition to inflammatory cytokine gene expression resulting from immune responses during heat stress and EHS, heat-inducible heat shock protein (Hsp72) of the 70 kilodalton (kD) family (Hsp70) is expressed. Hsp72 is critical to the cellular heat shock response [40] but has different roles intracellularly versus extracellularly [41], though much remains unknown about the diverse functions of Hsp70 family members. Hsp72 is regulated by many factors, including TLR4 signaling, and this is powerfully demonstrated by the increases in expression of Hsp70 (estimate of Hsp72) in mice challenged with both hyperthermia and LPS (vs. either treatment alone) [34, 35]. The presence of Hsp72, through transcription factor known as NF-κB (nuclear factor kappa-light-chain-enhancer of activated B cells), positively feeds back and increases inflammatory cytokine gene expression through TLR4 as shown in clinical inflammatory conditions (not EHS) [42, 43]. In TLR4 null mutants, the effects of Hsp72 on cytokine expression, such as that of interleukin 8 (IL-8), are reduced [42], supporting the notion that the cellular Hsp response and TLR4 signaling are directly linked to promote inflammation during clinical conditions and perhaps during EHS.

Hsp treatment [44], transgenic expression of porcine Hsp70 [45] (i.e., Hsp72), overexpression of Hsp72 [46], and exercise preconditioning to induce Hsp72 [47] have all been shown to reduce symptoms and severity of EHS. Well-controlled animal work has demonstrated that genotypes associated with Hsp70/72 may be linked to thermal tolerance [48–50], but very little has demonstrated that Hsp72 genotypes are linked to Malignant Hyperthermia (MH) or EHS susceptibility. We speculate that although Hsp72 has such a critical role in the molecular mechanisms of heat stress response and EHS, it is difficult to associate genotypically with the condition because of its fundamental, diverse, and pleiotropic roles in physiology.

Pharmacological Treatments Reveal Pathophysiological Molecular Mechanisms

Much remains unknown about non-sepsis-related molecular/cellular contributors to EHS susceptibility and pathophysiology. Studies of pharmacological agents used to treat symptoms or severity of heat stroke are revealing. For example, despite evidence that glucocorticoid (dexamethasone) treatment in baboons does not protect and may exacerbate heat stroke [51], promising evidence suggests that glucocorticoid administration helps reduce symptom heat stroke lethality, symptom severity, and recovery time [52–54]. It is not clear whether the anti-inflammatory effects of glucocorticoids or another mechanism is involved in this endocrine factor in heat stroke pathophysiology. Additionally, whether these treatments are translatable to pre- or posttreatment of EHS is not clear from the current literature base.

Similarly, melatonin, a multifunctional, potential antioxidant treatment, appears to reduce lung damage [55] and brain damage [56] in animal models of heat stroke. Two key reviews have determined that multiple pharmacological agents with antioxidant, stem cell, anti-inflammatory, endocrine, and antihypertensive functions were effective in reducing hypothalamic damage during heat stroke [5, 57].

These studies indicate possible pathways to explore for molecular mechanisms of EHS development. Genotypes associated with variants in proteins associated with these pathways are not associated clearly with susceptibility to EHS or thermal intolerance. In many cases, identifying genotypes in these pathways may be difficult to relate to heat stroke susceptibility because of the fundamental and pleiotropic roles of many of these molecular factors. At the protein/molecular level, these can be targeted with pharmacological treatments, and additional research on genotypes clearly associated with EHS risk may be complimentary to such therapy options.

Genotypes Associated with Risk for EHI and EHS

Malignant Hyperthermia (MH) and EHS Share Genotype-Associated Susceptibility

A remarkable case study presented identical twins who experienced exertional heat stroke during the same race in which there were ~14 EHS cases among 38,000 competitors [58]; that there is a genetic link to thermal tolerance and EHS susceptibility is clear, although the nature of that link remains undefined. Heritable genetic variants associated with anesthetic-triggered hyperthermia, metabolic disturbances, and altered hematology are among those considered to be related to increased risk for exertional heat stroke (EHS) (Table 8.2). Among these genetic variants include those relevant to malignant hyperthermia (MH), a skeletal muscle disorder [59]. Malignant hyperthermia is associated with most commonly (>70% of cases) [60] a heterozygous mutation in the gene coding for the ryanodine receptor RYR1, a calcium channel in the membrane of the sarcoplasmic reticulum, which is responsible for the release of calcium during muscle contractions [61]. Inappropriately timed releases of calcium from intermuscular calcium stores can occur in susceptible individuals as a result of exposure to anesthetic agents or muscle relaxants such as succinylcholine [62]. MH susceptibility is tested functionally by an in vitro contracture test (IVCT), a highly invasive procedure that exposes muscle fibers to halothane and caffeine to measure a response [62, 63]. The subsequent contraction of the muscle results in muscle rigidity, large increases in the production of metabolic heat leading to hyperthermia, metabolic and respiratory acidosis, and rhabdomyolysis. The test is 97–99% sensitive and 78–94% specific [64, 65].

Among individuals with genetic susceptibility to MH, there are those who appear to be at risk also for what is termed "awake" or nonanesthetic malignant hyperthermia that was defined early on as porcine stress syndrome in the 1960s and linked to human conditions [66, 67]. More than 50 years later, EHS links to MH have been more specifically defined with terminology such as "MH-like syndrome" to address possible variations of the syndromes [59]. Novel variants or presence of two mutations on different alleles [68] may decrease the thermal tolerance of an individual to environmental conditions, exercise, infection, and any drugs that affect heat balance. Data confirm the likelihood of relationships between MH-related genotypes and exertional heat stroke or sensitivity to exercise-heat stress. Strenuous treadmill running induces hyperthermia and rhabdomyolysis in mice with altered RYR1 genes [65]. Researchers have performed diagnostic contracture tests on individuals who have collapsed with EHS [69], observing that up to 45.6% of EHS survivors were positive for an in vitro contracture test, indicating MH susceptibility [63]. Multiple case reports have described cases in which individuals who suffer from an exertional heat stroke respond positively to an IVCT [10, 11]. Wappler et al. identified 10 out of 12 patients presenting with EHS symptoms to also be MH-susceptible. Three of these ten had candidate *ryr1* variants [70]]. Bendahan et al. diagnosed 26 with EHS and all of them were positive for an IVCT test [71].

A dysfunctional *RYR1* variant confirms a diagnosis of MH in conjunction to an IVCT, but MHS (malignant hyperthermia susceptibility) is genetically heterogeneous [69]. Genetic variants other than those associated with *RYR1* are associated with different forms of MH and thus perhaps with EHI/EHS susceptibility. Among MH cases not associated with RYR1 variants, ~1% [60] (MH5) are associated with defects in the CACNA1S gene. CACNA1S encodes the alpha-1 subunit of an L-type voltage-gated calcium channel in skeletal muscle that responds to a depolarizing stimulus [61, 72]. Another calcium channel gene associated with MH, CACNA2D1 [73, 74], encodes the subunit of a calcium channel in the skeletal muscle that is

Table 8.2 Genes associated with variants that reduce exercise and thermal tolerance and likely increase exertional heat stroke (EHS) susceptibility

Disease	Affected gene		Gene location	Effect
Malignant hyperthermia	*RYR1*	Ryanodine receptor 1, skeletal muscle sarcoplasmic metabolism	19q13.2	Increase in intramuscular calcium in response to anesthetic agents
	CACNA1S	Alpha-1 subunit, L-type voltage-gated calcium channel	1q32.1	Increase in intramuscular calcium in response to a depolarizing stimulus
	SCN4A	Alpha subunit, type 4 voltage-gated sodium channel	17q	Typically associated with hyperkalemic paralysis, MH susceptibility
	CACNA2D1, non-coding region	Alpha-2 subunit, L-type voltage-gated calcium channel	7q21-q22	Affects *RYR1* function at triadic junctions, increases intramuscular calcium
	CASQ1	Calsequestrin 1, Ca2+ binding protein	1q23.2	Main Ca2+ buffer of the sarcoplasmic reticulum of cardiac and skeletal muscle
	TRPV1	Transient receptor potential cation channel subfamily V, member 1	17p13.2	Nonselective cation channel activated by noxious stimuli to central nervous system (pain, temperature)
Catechol-aminergic ventricular tachycardia	*RYR2*	Ryanodine receptor 2, cardiac muscle sarcoplasmic reticulum		Increase in intramuscular calcium, resulting in tachycardia and cardiac dysfunction
Sickle cell trait	*HBB*	Hemoglobin beta-chain	11p15.4	Polymerization of hemoglobin β-chains
Carnitine palmito-yltransferase II deficiency	*CPTII*	Carnitine palmitoyltransferase II, inner membrane of mitochondria	1p32.3	Inability to bring fatty acids into mitochondria for beta-oxidation
Very long-chain acetyl-CoA dehydrogenase deficiency	*VLCAD*	Very long-chain acetyl-CoA dehydrogenase, helps catalyze beta-oxidation	17p13.1	Very long-chain fatty acid beta-oxidation is decreased
McArdle disease	*PYGM*	Muscle glycogen phosphorylase	11q13.1	Inability to breakdown muscle glycogen
Glycogen storage disease VII	*PFKM*	Muscle phosphofructokinase, a regulatory enzyme required for glycolysis	12q13.11	Impaired glycolysis, resulting in exertional myopathy, muscle cramping, myoglobinuria
Glycogen storage disease XI	*LDHA*	Lactate dehydrogenase A	11p15.1	Decreased interconversion of lactate and pyruvate. Results in low exercise tolerance and myoglobinuria

associated with RYR1 at triadic junctions. These and other genetic variants associated with less common types of malignant hyperthermia (MH2–6) exhibit clinical manifestations that may be related to thermal intolerance and risk for exertional heat complications, but no consistent and direct link has been found between many of these variants and risk for EHS or thermal intolerance in exercise-heat stress settings. Studies of MH and EHI/EHS patients have revealed isolated cases of individuals positive for mutations in CACNA1S and CACNA2D1 [75, 76].

Other proteins such as calsequestrin-1 (CASQ1) have also been explored as candidate genes for MH and EHS susceptibility [77, 78]. CASQ1 encodes a protein that regulates RYR1-mediated calcium release. In 2009, researchers [77] created a CASQ1 knockout model in mice and observed that these mice had increased susceptibility to and spontaneous mortality during halothane anesthetic administration and heat stress. CASQ1 null mice experienced hyperthermia and rhabdomyolysis during heat stress and were successfully treated if administered with dantrolene, a drug that is known to reduce RyR1 calcium release and is used to treat malignant hyperthermia. In a study of 75 MH-susceptible (MHS) individuals diagnosed by positive IVCT, clinicians and researchers determined that a CASQ1 variant (c.260 T > C) was present in 6 heterozygous individuals also carrying an MH-causative mutation in RYR1; further analysis of 130 additional patients with MH susceptibility (positive IVCT and causative RYR1 mutation) revealed 9 additional heterozygous individuals for the CASQ1 variant. However, based on analysis of additional MHS and MHS-negative samples, researchers determined that the CASQ1 variant they observed was not likely to be a major MHS locus in the North American population [79]. Other investigators [78] have identified additional CASQ1 variants that appear to be linked to heat stroke patients in populations outside North America and further identified other possible genetic links to heat intolerance and heat stroke susceptibility and pathophysiology.

Gene variants associated with additional MHS classifications have not been as well-studied with respect to EHS susceptibility, but they are considered candidate genes to explore in the future. MHS2 is a form of malignant hyperthermia that stems from a mutation on the gene coding for the voltage-gated sodium channel SCNA4 on chromosome 17q [80, 81]. Problems with this channel typically result in hyperkalemic periodic paralysis, but Olckers et al. [81] felt there was enough evidence to link mutations in the SCNA4 gene to malignant hyperthermia susceptibility. MHS4 was determined to exist in a single German family by Sudbrak et al. (1995). They linked markers defining a 1-cM interval on chromosome 3q13.1. They confirmed the MH phenotype via an in vitro contracture test [82]. MHS6 was discovered in 1997 by Robinson et al. A genome-wide search of a Belgian family with MH revealed linkage to a region on chromosome 5p. Robinson et al. concluded their study by suggesting that there is at least one more MHS locus [72].

Novel genes not yet associated with specific MH subtypes also are interesting candidates to consider in EHS susceptibility. One recent target is the TRPV1 (transient receptor potential vanilloid 1) nonselective cation channel which is responsible for sensing noxious stimuli in the nervous system. This receptor which is capable of detecting temperature, pain, and other stimuli can vary among individuals and appears to be affected by the hypermetabolic state in MH. One comprehensive study in 2018 [83] identified that TRPV1 is activated by anesthetics in cell culture models of MH. More compelling are their findings that of 28 MH patients, 2 unrelated patients possessed rare genetic TRPV1 variants; transfection of these variants into cell culture affected calcium signaling and response to anesthetic-induced events in vitro/in situ. Treatment of animal models of heat stroke with GSK2193874, a TRPV4 channel, was not prophylactically effective but was effective in reducing heat stroke-related injury when administered at the onset of heat stroke [84]. Physiological, tissue-level, biomarker, and lethality outcomes were improved with the administration of this drug [84], contributing to the evidence that this may also be a novel MHS genotype that can be further explored in future EHS research. There are likely other heritable factors that contribute to different classifications of MH and may be associated with EHS but much remains unknown in this area.

Non-MH Related Heritability Is Associated with Exercise-Heat Intolerance

Data linking MH and EHI/EHS are compelling. Less understood is how genotypes associated with other clinical conditions are related to high incidence of intolerance to exercise-heat stress. For example, mutations in gene coding for RYR2, a ryanodine receptor found in cardiac muscle, can lead to sudden, exercise-induced death (catecholaminergic ventricular tachycardia). There are two proposed mechanisms. The first is that a decreased concentration of channel stabilizing protein calstabin-2, which binds and stabilizes the "closed" state of RYR2, causes a calcium leak into the cardiac tissue, triggering cardiac arrhythmias. The second mechanism purports that during exercise, RYR2 is phosphorylated by PKA, causing dissociation of the binding protein FKBP12.6. In patients with stress-induced polymorphic ventricular tachycardia, mutations in the genes coding for RYR2 resulted in a decrease in affinity for FKBP12.6. Similar to the first mechanism, this dissociation causes an increase in intercellular calcium, resulting in cardiac dysfunction [85].

Another example of a heritable condition increasing susceptibility to exercise-heat stress is sickle cell trait/disease. Individuals with sickle cell trait (SCT) are already at a greater risk of exercise-induced death illness given the nature of the disease. Exertional sickling can be compounded by high heat, humidity, and dehydration, coupled with intense bouts of exercise in which blood oxygen is reduced [85].

SCT is no longer considered a result of one genetic mutation but rather a combination of multiple genotypes that determine the severity of an individual's disease [86, 87]. Hemoglobin, the oxygen-carrying protein in red blood cells, comprises two α- and two β-subunits. Fetal hemoglobin contains γ-subunits instead of β-subunits. Sickle cell hemoglobin (HbS) is monogenetically inherited and is common across all phenotypes. A single nucleotide substitution occurs on chromosome 11p15.5 and results in hydrophobic valine replacing hydrophilic glutamic acid in the β-subunit of hemoglobin (Hb), denoted as $β^S$ [88]. This mutation can interact with other β-subunit mutations to produce varying severities of sickle cell disease. Other genotypes can influence sickle cell aggregation to the endothelial cells, the degree of sickling, and the concentration of fetal hemoglobin. Homozygotes for β^S, which lead to a condition known as sickle cell anemia (HbSS), demonstrate the most severe phenotype, which manifests almost identically to another genotype, heterozygous HbS/β^0 thalassemia. β^0 thalassemia is a condition in which no β-subunits are produced. HbS/β^+ thalassemia is a heterozygotic disease in which β-subunits are produced, but in lower amounts, and phenotypically is much less severe [89]. Individuals with HbS combined with a hereditary persistence of fetal Hb demonstrate a mild phenotype or are symptom-free [87, 88].

Healthy erythrocytes have a high degree of deformability, allowing them to traverse small arterioles and capillaries. In individuals with sickle cell trait, stress (e.g., low oxygen, dehydrated, high temperature, low pH) induces HbS polymerization and erythrocyte sickling [87]. Sickled red blood cells [26, 27] become trapped resulting in vaso-occlusion and reduced blood flow to tissues including skeletal muscle. Other events compounding this include adhesion of erythrocytes to the epithelium and the binding of leukocytes to the sickled cells [27]. The presence of epinephrine can also exacerbate the adhesion of sickled cells [88]. Local inflammatory responses continue to aggravate the adhesion and the binding of immune cells, and the local hypoxic environment caused by the vaso-occlusion contributes to further sickling of cells. This causes a positive feedback loop that ultimately results in the "metabolic failure" of exercising muscle [87].

The risk of death from exertional sickling is greatly elevated in both athletes and military personnel [90, 91]. Most reported cases of exertional collapse associated with sickle cell trait (ECAST) occur during preseason training, or after return from injury. Other musculoskeletal stresses, especially those which have been shown to lead to exertional rhabdomyolysis (ER), can decrease the "threshold" required for a severe ECAST [92].

Of note, while many case studies examine exertional sickling, rhabdomyolysis, and exertional heat stroke during the football preseason when athletes are exposed to hot and humid environmental conditions in an unacclimatized state, high temperatures are not a prerequisite for exertional sickling. Individuals will often have an ECAST episode early enough during the exercise without core body temperature reaching pathologically high levels. Thus, patients lack the elevated core temperature found in EHS patients and do not have impaired CNS function [92, 93]. It is thought that leading cause of exertional sickling is exercise intensity [93]. The link between SCT and EHS genetic susceptibilities is thus not entirely clear, though data linking SCT and EHI/EHS is suggestive, both in military and athlete populations [94–96].

Metabolic Disturbances Likely Reduce Tolerance to Exercise-Heat Stress

Rhabdomyolysis is a condition during which striated muscle, typically skeletal muscle, breaks down due to high mechanical and metabolic stress. The consequent release of the muscle contents can lead to myoglobinuria, acute kidney injuries, acute compartment syndrome, and, in extreme cases, arrhythmias and death [97].

Exertional rhabdomyolysis (ER) is a pathological condition where muscle breakdown occurs after a bout of exercise. In most cases, ER occurs as a result of excessive, prolonged, or repeated eccentric exercises [97, 98]. Individuals with a low baseline fitness level or low heat tolerance are also at risk for ER [29]. There are several inherited skeletal muscle metabolic disorders that increase the risk of developing ER as a result of intense exercise.

Carnitine palmitoyltransferase (CPT) II is an enzyme located on the inner mitochondrial membrane that catalyzes the formation of fatty acyl co-A. The CPT system facilitates long-chain fatty acid transport into the mitochondria. Mutations in the gene coding for CPT II can cause deficiency of the enzyme, though the degree of disease caused by CPT II deficiency is variable [32]. Nonfatal forms of the disease are characterized by exercise-induced muscle pain, rhabdomyolysis, and myoglobinuria [99]. A Japanese study [100] of 24 heat stroke (non-exertional) patients revealed a common CPTII variant (F352C) in 11 patients that was associated with greater JAAM DIC diagnostic criteria score and SOFA indicating greater coagulopathy and organ dysfunction that was associated with double mean hospital stays (21.5 ± 23.0 vs. 9.5 ± 13.2 days). All other aspects of acute illness including body temperature, albumin, and creatine kinase, were similar between those with F352C variant and control patients.

Very long-chain acetyl-CoA dehydrogenase deficiency (VLCAD) is an inherited metabolic disease of fatty acid beta-oxidation. Clinically, VLCAD deficiency manifests in one of three ways: (1) early onset, which is very severe and has a high mortality rate, (2) childhood onset with intermediate severity and a more favorable outcome, and (3) adult onset, which is usually characterized by rhabdomyolysis and myoglobinuria after exercise [101]. The disease is the result of a homozygous mutation in the gene coding for very long-chain acyl-CoA dehydrogenase on chromosome 17p13 [101]. Other common inherited fatty acid metabolic disorders leading to rhabdomyolysis are medium-chain acyl-CoA dehydrogenase (MCAD) and trifunctional enzyme deficiency [102, 103].

McArdle disease, or glycogen storage deficiency V is another heritable metabolic disease that increases susceptibility to rhabdomyolysis. GSD5 is caused by a homozygous mutation in the genes coding for muscle glycogen phosphorylase, at chromosome 11q13 [104]. Affected individuals are unable to mobilize muscle glycogen stores [105]. During exercise, patients experience muscle cramps, weakness, and myalgia [35]. Transient episodes of myoglobinuria can occur as a result of rhabdomyolysis, and severe myoglobinuria can lead to kidney failure [104, 106].

Other forms of glycogen storage deficiencies can lead to an increased risk of exertional myopathies. GSD7 is an autosomal recessive disorder and comes from a mutation on chromosome 12q13, the gene coding for muscle phosphofructokinase (PFK) [106]. Symptoms include muscle cramping, exercise intolerance, and exertional myopathies such as a rhabdomyolysis. In severe cases, myoglobinuria occurs as a result of muscle damage. Unique to GSD7 are a partial loss of muscle PFK and partial loss of red cell PFK activity [107]. GSD11 is caused by a mutation in the gene coding for muscle lactate dehydrogenase (LDHM), on chromosome 11p15. As with other glycogen storage deficiencies, patients complain of exercise intolerance and myoglobinuria. GSD11 has been documented only in the Japanese populations, thus far, and is relatively rare [108]. In many cases, glycogen storage deficiencies are mild, and many patients do not seek medical attention [107].

The link between rhabdomyolysis and exertional heat stroke is complex though the conditions often occur concurrently due to MOD and specifically muscle tissue damage often seen in EHS. However, individuals with genetic predisposition to rhabdomyolysis and other muscle disorders often present exercise intolerance as a symptom, due to factors like ineffective fatty acid metabolism and issues related to glycogen storage and use. This could limit the ability of an athlete to exercise effectively in the hot conditions.

Summary and Conclusions

Current understanding is limited regarding genetic predispositions for EHI/ EHS. Known mechanisms of cellular/molecular mechanisms of thermal tolerance have given scientists and clinicians an indication of where to look for potential factors in EHS susceptibility, but thermoregulation, cellular/molecular thermal tolerance, and EHS pathophysiology are all independently complex with some, and to what degree, unknown overlap. For example, Hsp72 is known to be critical for cellular recovery from heat stress and cytoprotection from subsequent heat insults. However, on a whole-body level, although Hsp72 is elevated in response to exercise-heat stress, there is little evidence that Hsp72 treatment clinically would prevent or treat EHS. Researchers and clinicians should acknowledge that it is improbable that manipulating a single cytoprotective molecule will prevent a systemic EHS event in every individual. In considering the biological importance of Hsp72, much additional research should be done to explore either genetic knockout/knockdown models, individual Hsp72 variants, pharmacological treatments with Hsp72, and expression of Hsp72, in human studies and ideally in EHS patients. To truly pursue discovery of molecular and cellular mechanisms that might have practical application in EHS treatment and prevention, scientists and clinicians must collaborate in a multidisciplinary fashion. Clearly defining mechanisms that contribute to thermal tolerance while concurrently exploring ways to manipulate those mechanisms in a practically meaningful way for clinicians will support forward progress in the field.

1. Cellular and whole-body thermal tolerance should be considered separately and differently when seeking markers for EHS susceptibility. Not all cellular stress responses are detectable systemically, and often, as in the case of Hsp72, intracellular and extracellular forms of the protein have different physiological roles and consequences.
2. Pathophysiology that occurs during EHS may not be linked to genotypes associated with EHS susceptibility, and thus also pathophysiology and genotype-associated risk factors should be considered in their appropriate contexts. For example, although endotoxemia and sepsis mediated by TLR4 and Hsp72 are directly implicated in EHS pathophysiology, there is little data to suggest that in

humans, genotypic variants associated with components in these pathways are consistent and clear factors in EHS susceptibility or exercise/heat intolerance.

3. Complexity in molecular mechanisms associated with cellular and systemic response to heat and resulting tolerance or EHS is vast. Our current understanding is limited and thus limits our ability to clearly define specific factors or combinations of factors that allow us to predict thermotolerance and EHS.

4. Promising targets for future research in the area of biomarkers and predisposing factors include multiple levels of physiological function, inflammation, heat shock response, skeletal and cardiac muscle function, calcium signaling, and most relatively unstudied, is how all these functions impact neuronal tissue.

References

1. Casa DJ, DeMartini JK, Bergeron MF, Csillan D, Eichner ER, Lopez RM, et al. National Athletic Trainers' Association position statement: exertional heat illnesses. J Athl Train. 2015;50(9):986–1000.

2. Armstrong LE, Lee EC, Armstrong EM. Interactions of gut microbiota, endotoxemia, immune function, and diet in exertional heatstroke. J Sports Med (Hindawi Publ Corp). 2018;2018:5724575.

3. Bouchama A, Knochel P. Heat stroke. N Engl J Med. 2002;346(25):1978–88.

4. Lim CL, Mackinnon LT. The roles of exercise-induced immune system disturbances in the pathology of heat stroke. Sports Med. 2006;36(1):39–64.

5. Lim C. Heat Sepsis precedes heat toxicity in the pathophysiology of heat stroke—a new paradigm on an ancient disease. Antioxidants. 2018;7(11):149.

6. Maron MB, Wagner JA, Horvath SM. Thermoregulatory responses during competitive marathon running. J Appl Physiol. 1977;42(6):909–14.

7. Byrne C, Lee JK, Chew SA, Lim CL, Tan EY. Continuous thermoregulatory responses to mass-participation distance running in heat. Med Sci Sports Exerc. 2006;38(5):803–10.

8. Sithinamsuwan P, Piyavechviratana K, Kitthaweesin T, Chusri W, Orrawanhanothai P, Wongsa A, et al.; Phramongkutklao Army Hospital Exertional Heatstroke Study Team. Exertional heatstroke: early recognition and outcome with aggressive combined cooling—a 12-year experience. Mil Med 2009;174(5):496–502.

9. Binkley HM, Beckett J, Casa DJ, Kleiner DM, Plummer PE. National Athletic Trainers' association position statement: exertional heat illnesses. J Athl Train. 2002;37(3):329–43.

10. Cleary M. Predisposing risk factors on susceptibility to exertional heat illness: clinical decision-making considerations. J Sport Rehabil. 2007;16(3):204–14.

11. Navarro CS, Casa DJ, Belval LN, Nye NS. Exertional heat stroke. Curr Sports Med Rep. 2017;16(5):304–5.

12. Hifumi T, Kondo Y, Shimazaki J, Oda Y, Shiraishi S, Wakasugi M, et al. Prognostic significance of disseminated intravascular coagulation in patients with heat stroke in a nationwide registry. J Crit Care. 2018;44:306–11.

13. Hifumi T, Kondo Y, Shimizu K, Miyake Y. Heat stroke. J Intensive Care. 2018;6:30. https://doi.org/10.1186/s40560-018-0298-4. Review

14. Snipe RMJ, Khoo A, Kitic CM, Gibson PR, Costa RJS. The impact of mild heat stress during prolonged running on gastrointestinal integrity, gastrointestinal symptoms, systemic endotoxin and cytokine profiles. Int J Sports Med. 2018;39:255. https://doi.org/10.1055/s-0043-122742. [Epub ahead of print].

15. Singer M, Deutschman CS, Seymour CW, Shankar-Hari M, Annane D, Bauer M, et al. The third international consensus definitions for sepsis and septic shock (sepsis-3). JAMA. 2016;315(8):801–10.

16. Costrini AM, Pitt HA, Gustafson AB, Uddin DE. Cardiovascular and metabolic manifestations of heat stroke and severe heat exhaustion. Am J Med. 1979;66(2):296–302.

17. Lambert GP. Intestinal barrier dysfunction, endotoxemia, and gastrointestinal symptoms: the 'canary in the coal mine' during exercise-heat stress? Med Sport Sci. 2008;53:61–73.

18. Leon LR, Helwig BG. Heat stroke: role of the systemic inflammatory response. J Appl Physiol (1985). 2010;109(6):1980–8.

19. Assimakopoulos SF, Triantos C, Thomopoulos K, Fligou F, Maroulis I, Marangos M, Gogos CA. Gut-origin sepsis in the critically ill patient: pathophysiology and treatment. Infection. 2018;46(6):751–60.

20. Dokladny K, Zuhl MN, Moseley PL. Intestinal epithelial barrier function and tight junction proteins with heat and exercise. J Appl Physiol (1985). 2016;120(6):692–701.

21. Nutsch KM, Hsieh CS. T cell tolerance and immunity to commensal bacteria. Curr Opin Immunol. 2012;24(4):385–91.

22. Hall DM, Baumgardner KR, Oberley TD, Gisolfi CV. Splanchnic tissues undergo hypoxic stress during whole body hyperthermia. Am J Physiol. 1999;276(5):G1195–203.

23. Mercer DW, Smith GS, Cross JM, Russell DH, Chang L, Cacioppo J. Effects of lipopolysaccharide on intestinal injury: potential role of nitric oxide and lipid peroxidation. J Surg Res. 1996;63(1):185–92.20.

24. Costa RJS, Snipe RMJ, Kitic CM, Gibson PR. Systematic review: exercise-induced gastrointestinal syndrome-implications for health and intestinal disease. Aliment Pharmacol Ther. 2017;46(3):246–65.

25. Lambert GP, Boylan M, Laventure JP, Bull A, Lanspa S. Effect of aspirin and ibuprofen on GI permeability during exercise. Int J Sports Med. 2007;28(9):722–6.

26. Guy J, Vincent G. Nutrition and supplementation considerations to limit endotoxemia when exercising in the heat. Sports (Basel). 2018;6(1):pii: E12. https://doi.org/10.3390/sports6010012.

27. Boutagy NE, McMillan RP, Frisard MI, Hulver MW. Metabolic endotoxemia with obesity: is it real and is it relevant? Biochimie. 2016;124:11–20.

28. Viswanathan VK, Hodges K, Hecht G. Enteric infection meets intestinal function:how bacterial pathogens cause diarrhoea. Nat Rev Microbiol. 2009;7(2):110–9.

29. Turner JR. Intestinal mucosal barrier function in health and disease. Nat Rev Immunol. 2009;9(11):799–809.

30. Wiersinga WJ, Leopold SJ, Cranendonk DR, van der Poll T. Host innate immune responses to sepsis. Virulence. 2014;5(1):36–44.

31. Goh J, Behringer M. Exercise alarms the immune system: a HMGB1 perspective. Cytokine. 2018;110:222–5.

32. Seys SF, Hox V, Van Gerven L, Dilissen E, Marijsse G, Peeters E, et al. Damage-associated molecular pattern and innate cytokine release in the airways of competitive swimmers. Allergy. 2015;70(2):187–94.

33. Pfalzgraff A, Weindl G. Intracellular lipopolysaccharide sensing as a potential therapeutic target for sepsis. Trends Pharmacol Sci. 2019;40(3):187–97.

34. Gupta A, Cooper ZA, Tulapurkar ME, Potla R, Maity T, Hasday JD, Singh IS. Toll-like receptor agonists and febrile range hyperthermia synergize to induce heat shock protein 70 expression and extracellular release. J Biol Chem. 2013;288(4):2756–66.

35. Tulapurkar ME, Ramarathnam A, Hasday JD, Singh IS. Bacterial lipopolysaccharide augments febrile-range hyperthermia-induced heat shock protein 70 expression and extracellular release in human THP1 cells. PLoS One. 2015;10(2):e0118010.

36. Cooper ZA, Ghosh A, Gupta A, Maity T, Benjamin IJ, Vogel SN, et al. Febrile-range temperature modifies cytokine gene expression in LPS-stimulated macrophages by differentially modifying NF-{kappa}B recruitment to cytokine gene promoters. Am J Physiol Cell Physiol. 2010;298(1):C171–81.

37. Cooper ZA, Singh IS, Hasday JD. Febrile range temperature represses TNF-alpha gene expression in LPS-stimulated macrophages by selectively blocking recruitment of Sp1 to the TNF-alpha promoter. Cell Stress Chaperones. 2010;15(5):665–73.

38. Kayagaki N, Wong MT, Stowe IB, Ramani SR, Gonzalez LC, Akashi-Takamura S, et al. Noncanonical inflammasome activation by intracellular LPS independent of TLR4. Science. 2013;341(6151):1246–9.
39. Wacker MA, Teghanemt A, Weiss JP, Barker JH. High-affinity caspase-4 binding to LPS presented as high molecular mass aggregates or in outer membrane vesicles. Innate Immun. 2017;23(4):336–44.
40. Lindquist S, Craig EA. The heat-shock proteins. Annu Rev Genet. 1988;22:631–77.
41. Lee EC, Muñoz CX, McDermott BP, Beasley KN, Yamamoto LM, Hom LL, et al. Extracellular and cellular Hsp72 differ as biomarkers in acute exercise/environmental stress and recovery. Scand J Med Sci Sports. 2017;27(1):66–74.
42. Chase MA, Wheeler DS, Lierl KM, Hughes VS, Wong HR, Page K. Hsp72 induces inflammation and regulates cytokine production in airway epithelium through a TLR4- and NF-kappaB-dependent mechanism. J Immunol. 2007;179(9):6318–24.
43. Wheeler DS, Chase MA, Senft AP, Poynter SE, Wong HR, Page K. Extracellular Hsp72, an endogenous DAMP, is released by virally infected airway epithelial cells and activates neutrophils via Toll-like receptor (TLR)-4. Respir Res. 2009;10:31. https://doi.org/10.1186/1465-9921-10-31.
44. Kourtis N, Nikoletopoulou V, Tavernarakis N. Small heat-shock proteins protect from heat stroke-associated neurodegeneration. Nature. 2012;490(7419):213–8.
45. Chen ZC, Wu WS, Lin MT, Hsu CC. Protective effect of transgenic expression of porcine heat shock protein 70 on hypothalamic ischemic and oxidative damage in a mouse model of heatstroke. BMC Neurosci. 2009;10:111. https://doi.org/10.1186/1471-2202-10-111.
46. Lee WC, Wen HC, Chang CP, Chen MY, Lin MT. Heat shock protein 72 overexpression protects against hyperthermia, circulatory shock, and cerebral ischemia during heatstroke. J Appl Physiol (1985). 2006;100(6):2073–82.
47. Hung CH, Chang NC, Cheng BC, Lin MT. Progressive exercise preconditioning protects against circulatory shock during experimental heatstroke. Shock. 2005;23(5):426–33.
48. Basiricò L, Morera P, Primi V, Lacetera N, Nardone A, Bernabucci U. Cellular thermotolerance is associated with heat shock protein 70.1 genetic polymorphisms in Holstein lactating cows. Cell Stress Chaperones. 2011;16(4):441–8.
49. Lockwood B, Julick CR, Montooth KL. Maternal loading of a small heat shock protein increases embryo thermal tolerance in *Drosophila melanogaster*. J Exp Biol. 2017;220(Pt 23):4492–501.
50. Sodhi M, Mukesh M, Kishore A, Mishra BP, Kataria RS, Joshi BK. Novel polymorphisms in UTR and coding region of inducible heat shock protein 70.1 gene in tropically adapted Indian zebu cattle (*Bos indicus*) and riverine buffalo (*Bubalus bubalis*). Gene. 2013;527(2):606–15.
51. Bouchama A, Kwaasi A, Dehbi M, Al Mohanna F, Eldali A, El-Sayed R, et al. Glucocorticoids do not protect against the lethal effects of experimental heatstroke in baboons. Shock. 2007;27(5):578–83.
52. Gathiram P, Wells MT, Brock-Utne JG, Gaffin SL. Prophylactic corticosteroid increases survival in experimental heat stroke in primates. Aviat Space Environ Med. 1988;59(4):352–5.
53. Lim CL, Wilson G, Brown L, Coombes JS, Mackinnon LT. Pre-existing inflammatory state compromises heat tolerance in rats exposed to heat stress. Am J Physiol Regul Integr Comp Physiol. 2007;292(1):R186–94.
54. Liu CC, Chien CH, Lin MT. Glucocorticoids reduce interleukin-1 concentration and result in neuroprotective effects in rat heatstroke. J Physiol. 2000;527(Pt 2):333–43.
55. Wu WS, Chou MT, Chao CM, Chang CK, Lin MT, Chang CP. Melatonin reduces acute lung inflammation, edema, and hemorrhage in heatstroke rats. Acta Pharmacol Sin. 2012;33(6):775–82.
56. Tian YF, Lin CH, Hsu SF, Lin MT. Melatonin improves outcomes of heatstroke in mice by reducing brain inflammation and oxidative damage and multiple organ dysfunction. Mediators Inflamm. 2013;2013:349280.
57. Chen SH, Lin MT, Chang CP. Ischemic and oxidative damage to the hypothalamus may be responsible for heat stroke. Curr Neuropharmacol. 2013;11(2):129–40.

58. Smith R, Jones N, Martin D, Kipps C. 'Too much of a coincidence': identical twins with exertional heatstroke in the same race. BMJ Case Rep. 2016;2016 https://doi.org/10.1136/bcr-2015-212592.

59. Hosokawa Y, Casa DJ, Rosenberg H, Capacchione JF, Sagui E, Riazi S, et al. Round table on malignant hyperthermia in physically active populations: meeting proceedings. J Athl Train. 2017;52(4):377–83.

60. Rosenberg H, Sambuughin N, Riazi S, Dirksen R. Malignant hypertermia susceptibility. In: Adam MP, Ardinger HH, Pagon RA, Wallace SE, LJH B, Stephens K, Amemiya A, editors. GeneReviews® [Internet]. Seattle: University of Washington, Seattle; 1993–2019.

61. Monnier N, Procaccio V, Stieglitz P, Lunardi J. Malignant-hyperthermia susceptibility is associated with a mutation of the alpha 1-subunit of the human dihydropyridine-sensitive L-type voltage-dependent calcium-channel receptor in skeletal muscle. Am J Hum Genet. 1997;60(6):1316–25.

62. Heytens K, De Bleecker J, Verbrugghe W, Baets J, Heytens L. Exertional rhabdomyolysis and heat stroke: beware of volatile anesthetic sedation. World J Crit Care Med. 2017;6(1):21–7.

63. Sagui E, Montigon C, Abriat A, Jouvion A, Duron-Martinaud S, Canini F, et al. Is there a link between exertional heat stroke and susceptibility to malignant hyperthermia? PLoS One. 2015;10(8):e0135496.

64. Thomas J, Crowhurst T. Exertional heat stroke, rhabdomyolysis and susceptibility to malignant hyperthermia. Intern Med J. 2013;43(9):1035–8.

65. Capacchione JF, Muldoon SM. The relationship between exertional heat illness, exertional rhabdomyolysis, and malignant hyperthermia. Anesth Analg. 2009;109(4):1065–9.

66. Gronert GA, Thompson RL, Onofrio BM. Human malignant hyperthermia: awake episodes and correction by dantrolene. Anesth Analg. 1980;59(5):377–8.

67. Lister D, Hall GM, Lucke JN. Letter: malignant hyperthermia: a human and procine stress syndrome? Lancet. 1975;305(7905):519.

68. Groom L, Muldoon SM, Tang ZZ, Brandom BW, Bayarsaikhan M, Bina S, et al. Identical de novo mutation in the type 1 ryanodine receptor gene associated with fatal, stress-induced malignant hyperthermia in two unrelated families. Anesthesiology. 2011;115(5):938–45.

69. Muldoon S, Deuster P, Brandom B, Bunger R. Is there a link between malignant hyperthermia and exertional heat illness? Exerc Sport Sci Rev. 2004;32(4):174–9.

70. Wappler F, Fiege M, Antz M, Schulte am Esch J. Hemodynamic and metabolic alterations in response to graded exercise in a patient susceptible to malignant hyperthermia. Anesthesiology. 2000;92(1):268–72.

71. Bendahan D, Kozak-Ribbens G, Confort-Gouny S, Ghattas B, Figarella-Branger D, Aubert M, Cozzone PJ. A noninvasive investigation of muscle energetics supports similarities between exertional heat stroke and malignant hyperthermia. Anesth Analg. 2001;93(3):683–9.

72. Robinson RL, Monnier N, Wolz W, Jung M, Reis A, Nuernberg G, et al. A genome wide search for susceptibility loci in three European malignant hyperthermia pedigrees. Hum Mol Genet. 1997;6(6):953–61.

73. Iles DE, Lehmann-Horn F, Scherer SW, Tsui LC, Olde Weghuis D, Suijkerbuijk RF, et al. Localization of the gene encoding the alpha 2/delta-subunits of the L-type voltage-dependent calcium channel to chromosome 7q and analysis of the segregation of flanking markers in malignant hyperthermia susceptible families. Hum Mol Genet. 1994;3(6):969–75.

74. Sudbrak R, Golla A, Hogan K, Powers P, Gregg R, Du Chesne I, et al. Exclusion of malignant hyperthermia susceptibility (MHS) from a putative MHS2 locus on chromosome 17q and of the alpha 1, beta 1, and gamma subunits of the dihydropyridine receptor calcium channel as candidates for the molecular defect. Hum Mol Genet. 1993;2(7):857–62.

75. Fiszer D, Shaw MA, Fisher NA, Carr IM, Gupta PK, Watkins EJ, et al. Next-generation sequencing of *RYR1* and *CACNA1S* in malignant hyperthermia and exertional heat illness. Anesthesiology. 2015;122(5):1033–46.

76. Roux-Buisson N, Monnier N, Sagui E, Abriat A, Brosset C, Bendahan D, et al. Identification of variants of the ryanodine receptor type 1 in patients with exertional heat stroke and

positive response to the malignant hyperthermia in vitro contracture test. Br J Anaesth. 2016;116(4):566–8.

77. Protasi F, Paolini C, Dainese M. Calsequestrin-1: a new candidate gene for malignant hyperthermia and exertional/environmental heat stroke. J Physiol. 2009;587(Pt 13):3095–100.

78. Li Y, Wang Y, Ma L. An association study of CASQ1 gene polymorphisms and heat stroke. Genomics Proteomics Bioinformatics. 2014;12(3):127–32.

79. Kraeva N, Zvaritch E, Frodis W, Sizova O, Kraev A, MacLennan DH, Riazi S. *CASQ1* gene is an unlikely candidate for malignant hyperthermia susceptibility in the North American population. Anesthesiology. 2013;118(2):344–9.

80. Levitt RC, Nouri N, Jedlicka AE, McKusick VA, Marks AR, Shutack JG, et al. Evidence for genetic heterogeneity in malignant hyperthermia susceptibility. Genomics. 1991;11(3):543–7.

81. Olckers A, Meyers DA, Meyers S, Taylor EW, Fletcher JE, Rosenberg H, et al. Adult muscle sodium channel alpha-subunit is a gene candidate for malignant hyperthermia susceptibility. Genomics. 1992;14(3):829–31.

82. Sudbrak R, Procaccio V, Klausnitzer M, Curran JL, Monsieurs K, van Broeckhoven C, et al. Mapping of a further malignant hyperthermia susceptibility locus to chromosome 3q13.1. Am J Hum Genet. 1995;56(3):684–91.

83. Abeele FV, Lotteau S, Ducreux S, Dubois C, Monnier N, Hanna A, et al. *TRPV1* variants impair intracellular Ca2+ signaling and may confer susceptibility to malignant hyperthermia. Genet Med. 2019;21(2):441–50.

84. Zhu YH, Pei ZM. GSK2193874 treatment at heatstroke onset reduced cell apoptosis in heatstroke mice. Cell Mol Biol (Noisy-le-Grand). 2018;64(7):36–42.

85. Bhuiyan ZA, van den Berg MP, van Tintelen JP, Bink-Boelkens MT, Wiesfeld AC, Alders M, et al. Expanding spectrum of human RYR2-related disease: new electrocardiographic, structural, and genetic features. Circulation. 2007;116(14):1569–76.

86. Chui DH, Dover GJ. Sickle cell disease: no longer a single gene disorder. Curr Opin Pediatr. 2001;13(1):22–7.

87. Loosemore M, Walsh SB, Morris E, Stewart G, Porter JB, Montgomery H. Sudden exertional death in sickle cell trait. Br J Sports Med. 2012;46(5):312–4.

88. Stuart MJ, Nagel RL. Sickle-cell disease. Lancet. 2004;364(9442):1343–60.

89. Cao A, Galanello R. Beta-thalassemia. Genet Med. 2010;12(2):61–76.

90. Harmon KG, Drezner JA, Klossner D, Asif IM. Sickle cell trait associated with a RR of death of 37 times in National Collegiate Athletic Association football athletes: a database with 2 million athlete-years as the denominator. Br J Sports Med. 2012;46(5):25–30.

91. Kark JA, Posey DM, Schumacher HR, Ruehle CJ. Sickle-cell trait as a risk factor for sudden death in physical training. N Engl J Med. 1987;317(13):781–7.

92. Asplund CA, O'Connor FH. Challenging return to play decisions: heat stroke, exertional rhabdomyolysis, and exertional collapse associated with sickle cell trait. Sports Health. 2016;8(2):117–25.

93. Eichner ER. Sickle cell considerations in athletes. Clin Sports Med. 2011;30(3):537–49.

94. Nelson DA, Deuster PA, O'Connor FG, Kurina LM. Sickle cell trait and heat injury among US army soldiers. Am J Epidemiol. 2018;187(3):523–8.

95. Pretzlaff RK. Death of an adolescent athlete with sickle cell trait caused by exertional heat stroke. Pediatr Crit Care Med. 2002;3(3):308–10.

96. Singer DE, Byrne C, Chen L, Shao S, Goldsmith J, Niebuhr DW. Risk of exertional heat illnesses associated with sickle cell trait in U.S. military. Mil Med. 2018;183(7–8):e310–7.

97. Szczepanik ME, Heled Y, Capacchione J, Campbell W, Deuster P, O'Connor FG. Exertional rhabdomyolysis: identification and evaluation of the athlete at risk for recurrence. Curr Sports Med Rep. 2014;13(2):113–9.

98. Kenney K, Landau ME, Gonzalez RS, Hundertmark J, O'Brien K, Campbell WW. Serum creatine kinase after exercise: drawing the line between physiological response and exertional rhabdomyolysis. Muscle Nerve. 2012;45(3):356–62.

99. Deschauer M, Wieser T, Zierz S. Muscle carnitine palmitoyltransferase II deficiency: clinical and molecular genetic features and diagnostic aspects. Arch Neurol. 2005;62(1):37–41.

100. Oda J, Yukioka T, Azuma K, Arai T, Chida J, Kido H. Endogenous genetic risk factor for serious heatstroke: the thermolabile phenotype of carnitine palmitoyltransferase II variant. Acute Med Surg. 2019;6(1):25–9.

101. Andresen BS, Olpin S, Poorthuis BJ, Scholte HR, Vianey-Saban C, Wanders R, et al. Clear correlation of genotype with disease phenotype in very-long-chain acyl-CoA dehydrogenase deficiency. Am J Hum Genet. 1999;64(2):479–94.

102. Shirao K, Okada S, Tajima G, Tsumura M, Hara K, Yasunaga S, et al. Molecular pathogenesis of a novel mutation, G108D, in short-chain acyl-CoA dehydrogenase identified in subjects with short-chain acyl-CoA dehydrogenase deficiency. Hum Genet. 2010;127(6):619–28.

103. Matsubara Y, Kraus JP, Yang-Feng TL, Francke U, Rosenberg LE, Tanaka K. Molecular cloning of cDNAs encoding rat and human medium-chain acyl-CoA dehydrogenase and assignment of the gene to human chromosome 1. Proc Natl Acad Sci U S A. 1986;83(17):6543–7.

104. Chen YT. Glycogen storage diseases. In: Scriver CR, Beaudet AL, Sly WS, Vale D, Childs B, et al., editors. The metabolic & molecular basis of inherited diseases. New York: McGraw-Hill; 2001. p. 1521–52.

105. Mommaerts WF, Illingworth B, Pearson CM, Guillory RJ, Seraydarian K. A functional disorder of muscle associated with the absence of phosphorylase. Proc Natl Acad Sci U S A. 1959;45(6):791–7.

106. Quinlivan R, Buckley J, James M, Twist A, Ball S, Duno M, et al. McArdle disease: a clinical review. J Neurol Neurosurg Psychiatry. 2010;81(11):1182–8.

107. Raben N, Sherman JB. Mutations in muscle phosphofructokinase gene. Hum Mutat. 1995;6(1):1–6.

108. Maekawa M, Kanda S, Sudo K, Kanno T. Estimation of the gene frequency of lactate dehydrogenase subunit deficiencies. Am J Hum Genet. 1984;36(6):1204–14.

Chapter 9
Management of Exertional Heat Stroke in Athletics: Interdisciplinary Medical Care

Yuri Hosokawa

Introduction

Exertional heat stroke (EHS) is one of the leading causes of death in sport and is the most severe form of exertional heat illness [1, 2]. Although it is not uncommon for athletes to reach a state of hyperthermia during exercise (i.e., exercise-induced hyperthermia [38.5–41.5 °C]) [3, 4], physiological [5] and behavioral [6] methods of thermoregulation can aid in protecting humans from experiencing sustained heat stress that can damage the body. However, in the context of athletics, varying organizational, administrative, and environmental factors may hinder athletes from controlling thermal strain at their own pace, predisposing vulnerable individuals to EHS. EHS is defined by high internal body temperature exceeding 40 °C with signs of central nervous dysfunction such as delirium, altered mental status, and changes in personality (e.g., aggression, hysteria) [1, 7]. Sustained thermal stress (≥ 40.5 °C for 30 minutes or longer) may lead to denaturation of cells, and end-organ dysfunction will ensue if external cooling is not provided to reduce the internal body temperature below 39 °C within 30 minutes of the collapse [8]. Therefore, prognosis from EHS depends on the early recognition, rapid assessment, rapid cooling, and rapid advanced care (Fig. 9.1) [9].

Medical professionals in athletic settings are faced with unique challenges for managing EHS. For example, the need for early recognition and assessment of EHS warrant qualified medical personnel (e.g., athletic trainer) to be on-site at athletic fields, which may not be feasible in some settings. Optimal EHS triage also asks to prioritize on-site treatment (i.e., aggressive, whole-body cooling) over transportation to an advanced medical facility, which may not be intuitive for many medical professionals, considering that most injuries are treated after the patient has been transported to the hospital [9]. Thus, successful management of EHS in

Y. Hosokawa (✉)
Faculty of Sport Sciences, Waseda University, Tokorozawa, Saitama, Japan

© Springer Nature Switzerland AG 2020
W. M. Adams, J. F. Jardine (eds.), *Exertional Heat Illness*,
https://doi.org/10.1007/978-3-030-27805-2_9

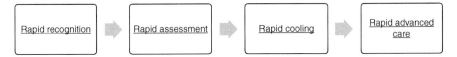

Fig. 9.1 Basic paradigm for the care of exertional heat stroke. (From Belval et al. [9], with permission)

athletics requires a well-established network of nonmedical and medical personnel to seamlessly deliver best practice in prevention, pre-hospital care, transport, and in-hospital care. This chapter will summarize key aspects of optimal EHS management while identifying key individuals (e.g., administrators, coaches, parents, athletic trainers, emergency medical service [EMS], physicians) who are responsible for carrying out the tasks needed to build an interdisciplinary network to successfully treat an athlete with EHS. In addition to local (i.e., team based) efforts, policy-based interventions can influence society at large and may be a useful method to establish a consensus across differing level of societal influence (e.g., team, school, region, state, league, nation) [10]. Policies introduced in the last decade pertaining to optimal prevention and treatment of EHS have shown favorable results to suggest that policy-based effort can promote both global and local changes. These successes in systematically overhauling the EHS management through policy-based interventions will also be discussed in the chapter.

Chain of Exertional Heat Stroke Prevention and Survival

Prevention

The first step in EHS management is prevention. Prevention strategies can be classified into those that can help, first, to identify and, second, to reduce risks. For example, preseason screening such as what occurs during an athlete's pre-participation examination and daily wellness logs can identify intrinsic risk factors that are associated with EHS, such as a history of exertional heat illness, poor fitness level, lack of heat acclimatization, dehydration, recent illness, level of fatigue, and sleep deprivation [2]. Athletes and parents (if the athletes are minors) have the responsibility to report accurate information about their health status so that appropriate risk mitigation plans can be implemented. Such plans include selecting exercise that matches one's physical fitness, implementing a team-wide heat acclimatization program, providing unlimited access to water to maintain proper hydration, and promoting adequate recovery before sport participation [1, 11]. When risk factors are known, qualified on-site medical personnel (e.g., athletic trainer, physiotherapist) and coaches also have the duties to share the information among each other so that informed decisions can be made when programming exercise mode, duration and intensity. It has been suggested that the presence of multiple risk factors heightens the risk of EHS [12]. Therefore, addressing as many modifiable risk factors identified in the preseason screening and daily wellness logs can be considered as the first line of defense in EHS prevention. A summary of existing literature about risk factors of EHS is further discussed in Chap. 3.

Environmental monitoring can also help identify EHS risk, where studies have shown increased prevalence of EHS fatalities when the environmental conditions are uncharacteristically hot for that specific region [13, 14]. These data support the use of injury surveillance and daily environmental monitoring as tools to determine high risk days for EHS, which can be led by coaches and athletic trainers. They should also determine the level of physical activity according to the wet-bulb globe temperature (WBGT), an index used to quantify the amount of environmental heat stress by incorporating the influence from solar radiation, air temperature, humidity, and wind speed [11, 14]. It is also important for administrators to reinforce WBGT-based activity modification guidelines to support decisions for shortening or cancelling of physical activity during extreme heat as these decisions can become hard for coaches in the face of competitive athleticism.

Methods that can directly reduce the risk of EHS include heat acclimatization and body cooling [2, 15–18]. Qualified on-site medical personnel should exercise due diligence to educate the benefits and importance of these methods to coaches and administrators to receive organizational support. In order to purposefully induce heat acclimatization, a heat acclimatization program must be incorporated within the training periodization to ensure that adequate amount of stress is applied to induce physiological adaptations. In the United States, an Inter-Association Task Force released a set of evidence-based guidelines regarding heat acclimatization in 2009, with the aim to reduce exertional heat illness risk during the summer months, particularly in the American football [19]. Since its introduction, eight states have mandated the implementation of preseason heat acclimatization in secondary school American football, which resulted in a 55% reduction in exertional heat illness (95% confidence interval: 13, 77%) [18]. Heat acclimatization process generally takes 10–14 days [17] and is recommended to be conducted during preseason (i.e., early spring or summer) to allow for gradual progression in physical and thermal loads placed on the body [20]. Heat acclimatization is also a useful method to prepare athletes who have scheduled competitions in regions where the weather conditions are warmer than their home. This not only helps reduce the risk of EHS but also optimizes athletic performance in heat [21].

Pre- (i.e., before activity) and per-cooling (i.e., during activity) are other useful methods to reduce the risk of EHS by directly lowering one's baseline internal body temperature prior to activity or by attenuating the rise in body temperature during activity, respectively [2, 15]. Since practical cooling strategies vary by setting and sport (i.e., American football is equipment laden but has unlimited number of substitutions, while soccer has a no re-entry rule for substitutions, limiting the opportunity for cooling during pregame and during halftime) [16], it is necessary for coaches and medical personnel to evaluate cooling methods that can be implemented readily. Lastly, it is important to educate coaches about the ergogenic benefits of heat acclimatization for enhancing cardiovascular fitness [17] and body cooling for endurance performance [21]. Coaches should realize that performance optimization in the heat can simultaneously facilitate EHS prevention and performance enhancement.

Pre-hospital Care

When EHS occurs, despite aforementioned prevention efforts, rapid recognition, rapid assessment, and rapid cooling must be carried out to avoid poor prognosis (see Fig. 9.1). Ideally, the pre-hospital care of EHS patients in athletics settings should be led by qualified medical personnel, such as an athletic trainer, as they are trained to recognize early signs and symptoms of EHS, use rectal thermometry to obtain an accurate internal body temperature, and administer cold water immersion to rapidly cool the body below 39 °C while continuously monitoring the internal body temperature [1]. When these steps are followed within the first 30 minutes of collapse, prognosis from EHS is promising [9]. Proper recognition and length of whole-body cooling rely on an accurate temperature assessment using rectal thermometry. However, Mazerolle et al. [22] found lack of rectal thermometry usage by college and high school athletic trainers due to insecurities, organizational barriers, and lack of resources. In such cases, clinicians and administrators should realize the legal implications for not using rectal thermometry since other methods of body temperature assessment (e.g., temporal, tympanic, oral, axillary, skin temperature) have been shown to be invalid for measuring the internal body temperature in individuals during or immediately after exercise [23, 24]. Therefore, both sports medicine and administrative staff members of an athletic team need to understand the essential use of rectal thermometry to accurately diagnose EHS and properly identify the duration of treatment. Information pertaining to the pre-hospital care of EHS patients should be documented in the form of a policies and procedures manual for the sports medicine team and a site-specific emergency action plan (EAP) to effectively carry out these procedures. Policies and procedures will help establish the consensus, while the EAP provides step-by-step process to recognize the condition, to initiate the pre-hospital care, and to transfer the patient to advanced medical facility once the hypothermia has been controlled.

In the absence of athletic trainers or other qualified medical personnel, coaches must rely on context-based inference to determine the presence of EHS since they may not be qualified or trained to use rectal thermometry. For that reason, it is imperative to educate coaches about common risk factors and clinical presentation of signs and symptoms of EHS and draft an EAP for nonmedical personnel so that they can initiate appropriate first aid (i.e., body cooling) and communicate clinical presentations to EMS [25].

Transport

Unlike other medical conditions, EHS requires rapid, on-site treatment (i.e., body cooling), prior to transport to higher level medical care. The key doctrine for EHS survival is "cool first, transport second" [8], and it is important to pre-establish a consensus about the need to prioritize on-site treatment over rapid transport among

Table 9.1 List of exertional heat stroke (EHS)-specific information to document on the patient's medical chart

Time of collapse
Environmental conditions
Wet-bulb globe temperature
Air temperature
Relative humidity
Wind speed
Signs and symptoms of EHS
Altered mental status
Aggression
Lethargy
Loss of memory
Profuse sweating
Activity type
Time of rectal temperature measurement
Initial and subsequent log of rectal temperature
Time to start cooling
Cooling method used for treatment
Ability to hydrate
Previous history of EHS
Personal or family history of malignant hyperthermia
Hematuria
Recent illness

the sports medicine team. Specifically, EMS are accustomed to quickly transporting patients to advanced care. Therefore, it is imperative for them to understand the significance of minimizing the duration of extreme hyperthermia since the extent of thermal stress can directly impact the severity of EHS and patient outcomes [26]. When EMS is the first medical responder on-site (i.e., no athletic trainer on-site), EMS should obtain a rectal temperature and actively cool the patient on-site or en route to the hospital. As it may be technically difficult to administer effective cooling modalities in a moving ambulance, on-site cooling to a safer core temperature (<39 °C) is preferred. At the time of transport, it is also important to document EHS-specific information in addition to the standard medical record information (Table 9.1). This information will become useful when retrospectively assessing the cause of EHS and identifying individualized plan for return to activity.

In-Hospital Care and Return to Physical Activity

In ideal conditions, patients will be transported to the hospital following on-site cooling. However, patients may arrive to the hospital's emergency department (ED) by private vehicle or ambulance with little or no attempt at pre-hospital cooling.

Rapid recognition, assessment, and cooling remain the priority for the ED staff. Vital signs including rectal temperature, blood pressure, heart rate, and respiratory rate should be assessed. In the acute phase, tachycardia and hyperventilation is usually observed in EHS patients. For those patients that receive pre-hospital cooling, these values may have returned to the normal range [27]. Cold water immersion in an ED may be challenging due to space and equipment (i.e., tubs, large quantities of ice and water) constraints. Other cooling modalities such as rotating ice water-soaked towels [28] or tarp-assisted cooling [29] may be substituted as effective cooling modalities.

Upon arrival to the ED, EHS patients may be dehydrated and exhibit signs of hypotension and hemoconcentration and hypercalcemia and hyperproteinemia [27]. Oral (if tolerated) or IV fluids may be necessary to restore fluid and electrolyte losses in these instances. In EHS patients, it is also not uncommon to observe a hypothermic overshoot following treatment [12]. The chance of a drastic drop in internal body temperature from pre-hospital treatment and patient's inability to restore normal body temperature ($\approx$36–37 °C) requires direct (e.g., rectal temperature) and continuous monitoring of internal body temperature. It should be noted that hypothermic patients may need rewarming as the ability to regulate body temperature may be altered in some patients. On the contrary, in the event that a patient's temperature begins to rise, cooling should be re-instituted. In addition, even after the internal body temperature is stabilized, the inflammatory response and blood coagulation may continue [27]. Blood tests such as blood urea nitrogen (BUN), creatinine (Cr), creatine phosphokinase (CPK), alanine aminotransferase (ALT), and aspartate aminotransferase (AST) levels should be obtained to quantify the level of muscle damage and monitor renal and liver functions, which are commonly affected in EHS patients [26, 27].

A physician may clear the athlete to low-intensity activity only when full recovery of organ function is confirmed via blood work and subjective symptoms (e.g., 7–21 days post EHS incident) [30]. The progression for return to activity should be supervised by trained personnel (e.g., team physician, primary care physician, athletic trainer, etc.), starting from low-intensity exercise in cool environment to gradually transitioning the intensity and environmental condition to mimic a traditional heat acclimatization protocol [30, 31]. Upon receiving the collapsed athlete's permission, it is ideal for the medical records taken at the time of hospital admittance be shared with qualified medical personnel who will have daily contact with the athlete during the return to activity progression to gauge the extent of initial damage incurred by the body. When the athlete has regained adequate physical fitness and heat tolerance, a standardized heat tolerance test [30, 32] can be prescribed to assess the athlete's ability to withstand a fixed exercise protocol in heat. Medical lab results, changes in clinical symptoms (e.g., lethargy, weakness), and heat tolerance test results should be evaluated together by the physician and/or athletic trainer, to comprehensively evaluate the athlete's readiness to return to full activity.

Policy-Based Intervention

Optimization of EHS management requires the sports medicine team (e.g., team physician, athletic trainer, physiotherapist) to recognize and understand the need to implement evidence-based best practices for the prevention, recognition, and management of this condition. The sports medicine team should have the autonomous and independent authority to make the necessary medical decisions to ensure survival from EHS without organizational conflicts that may stem from lack of understanding and/or support from coaches and administrators [22]. For example, coaches and administrators may perceive the reduction in training duration or exercise intensity due to high environmental heat as hindrance to their planned training schedule. In the secondary school setting, athletic directors may oppose the use of rectal thermometry in minors from perceived uneasiness about the topic. These misconceptions and apprehensions are common unless the sports medicine team initiates the proper dialogue to inform and educate them of the current medical standard of care of this condition. Therefore, the sports medicine team should work collaboratively with coaches and administrators to cultivate a cultural norm that supports the need to implement evidence-based best practices [33]. This may require persistent education on appropriate EHS management practices to the nonmedical stakeholders of the athletic team (e.g., coaches, administrators, parents). Use of policy statements by various governing organizations (e.g., state high school association, state legislation, sports medicine advisory board of a sport association) that are developed using recommendations established by the leading sports medicine associations (e.g., American Medical Society for Sports Medicine, American College of Sports Medicine, National Athletic Trainers' Association) may help facilitate this process, especially when they are required to be followed by the former entities [10, 18]. Following current guidelines that are endorsed by sports medicine associations will also ensure that these guidelines are based on current best practice and evidence.

Several consensus statements have been published to address the need to implement best practice policies pertaining to EHS prevention and management [20, 34, 35]. In 2017, Huggins et al. [36], summarizing position statements published by the National Athletic Trainers' Association [1] and the American College of Sports Medicine [11], outlined the best safety practice recommendations for EHS management in youth athletics' settings (Table 9.2). These recommendations can serve as the foundation for local policies, if evidence-based best practices have yet to be adopted.

The greatest benefit of endorsing best practice through policy implementation is its ability to disseminate a common consensus across a large population. However, policy implementation, especially a mandated policy, is often a reaction to tragedy instead of a proactive intervention [33]. For example, in 2011, the state of Arkansas, USA, experienced one of the hottest summers on record. Two secondary school American football players, Will James and Tyler Davenport, collapsed due to EHS with contrasting outcomes [37]. James was immediately treated by an athletic trainer

Table 9.2 Best safety practice recommendations for exertional heat stroke (EHS) management [36]

Rapid recognition	Athletes who demonstrate confusion, nausea, dizziness, altered consciousness, combativeness, other unusual behaviors, or staggering during walking or running or collapse while exercising should be suspected of having a heat-related injury
	Educate on the prompt recognition of EHS, activation of emergency medical service, importance of immediate cooling, and transport of the athlete to the hospital
Rapid assessment	A rectal thermometer is required for the accurate assessment of core body temperature (for use by medical personnel only). All other on-field temperature assessment techniques (e.g., mouth, ear, forehead, armpit) are inaccurate and should be avoided
Rapid cooling	The athlete with a suspected heat illness who has collapsed or is unresponsive but is breathing and has a heartbeat should be immediately cooled via cold water immersion in a tub of ice water or the rotation of ice towels over the entire body while 911 is called
	Excess clothing and equipment should be removed from the athlete to help with the dissipation of heat. During cooling, the athlete should be moved from direct sunlight into shade if possible
	A large tub, plastic tarp, kiddie pool, or empty trash barrel are all options to hold ice and water for the athlete who needs rapid and immediate cooling
	A water source, extra water cooler(s), access to a locker room with shower, ice chest(s), and towels or sheets are recommended to assist in the rapid cooling of the athlete
	If medical personnel (e.g., physician, athletic trainer, or other medical personnel trained in heat illnesses) and equipment (e.g., rectal thermometer, cold tub, plastic tarp, kiddie pool, shower, access to water and ice, towels) are on-site, "cool first, transport second" should be implemented, and cooling should continue uninterrupted until the athlete's core body temperature is less than 38.9 °C
Rapid advanced care	If medical personnel are *not* on-site, call 911 (i.e., activate emergency action plan) while simultaneously pursuing rapid cooling. Until medical personnel arrive, continue to cool and monitor the athlete

with aggressive cooling on-site, whereas Davenport's internal body temperature reached 42.2 °C due to an absence of immediate treatment, and he ultimately lost his life due to multi-organ dysfunction that ensued following his injury [37]. This tragedy enabled the state to pass legislation (Act 1214) in 2011 requiring the implementation of an EAP and education about best safety practices for coaches at the secondary school athletics level [38]. In the following year (2012), the Arkansas Department of Health mandated the assessment of rectal temperature by EMS personnel when EHS is suspected and the use of aggressive cooling before transporting to an advanced care [39]. Although these changes were a reaction to the prior tragedy, Arkansas swiftly became one of the leaders in evidence-based EHS management [33].

Despite the lessons learned in Arkansas, a majority of US states still lack appropriate statewide policies to safeguard student athletes from sudden death and catastrophic injuries in secondary school-organized sports [40]. According to Adams et al. [40], the median score of a state-level policy implementation rubric, which was created using existing scientific and medical literature, was only 47.1% (range, 23.0% to 78.7%). This variability and lack of full compliance to evidence-based best practice may be due to barriers faced by states that fit in multiple levels of socioecological framework (e.g., interpersonal, organizational, environmental) [10]. For example, a previous study has identified that an athletic trainers' lack of knowledge, lack of initiative, lack of equipment, fear of liability, and lack of comfort level were associated with barriers in implementing evidence-based practice for EHS [41]. A similar investigation was conducted among state high school athletics association leaders and sports medicine advisory committee members (i.e., administrative stakeholders) to identify their barriers toward health and safety policy implementation [42]. The study revealed that administrative stakeholders viewed cost as the major organizational barrier, while also identifying the lack of understanding and misconception regarding the role of policy in enhancing athletic safety [42]. These barriers reported by both medical and nonmedical personnel hinder the implementation of evidence-based practices for EHS. As stakeholders of athlete health and safety, team physicians and other qualified medical personnel have the responsibility to acquire contemporary expertise as it relates to the management and care of EHS and serve as the hub for delivering relevant information to nonmedical personnel. Concurrently, nonmedical personnel (e.g., coaches and administrators) must make the effort to provide medical personnel the autonomy in making medical decisions and identify opportunities for best practice policy implementation. These efforts are expected to gradually shift barriers perceived by interpersonal and organizational level and ultimately update policies and behaviors observed in the target community.

These barriers perceived by athletic trainers and administrators are not easy to overcome, but they may be addressed through accumulation of local data to support the effectiveness of policy implementation [43]. For example, the Georgia High School Association (Georgia, USA) developed activity modification guidelines aimed to prevent EHS during the fall preseason in American football by analyzing the pattern of heat-related injury occurrence in the state of Georgia for 3 years [43]. The creation of the guidelines from real data helped reduce skepticism from key stakeholders (e.g., administrators, coaches, members of the rules committee) who were not supportive implementing activity modification guidelines [43]. Since 2011, 14 states, including Georgia, have implemented heat acclimatization guidelines. When these guidelines were followed it totality, states recorded zero EHS deaths, which is a significant improvement from the average of 1.2 EHS deaths per year calculated from previous data [44]. In another study, Kerr et al. [18] found states that mandated heat acclimatization had lower rates of exertional heat illness when compared to those that did not mandate the policy (0.42 per 10,000 athlete exposures vs. 0.72 per 10,000 athlete exposures). Thus, continued efforts to collect data that are tangible for stakeholders may help persuade skeptics to alter their belief regarding policy implementation to optimize EHS management.

Conclusion

More than enough evidence and case reports exist to support the need for early recognition, rapid assessment, rapid cooling, and rapid advanced care in EHS survival [8, 9, 12, 20, 26, 27]. It should be emphasized that optimal EHS management in athletics settings entails a continuum of actions by medical and nonmedical stakeholders. These stakeholders also represent the different levels of socioecological framework, which may greatly influence the success of policy implementation at large [10]. The first step in optimal EHS management should start from medical professionals; athletic trainers and physicians must become the leaders in embodying evidence-based practice to propagate scientifically supported consensus across stakeholders.

References

1. Casa DJ, DeMartini JK, Bergeron MF, Csillan D, Eichner ER, Lopez RM, et al. National Athletic Trainers' Association position statement: exertional heat illnesses. J Athl Train. 2015;50(9):986–1000.
2. Hosokawa Y, Adams WM, Stearns RL, Casa DJ. Heat stroke in physical activity and sports. PENSAR EN MOVIMIENTO: Revista de Ciencias del Ejercicio y la Salud. 2014;12(2):1–22. http://www.redalyc.org/html/4420/442042967002/index.html.
3. Hosokawa Y, Adams WM, Stearns RL, Casa DJ. Comparison of gastrointestinal and rectal temperatures during recovery after a warm-weather road race. J Athl Train. 2016;51(5):382–8.
4. Racinais S, Moussay S, Nichols D, Travers G, Belfekih T, Schumacher YO, Periard JD. Core temperature up to 41.5oC during the UCI Road Cycling World Championships in the heat. Br J Sports Med. 2019;53(7):426–9.
5. Wingo JE, Crandall CG, Kenny GP. Human heat physiology. In: Casa DJ, editor. Sport and physical activity in the heat maximizing performance and safety. Cham: Springer; 2018. p. 15–30.
6. Schlader Z. The relative overlooking of human behavioral temperature regulation: an issue worth resolving. Temperature. 2014;1(1):20–1.
7. Binkley HM, Beckett J, Casa DJ, Kleiner DM, Plummer PE. National Athletic Trainers' Association Position Statement: Exertional Heat Illnesses. J Athl Train. 2002;37(3):329–43.
8. Casa DJ, McDermott BP, Lee EC, Yeargin SW, Armstrong LE, Maresh CM. Cold water immersion: the gold standard for exertional heatstroke treatment. Exerc Sport Sci Rev. 2007;35(3):141–9.
9. Belval LN, Casa DJ, Adams WM, et al. Consensus statement—prehospital care of exertional heat stroke. Prehosp Emerg Care. 2018;22(3):392–7.
10. Scarneo SE, Kerr ZY, Kroshus E, Register-Mihalik JK, Hosokawa Y, Stearns RL, et al. The socio-ecological framework: a multi-faceted approach to prevent sport-related death in high school sports. J Athl Train. 2019;54(4):356–60. https://doi.org/10.4085/1062-6050-173-18.
11. American College of Sports Medicine, Armstrong LE, Casa DJ, Millard-Stafford M, Moran DS, Pyne SW, Roberts WO. American College of Sports Medicine position stand. Exertional heat illness during training and competition. Med Sci Sports Exerc. 2007;39(3):556–72.
12. Adams WM, Hosokawa Y, Huggins RA, Mazerolle SM, Casa DJ. An exertional heat stroke survivor's return to running: an integrated approach on the treatment, recovery, and return to activity. J Sport Rehabil. 2016;25(3):280–7.
13. Grundstein AJ, Ramseyer C, Zhao F, Pesses JL, Akers P, Qureshi A, et al. A retrospective analysis of American football hyperthermia deaths in the United States. Int J Biometeorol. 2012;56(1):11–20.
14. Grundstein AJ, Hosokawa Y, Casa DJ. Fatal exertional heat stroke and American football players: the need for regional heat-safety guidelines. J Athl Train. 2018;53(1):43–50.
15. Pryor RR, Casa DJ, Adams WM, Belval LN, DeMartini JK, Huggins RA, et al. MSMaximizing athletic performance in the heat. Strength Cond J. 2013;35(6):24–33.

16. Adams WM, Hosokawa Y, Casa DJ. Body-cooling paradigm in sport: maximizing safety and performance during competition. J Sport Rehabil. 2016;25(4):382–94.
17. Armstrong LE, Maresh CM. The induction and decay of heat acclimatisation in trained athletes. Sports Med. 1991;12(5):302–12.
18. Kerr ZY, Register-Mihalik JK, Pryor RR, Pierpoint LA, Scarneo SE, Adams WM, et al. The association between mandated preseason heat acclimatization guidelines and exertional heat illness during preseason high school American football practices. Environ Health Perspect. 2019;127(4):47003.
19. Casa DJ, Csillan D; Inter-Association Task Force for Preseason Secondary School Athletics Participants, Armstrong LE, Baker LB, Bergeron MF, et al. Preseason heat-acclimatization guidelines for secondary school athletics. J Athl Train 2009;44(3):332–3.
20. Casa DJ, Guskiewicz KM, Anderson SA, Courson RW, Heck JF, Jimenez CC, et al. National Athletic Trainers' Association position statement: preventing sudden death in sports. J Athl Train. 2012;47(1):96–118.
21. Racinais S, Alonso JM, Coutts AJ, Flouris AD, Girard O, González-Alonso J, et al. Consensus recommendations on training and competing in the heat. Br J Sports Med. 2015;49(18):1164–73.
22. Mazerolle SM, Scruggs IC, Casa DJ, Burton LJ, McDermott BP, Armstrong LE, Maresh CM. Current knowledge, attitudes, and practices of certified athletic trainers regarding recognition and treatment of exertional heat stroke. J Athl Train. 2010;45(2):170–80.
23. Ganio MS, Brown CM, Casa DJ, et al. Validity and reliability of devices that assess body temperature during indoor exercise in the heat. J Athl Train. 2009;44(2):124–35.
24. Casa DJ, Becker SM, Ganio MS, Brown CM, Yeargin SW, Roti MW, et al. Validity of devices that assess body temperature during outdoor exercise in the heat. J Athl Train. 2007;42(3):333–42.
25. Adams WM. Exertional heat stroke within secondary school athletics. Curr Sports Med Rep. 2019;18(4):149–53.
26. Stearns RL, Casa DJ, O'Connor FG, Lopez RM. A tale of two heat strokes: a comparative case study. Curr Sports Med Rep. 2016;15(2):94–7.
27. Bouchama A, Knochel JP. Heat stroke. N Engl J Med. 2002;346(25):1978–88.
28. McDermott BP, Casa DJ, Ganio MS, Lopez RM, Yeargin SW, Armstrong LE, Maresh CM. Acute whole-body cooling for exercise-induced hyperthermia: a systematic review. J Athl Train. 2009;44(1):84–93.
29. Hosokawa Y, Adams WM, Belval LN, Vandermark LW, Casa DJ. Tarp-assisted cooling as a method of whole-body cooling in hyperthermic individuals. Ann Emerg Med. 2017;69(3):347–52.
30. Stearns RL, Deuster PA, Kazman JB, Heled Y, O'Connor FG. Heat tolerance testing. In: Casa DJ, editor. Sport and physical activity in the heat maximizing performance and safety. Cham: Springer; 2018. p. 213–27.
31. Adams WM, Belval LN. Return-to-activity following exertional heat stroke. Athl Train Sports Health Care. 2018;10(1):5–6.
32. Kazman JB, Heled Y, Lisman PJ, Druyan A, Deuster PA, O'Connor FG. Exertional heat illness: the role of heat tolerance testing. Curr Sports Med Rep. 2013;12(2):101–5.
33. Pagnotta KD, Mazerolle SM, Pitney WA, Burton LJ, Casa DJ. Implementing health and safety policy changes at the high school level from a leadership perspective. J Athl Train. 2016;51(4):291–302.
34. Casa DJ, Almquist J, Anderson SA, Baker L, Bergeron MF, Biagioli B, et al. The inter-association task force for preventing sudden death in secondary school athletics programs: best-practices recommendations. J Athl Train. 2013;48(4):546–53.
35. Casa DJ, Anderson SA, Baker L, Bennett S, Bergeron MF, Connolly D, et al. The inter-association task force for preventing sudden death in collegiate conditioning sessions: best practices recommendations. J Athl Train. 2012;47(4):477–80.
36. Huggins RA, Scarneo SE, Casa DJ, Belval LN, Carr KS, Chiampas G, et al. The inter-association task force document on emergency health and safety: best-practice recommendations for youth sports leagues. J Athl Train. 2017;52(4):384–400.

37. Arkansas Educational Television Network. 108°: critical response. https://www.aetn.org/programs/108degrees. Accessed 5 May 2019.
38. Ingram P. HB 1743; Act 1214. An act to promote the health and safety of students in public school athletic activities through the use of athletic trainers and professional development for coaches; and for other purposes. 28 Feb 2011. http://www.arkleg.state.ar.us/assembly/2011/2011R/Acts/Act1214.pdf. Accessed 29 Jan 2019.
39. Ferrara MS, Swearngin R, Adams WM, Casa DJ. Developing safety policies for organized sports. In: Casa DJ, Stearns RL, editors. Emergency management for sport and physical activity. Burlington, MA: Jones & Bartlett Learning; 2015. p. 1–16.
40. Adams WM, Scarneo SE, Casa DJ. State-level implementation of health and safety policies to prevent sudden death and catastrophic injuries within secondary school athletics. Orthop J Sports Med. 2017;5(9):2325967117727262.
41. Mazerolle SM, Pinkus DE, Casa DJ, McDermott BP, Pagnotta KD, Ruiz RC, et al. Evidence-based medicine and the recognition and treatment of exertional heat stroke, part ii: a perspective from the clinical athletic trainer. J Athl Train. 2011;46(5):533–42.
42. Pike AM, Adams WM, Huggins RA, Mazerolle SM, Casa DJ. Analysis of states' progress towards and barriers to health and safety policy implementation for secondary school athletics. J Athl Train. 2019;54(4):361–73.
43. Hosokawa Y, Grundstein AJ, Vanos JK, Cooper ER. Environmental condition and monitoring. In: Casa DJ, editor. Sport and physical activity in the heat maximizing performance and safety. Cham: Springer; 2018. p. 147–62.
44. Attanasio SM, Adams WM, Stearns RL, Huggins RA, Casa DJ. Occurrence of exertional heat stroke in high school football athletes before and after implementation of evidence-based heat acclimatization guidelines. J Athl Train. 2016;51(6):S–168.

Chapter 10
Exertional Heat Illness Considerations in the Military

Nathaniel S. Nye and Francis G. O'Connor

Warfighters, as tactical athletes on the modern-day battlefield, confront a variety of environmental challenges, in particular with the emergence of unconventional, asymmetric, and hybrid warfare. Accordingly, it is essential for the military medical officer (MMO) to understand the environmental threats that confront the warfighter and leverage strategies to mitigate these stressors that may impact performance on the battlefield. This chapter addresses the challenge of environmental heat as applied to today's warfighter, with a focus on enhancing performance in this setting. Specifically discussed are a review of relevant military history, epidemiology, and military-unique applied physiology, a detailed discussion of military special populations and risk factors, and finally military-unique prevention strategies, to include return to duty (RTD). Importantly, specific guidance and resources are provided to assist in the identification and prevention of environmental heat stress as applied to the warfighter.

History

Environmental extremes involving heat have plagued warfighters and commanders since the beginning of combatant events [1–3]. Biblical Old Testament authors documented the health risks of wearing heavy body armor in the heat posed to

The opinions and assertions contained herein are private views and are not to be construed as official or as reflecting the views of the US Army Medical Department, the US Air Force Medical Service, the Uniformed Services University, or the Department of Defense at large.

N. S. Nye (✉)
Sports Medicine Clinic, 559th Medical Group, Joint Base San Antonio-Lackland, TX, USA

F. G. O'Connor
Military and Emergency Medicine, Consortium for Health and Military Performance, Uniformed Services University of the Health Sciences, Bethesda, MD, USA

© Springer Nature Switzerland AG 2020
W. M. Adams, J. F. Jardine (eds.), *Exertional Heat Illness*,
https://doi.org/10.1007/978-3-030-27805-2_10

warfighters noting "when the sun stands still in the heavens," it helps the Hebrews fight the more heavily armored Canaanites. In 400 BC, in one of the first reliable reports on the effect of environmental heat on military operations, Herodotus described the effects of load carriage, protective clothing, and heat stress during an Athenian and Spartan conflict as both were worn out by the "thirst of the sun." In 325 BC, Alexander the Great, while returning home from his conquests along with 40,000 of his troops, exposed to 2 months of extreme heat and a lack of adequate water arrived home with only 5000 soldiers remaining. The Roman legionary leveraged knowledge of heat illness and associated risk factors to include load carriage and instituted effective mitigation strategies; headgear included the capability to insert "rushes" in the helmet that were to be kept wet with water to keep the legionnaires cool, and noncombatant auxiliaries were utilized to facilitate the legionnaire's load and complete digging so as to preserve the legionnaires for fighting.

The principle of heat acclimatization was fathomed as King Edward's heavily armored crusaders were defeated by lighter Arab horsemen in one of the final battles of the crusades; the loss was attributed to the advantage the native Arabs had by living regularly in the heat and utilizing appropriate clothing [1]. Military environmental casualties and loss of troop effectiveness have remained significant operational concerns in modern warfare; it is estimated that in the early period of World War II Pacific theater of operations, for every combat casualty, there were over 100 casualties from heat or illness.

Epidemiology

The Armed Forces Health Surveillance Center (AFHSC) publishes the monthly Medical Surveillance Monthly Report (MSMR), an important document for all MMOs to be familiar with as it regularly provides critical insight into disease trends in the US military. Figures 10.1 and 10.2 present patterns of heat stroke and heat exhaustion, respectively, over the period of 2013 through 2017 [4].

In 2016 alone, there were 2163 incident diagnoses of EHI (heat exhaustion and exertional heat stroke [EHS]) among active component service members (incidence rate: 1.79 cases per 1000 person-years [p-yrs]). The overall crude incidence rates of heat stroke and heat exhaustion were 0.38 and 1.41 per 1000 p-yrs, respectively. Subgroup-specific incidence rates of heat stroke were highest among males and service members aged 19 years or younger, Asian/Pacific Islanders, Marine Corps and Army members, recruit trainees, and those in combat-specific and "other" occupations [4].

Unfortunately, recent efforts to mitigate exertional heat stroke casualties have not proven to reduce injury rates. The annual rate (unadjusted) of cases of heat stroke in 2017 was slightly higher than in 2016 and 58% higher than in 2013. Heat stroke rates in the Marine Corps were 50% higher than in the Army; Army heat injury rates were more than ninefold those in the Air Force and Navy. Lastly, the incidence was 86% higher among males than females [4].

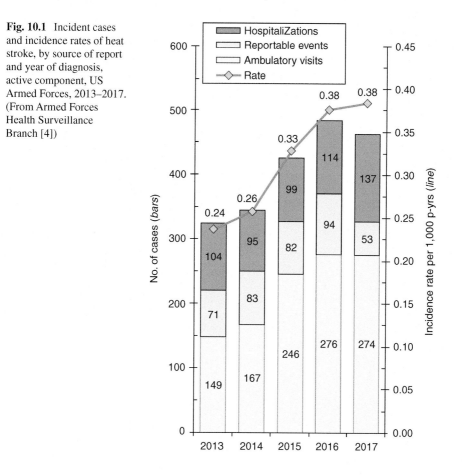

Fig. 10.1 Incident cases and incidence rates of heat stroke, by source of report and year of diagnosis, active component, US Armed Forces, 2013–2017. (From Armed Forces Health Surveillance Branch [4])

Military Unique Physiologic Considerations

Human performance is compromised with the extremes of temperature, as well as at depth and at increased altitudes above sea level. Understanding the basic principles of applied physiology that contribute to this performance decrement is critical for the MMO, who is frequently called upon for the proper interpretation of resources and guidelines that discuss environmental stress. Knowledge of physiology enables the MMO to identify and modify those factors that can be mitigated or leveraged for success in the military operational environment while promoting prevention by educating the individual warfighter as well as the unit leadership.

The human body has a remarkable thermoregulatory system, which helps maintain core temperature within a physiologically safe range. When the thermoregulatory system is overwhelmed, the human body demonstrates great resilience against cold temperature decrements, but it can tolerate only minor core temperature eleva-

Fig. 10.2 Incident cases and incidence rates of heat exhaustion, by source of report and year of diagnosis, active component, US Armed Forces, 2013–2017. (From Armed Forces Health Surveillance Branch [4])

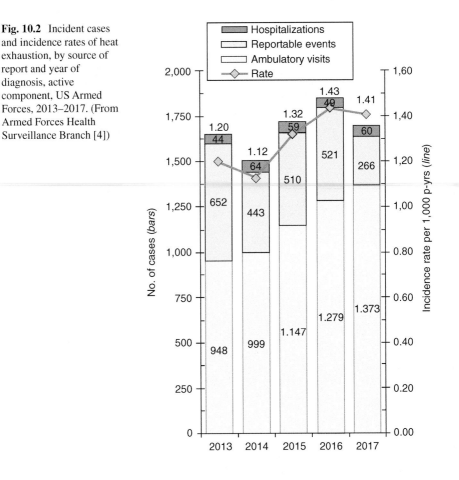

tions (5–7 °F or 2.8–3.9 °C) without developing systemic dysfunction, which ultimately leads to multi-organ failure and death if body temperature cannot be lowered [5, 6]. The human body utilizes multiple physiologic mechanisms to leverage heat dissipation via convection, conduction, radiation, and most importantly evaporation (Fig. 10.3).

During exercise, the human body acts to dissipate the excess heat generated by skeletal muscle; this requires an intact cardiovascular system that uses blood to transfer heat from the body core to the skin, where the mechanisms for dissipating heat can take effect. However, when the ambient temperature is higher than the body's core temperature, convection, conduction, and radiation are no longer effective. Environmental conditions also affect evaporative cooling. A water vapor pressure gradient must exist for sweat to evaporate and release heat into the environment. In high humidity (relative humidity >75%) or under occlusive clothing/gear, evaporation becomes ineffective for transferring heat. Thus, in hot and humid conditions, warfighters become susceptible to exertional heat illness.

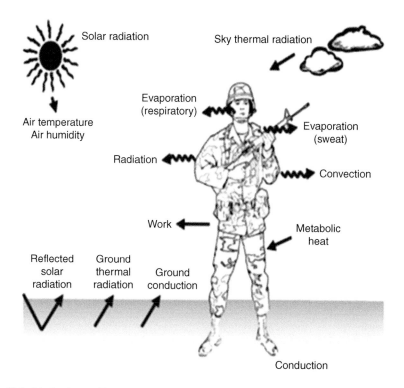

Fig. 10.3 Mechanisms of heat production/gain and heat dissipation/loss are illustrated as pertaining to the warfighter [6]

Limitations on heat dissipation in hot and humid weather are exacerbated during intense exercise by a finite supply of blood that must fulfill multiple functions, including meeting the metabolic demands of active skeletal muscle and transporting heat to the skin surface for cooling. Further complicating matter is the dehydration that develops in most individuals during intense exercise in the heat, which decreases plasma volume. Studies suggest that during intense exercise in the heat, for every 1% of body weight lost from dehydration, there is a concomitant increase in core body temperature of 0.22 °C (0.4 °F) [6]. In other words, other factors being equal, a warfighter who loses only 1% of body weight from dehydration during intense exercise in the heat would be 1 °C cooler compared to a buddy who loses 4% of body weight. This would equate to a temperature difference of approximately 39 °C (102 °F) versus 40 °C (104 °F) at the end of a training session. A number of additional factors influence the rate at which a person's core body temperature rises during vigorous activity, including fitness level, degree of acclimatization to heat, clothing/equipment, and use of certain types of nutritional supplements that affect physiologic response (e.g., metabolic rate, degree of tachycardia).

During exercise, the body temperature rises in response to the increase in metabolic heat production; a modest rise in temperature is thought to represent a favorable adjustment that optimizes physiologic functions and facilitates heat loss mechanisms as previously described. With compensated heat stress (CHS), the body achieves a new steady-state core temperature that is proportional to the increased metabolic rate and available means for dissipating heat. Studies in runners describe this mechanism as exercise-induced hyperthermia; acclimatized warfighters and athletes can complete events successfully with significantly elevated core temperatures (103–104°F) while remaining entirely asymptomatic [7]. Uncompensated heat stress (UCHS) results when cooling capacity is exceeded, and the warfighter or athlete cannot maintain a steady temperature. Continued exertion in the setting of UCHS increases heat retention, causing a progressive rise in core body temperature and increasing the risk for severe heat illness.

The understanding and identification of risk factors that can contribute to warfighters UCHS are critical to both the MMO and the Commander (Table 10.1). Body temperature, as previously identified, can increase through a number of mechanisms: exposure to environmental heat (impeded heat dissipation); physical exercise (increased heat production); and impaired thermoregulation due to medical conditions, certain medications, and individual factors such as sleep deprivation and low physical fitness. Due to operational requirements, warfighters do not always have time to properly acclimatize and may encounter scenarios where a failure to compensate may result in an exertional heat illness.

Importantly, febrile persons have accentuated elevations in core temperature when exposed to high ambient temperature, physical exercise, or both. Environmental temperature and humidity, medication, and exercise heat stress in turn challenge the cardiovascular system to provide high blood flow to the skin, where blood pools in warm, compliant vessels such as those found in the extremities. When blood flow is diverted to the skin, reduced perfusion of the intestines and other viscera can result in ischemia, endotoxemia, and oxidative stress [8]. In addition, excessively high tissue temperatures (heat shock: >41 ° C [105.8 ° F]) can produce direct tissue injury; the magnitude and duration of the heat shock influence whether cells respond by adaptation (acquired thermal tolerance), injury, or death (apoptotic or necrotic). Heat shock, ischemia, and systemic inflammatory responses can result in cellular dysfunction, disseminated intravascular coagulation, and multi-organ dysfunction syndrome. In addition, reduced cerebral blood flow, combined with abnormal local metabolism and coagulopathy, can lead to dysfunction of the central nervous system. The aforementioned illustrates UCHS, which can severely denigrate the warfighter's performance, and the process by which UCHS may progress to exertional heat stroke, which puts the individual at risk for significant morbidity and mortality and compromises the unit's mission.

Table 10.1 Factors predisposing to heat illness

Individual factors
Lack of acclimatization
Low physical fitness
Obesity
Dehydration
Sleep deprivation
Extremes of age (infants, elderly)
Genetics (*RYR1* mutation, *TLR4* polymorphisms)
Health conditions
Metabolic and thermoregulatory disorders: Febrile illness, insomnia/sleep deprivation, hyperthyroidism/thyroid storm, seizures, neuroleptic malignant syndrome, malignant hyperthermia
Disorders of skin and sweating: Extensive rash, sunburn, large areas of burned/scarred/grafted skin, diabetes mellitus, chronic anhidrosis, cystic fibrosis, ectodermal dysplasia
Unknown mechanism: Sickle cell trait
Drugs
Anticholinergics (e.g., meclizine, tolterodine, atropine)
Antiepileptics (e.g., lamotrigine, topiramate)
Antihistamines (e.g., diphenhydramine, loratadine)
Glutethimide (Doriden)
Phenothiazines (e.g., thioridazine, chlorpromazine, promethazine)
Tricyclic antidepressants
Amphetamines (e.g., Ritalin®, Ecstasy [*3,4-methylenedioxy-methamphetamine* (MDMA)])
Ergogenic stimulants (e.g., caffeine, pre-workout supplements, ephedrine, ephedra)
Lithium
Diuretics
β-Blockers and calcium channel blockers
Ethanol
Nonsteroidal anti-inflammatories
Environmental factors
High temperature
High humidity
Little air movement
Lack of shade
Physical exercise
Heavy clothing or gear
Prior compromised heat exposures

Military Unique Populations

Analogous to how athletes practice with their teams in order to prepare for game day, warfighters spend significant time training with their units on a day-to-day and month-to-month basis throughout their military careers. Each unit has a specific mission and must maintain readiness to execute that mission in combat operations when called upon. Several aspects of high-risk military training and operations will be discussed to illustrate how each is uniquely associated with heat illness risk.

Basic Training

The task of creating a lethal fighting force out of civilian volunteers drawn from an increasingly sedentary population carries many challenges and risks, among which is the risk of exertional heat illness. Each military component (Army, Navy, Air Force, Marine Corps, Coast Guard) maintains one or more locations dedicated to entry-level training, where civilian recruits are indoctrinated with basic military knowledge and skills. These include marching and drill, physical fitness, basic weapons skills, and proper usage of military gear (e.g., flak vests, helmets, rucksacks, gas masks), among many other tasks. While much of this training is only moderately strenuous, some aspects are quite physically intense or prolonged in nature. With this in mind, the primary risk of heat illness in basic military training stems from the fact that many recruits, just a few weeks or even days prior, were predominantly sedentary and spent most of their time seated indoors. Military training programs generally offer little to no acclimatization period or a progressive nature of training (varies by service and even, to some degree, by individual instructor). However, Air Force Basic Military Training has recently made changes to their physical training program to allow 10 days of acclimatization prior to any maximum effort fitness test.

Geography plays an important role in the warfighter's risk for exertional heat illness. Most military basic training installations lie in hot, humid regions of the USA, such as Ft. Jackson, SC (Army); Ft. Benning, GA, USA (Army); and Joint Base San Antonio—Lackland, TX, USA (Air Force). Marine Basic Training, generally acknowledged as the most physically intense of all enlisted basic training, occurs in similarly hot and humid locations: Marine Corps Recruit Depot (MCRD) Parris Island, on the coast of South Carolina, USA and MCRD San Diego in southern California, USA. Navy and Coast Guard recruits complete their basic training at Naval Station Great Lakes (near Chicago, IL, USA) and Training Center Cape May (New Jersey, USA), respectively, where the climate is more temperate on average than other US basic training sites. But even Great Lakes and Cape May can be quite hot and humid during summer months. Recruits arrive at these training bases from all over the country, many times leaving frigid winter weather to begin training in warmer climates the very next day.

In addition to these factors, the sheer volume of trainees at these installations increases the probability of heat illness in those with a genetic predisposition to heat intolerance. The Department of Defense trains just over 200 K new enlisted recruits annually, including active duty, guard, and reserve components. The Army leads the way with numbers (80–100 K), followed by Navy (40–45 K), Air Force (35–40 K), Marine Corps (30–35 K), and Coast Guard (3–4 K). Among numbers of that scale, it becomes likely that a few will be found with genetic predisposition for heat illness (such as *RYR1* gene mutation) or other risk factors, requiring medics to be always at the ready [9, 10].

Finally, there is an element of the traditional mentality or paradigm underlying the training. Each new generation of recruits is trained by a seasoned cadre of instructors who instill the warrior ethos and maintain strict military discipline, conducting training in much the same way they were trained themselves, passing on these military traditions, and ever vigilant to prevent the military from becoming too "soft." Though there may be operational benefits to this approach, this historical inertia may create resistance to risk reduction interventions (e.g., more gradual progression of training, longer acclimatization periods, more allowance for resting breaks) and promote individual recruit over-reaching.

Officer Training

Most of the considerations related to basic training pertain to officer training as well, with several important differences that will be discussed here. Many military officers are trained at one of the service academies, such as the US Military Academy at West Point (upstate New York, USA), the US Naval Academy (Annapolis, MD, USA), or the US Air Force Academy (Colorado Springs, CO, USA). While each of the academies enjoys a more temperate climate than most of the basic training sites, the risk of heat illness is nonetheless substantial. The overall physical intensity of training in each service academy is difficult to quantify or compare, but none would argue that certain phases of officer training are extremely physically intense. Perhaps the most notable example is that all US military service academies conduct high-intensity training each summer at the very beginning of the academic year with each incoming class of new cadets, though format and content differs. Risk of heat illness could potentially be elevated due to limited time for acclimatization prior to this early phase of training. Additionally, the culture of training and leadership paradigms in these officer training platforms may be more risk tolerant than basic training (if it is possible to generalize). Part of this relatively higher risk tolerance may be well founded, noting generally higher entry-level physical fitness of officer candidates. All service academy cadets must complete a physical fitness assessment prior to entry [11–13], whereas only the Marine Corps and Army conduct physical fitness assessments prior to entry into enlisted basic training [14, 15]. Additionally, officer training at the service academies lasts 4 years, which in theory allows more opportunity for acclimatization, but in reality, as noted above, some of the most physically intense training occurs in the first several weeks after each class of new cadets arrives to begin their freshman year.

Reserve Officer Training Corps (ROTC) programs are offered by most universities and serve as a large proportion of officer accessions. Without question, training at ROTC units is variable by location, some being large and well-reputed programs with intense and well-organized physical fitness curriculum. In contrast, some smaller ROTC programs may be less physically intense (perhaps lowering heat illness risk) but may also have fewer instructors and perhaps less subject matter expertise in physical fitness training or associated medical hazards.

The Marine Corps Officer Candidates School (OCS) merits separate discussion. This 10-week training program is located at Marine Corps Base Quantico (northern Virginia, USA) and records likely the highest incidence rates per capita of exertional heat stroke of any US military training activity. With an average of roughly 2700 total candidates per year (approx. 2400 graduates), OCS staff have reported 297 total heat strokes over calendar years 2016–2018, for an average just over 99 heat strokes per year. Seasoned OCS physicians attribute this high incidence rate to the extreme physical intensity of training in addition to the hot/humid climate during summer months, when most heat strokes occur [16].

Special Operations and Other High-Risk Military Populations

Upon completing basic military or officer training, the majority of military personnel proceed to career fields where physical fitness and exercise are largely self-paced and self-guided. However, those who go on to special operations career fields (e.g., Navy SEALs, Army Green Berets, Air Force Pararescue, and Combat Controllers, along with officer counterparts) must complete extremely strenuous training to join and maintain the ranks of these elite warrior athletes. Nearly every conceivable heat illness risk factor is at play in special operations (discussed further below), and these risks do not disappear upon completion of training, as operational missions are often even more demanding.

Other populations in the military also face significant heat stress, and it is not feasible to enumerate all of them due to the number and diversity of military units with their unique missions. Consider heat exposures experienced by the pilot in the cockpit, tank crew on extended missions, and disaster cleanup personnel who must wear full-body chemical protective suits and gas masks for hours at a time, just to name a few.

Military Unique Risk Factors of Heat-Related Illness

Much of the heat illness risk during military training and operations can be attributed to known risk factors. Some of these are modifiable, while others are not. (Please see Chap. 3 for more thorough discussion regarding the physiology and risk factors for exertional heat illness). In some military scenarios, mission requirements may take top priority, so it may not be feasible to modify certain factors, which in peacetime duties or civilian athletics may be easily modified (Table 10.2).

Table 10.2 Significance of military-specific risk factors

Military-specific risk factors	Significance
Gear and equipment	Body armor and gear often weigh 60–100 lbs., driving metabolic workload and barrier to heat dissipation Joint Service Lightweight Integrated Suit Technology (JS-LIST) incapacitates human thermoregulatory mechanisms
Dietary supplements	70% of military use dietary supplements, of which >10% use high-risk supplements such as pre-workout stimulants or anabolic agents
Intrinsic vs. extrinsic motivation	Training instructors provide powerful extrinsic motivation, while mission or "earning your beret" provides powerful intrinsic motivating forces
Sleep deprivation	Extended duty hours, limited opportunity to sleep. Depression and anxiety may lead to insomnia
Dehydration	Availability of water, palatability of water
Acclimatization	Warfighters deploy from home station in temperate climates to arrive in a hot, arid theater of combat; mission may allow little time to acclimatize
Solo training, remote operational missions	Altered mental status may not be detected, with none present to witness and respond. Cooling means not available in remote locations
Infectious diseases	Large group training and operations with closely shared lodging increase transmission of respiratory and gastrointestinal viruses
Leadership factors	Awareness and knowledge level of leadership with respect to heat stress informs their risk tolerance and training paradigms

Military Gear and Equipment

The military gear ensemble varies substantially depending on the unit and mission (especially combat vs. noncombat missions) but begins with the uniform. Combat uniforms typically consist of a durable, long sleeve, mostly-cotton shirt and cargo pants, but more modern combat uniforms feature more functional design and advanced nylon-cotton or other blended fabrics that are lighter, more breathable, ripstop, and in some cases flame-retardant. The combat boot has many varieties and come in hot-weather and cold-weather versions ranging from relatively stiff/heavy to flexible/lightweight construction. In addition to the uniform, combat personnel must wear body armor (tactical helmet, flak vest), eye protection, and duty gloves. Depending on the mission, most warfighters must also carry weapons and essential gear (radios, batteries, food/water, first aid kits, etc.). The metabolic workload of carrying the body armor and gear (often weighing 60–100 lbs.) is momentous, and these items also constitute a significant barrier to heat dissipation via sweat evaporation, convection, and radiation. However, of all gear and uniform items, perhaps the greatest heat stress comes with the Joint Service Lightweight Integrated Suit Technology (JS-LIST). This is a full-body suit with gas mask, which provides a complete, impermeable barrier to chemical, biological, radiological, and nuclear

(CBRN) warfare agents. It is used by all military services, and anyone who has performed any type of physical activity while wearing it (or similar gear) understands the extreme heat stress it brings. Sweat evaporation, the primary means of human thermoregulation, is basically impossible and completely ineffective. Heat dumping through convection, radiation, and evaporation with respiration is also severely impaired.

Dietary Supplements

Use of dietary supplements is rampant in the military, with approximately 70% of servicemembers using some form of dietary supplement regularly versus 50% of civilians. Most of these supplements are low-risk, such as protein, amino acids, and multivitamins, but at least 10% of military personnel (higher in certain subgroups) use high-risk supplements such as pre-workout stimulants or anabolic agents. There is minimal regulation or oversight of the dietary supplements industry, and product safety does not have to be proven before marketing and sale to consumers, raising serious concerns about potential harms. In response to serious adverse events (including multiple deaths) among servicemembers, the DoD has led the way by banning the sale of supplements containing certain ingredients (e.g., ephedra, ephedrine alkaloids, 1,3-dimethylamylamine, or DMAA) on military bases; these substances were later banned by the US Food and Drug Administration (FDA) [17]. Nonetheless, supplement manufacturers continue to sell products containing prohibited or dangerous substances through dishonest labeling and other means. Serious adverse events continue to occur among servicemembers, including heat illness, rhabdomyolysis, and liver/kidney injury, sometimes leading to hospitalization or even death. Efforts to educate warfighters, military leaders, and lawmakers must continue.

Intrinsic Versus Extrinsic Motivation

The protective effects of fatigue may at times be overridden by strong motivation to train and excel, which may be intrinsic or extrinsic. Classically, instructors in basic training (commonly known by the Army term "Drill Sergeant") and officer training are passionate, vocal, and strict, providing a strong extrinsic motivating force. Conversely, many trainees have more powerful intrinsic motivation. The classic example of this is special operations training, where many trainees have an intense desire to successfully complete training and attain status as an elite special operator (e.g., SEAL, Green Beret, Pararescueman), despite very high attrition rates due to high-intensity training.

Sleep Deprivation

Military training and operations may at times involve extended hours, very early mornings, and limited opportunity to sleep. Some special operations training involves "stress inoculation" with 24-hour training exercises or longer, mimicking combat operations that may involve round-the-clock tempo. In other instances, military personnel may suffer from insomnia related to anxiety, depression, and/or excessive use of caffeine and other stimulants. When physical exertion occurs in the setting of sleep deprivation, the risk of heat illness is increased.

Dehydration

Overall, most military units are very cognizant of the risks of dehydration and offer ample opportunity to hydrate. Dehydration remains a challenge, however, not so much due to availability of water but sometimes palatability of water (in some areas, the only water source is a large mobile water tank/trailer or "water buffalo," often left out in the sun causing the water to heat up).

Acclimatization

For various reasons, military training and operations often allow little to no time to acclimatize. Deployment is a good example, with warfighters leaving home station in potentially cool, temperate climates to arrive in a hot, arid theater of combat.

Solo Training/Remote Operational Missions

Military survival training, known as SERE (Survival, Evasion, Resistance, and Escape), includes many components of physically arduous and prolonged exertion, and some of this is done as a solo wilderness survival exercise. Solo training presents the threat that if one begins to succumb to heat stress, altered mental status may not be detected until it is too late, with none immediately present to witness and respond. At least one such case resulted in death due to probable exertional heat stroke in recent years. Remote operational missions present a similar difficulty, except that although heat illness may be identified, definitive cooling capability may be inaccessible. Furthermore, warfighters who become isolated from their unit in hostile territory may be required to survive and evade capture while navigating back to safer zones or to an optimal location for pickup by rescue teams. This may involve significant heat exposure and dehydration. If the isolated warfighter is solo, the risk of heat illness would be significantly higher.

Infectious Disease

Military training often occurs in large group settings, with personnel frequently housed in large barracks with shared bathroom facilities. These closely shared living and lodging situations increase transmission of respiratory and gastrointestinal viruses, which often results in fever, fatigue, and decreased ability to compensate for heat stress.

Leadership Factors

Paramount in heat illness prevention, leadership factors often distinguish units that have few heat casualties from those that have many. The awareness and knowledge level of leadership with respect to heat stress informs their risk tolerance and training paradigms. Sensible policy and well-trained personnel provide a very effective safety net against many threats, including heat illness.

Military Strategies for Prevention of Heat-Related Illness

As discussed above, military training and operations involve significant heat exposure. Efforts to minimize heat exposure and mitigate risk factors before the warfighter has been subjected to a heat load are considered primary prevention of heat illness. The military services systematically approach risk management for environmental stress comparable to approaches utilized for other stresses, utilizing a series of steps [18]. The five steps of operational risk management—identify the hazards, assess the hazards, develop controls and make risk decisions, implement controls, and supervise and evaluate—are used across the services to help them operate as a joint force and optimize readiness (Fig. 10.4) [18].

When leadership determines there is an environmental risk of EHI, the aforementioned risk management process is carefully planned to assess risk and implement strategies to mitigate that risk. Activities implemented to reduce risk include those previously discussed in this chapter: education, acclimatization, appropriate adjustment of activities to include work/rest and hydration strategies, and being prepared for early EHI management to mitigate the risk of EHS. Dependent upon the degree of assessed risk, leaders of increasing rank are required to review and sign off to approve training plans. Arguably the military's most important tool in preventing EHI is leadership; all leaders are expected to proactively implement

Fig. 10.4 The five-step
process of operational
risk management [18]

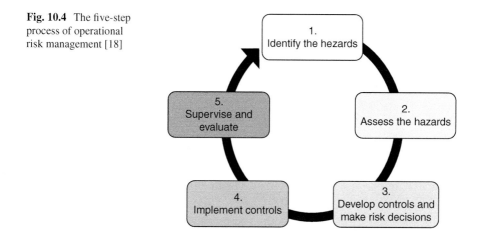

preventive measures to mitigate the threat of heat casualties. Some leaders are willing to accept a higher risk of heat casualties for the sake of higher-intensity training and operations; it must be remembered, however, that determining the appropriate balance between training intensity and health risk in order to optimize probability of mission success is a quintessential role and responsibility of the commander.

Primary Prevention

Tolerance of extreme heat and humidity depends upon a number of functional, acquired, and congenital factors, of which acclimatization is of great importance (Table 10.3) [19]. Acclimatization is the body's ability to improve its response and tolerance of heat stress over time and is the most important factor determining how well a warfighter withstands extreme heat. Thus, allowing sufficient time and using optimal training strategies that enable warfighters to acclimatize are critical for improving performance and mitigating the risk for EHI. Observational studies have found that the first week of training in high heat and humidity, for both warfighters and athletes, is the period of greatest risk for developing EHI [6, 20]. Acclimatization requires at least 1–2 weeks. However, any improved tolerance of heat stress generally dissipates within 2–3 weeks of returning to a more temperate environment. Acclimatization in warfighters is accomplished with a combination of environmental exposure with exercise; Technical Bulletin MED 507/Air Force Pamphlet 48–152, *Heat Stress Control and Heat Casualty Management*, details optimal acclimatization strategies [6].

The major physiologic adjustments that occur during heat and humidity acclimatization include plasma volume expansion, improved cutaneous blood flow, lower threshold for initiation of sweating, increased sweat output, lower salt concentration in sweat, and lower skin and core temperatures for a standard exercise [21]. These adaptations allow for better dissipation of heat during exercise and limit increases in

Table 10.3 Factors upon which tolerance of extreme heat and humidity depends

Congenital	Functional	Acquired
Malignant hyperthermia susceptibility (RYR1 mutation)	*Low physical fitness*	*Sweat gland dysfunction (large rash, diabetes mellitus, large thermal/radiation burns, or scarred/grafted skin area)*
	Lack of acclimatization	
	Low work efficiency	
Ectodermal dysplasia	*Reduced skin surface area-to-mass ratio (e.g., obesity)*	*Febrile illness*
Chronic idiopathic anhidrosis		*Previous heat stroke*
Cystic fibrosis	*Sleep deprivation*	*Medications, alcohol*
	Dehydration	

Table 10.4 Thermoregulatory benefits of of heat acclimatization

Thermal comfort improved	Exercise performance improved
Core temperature reduced	Cardiovascular stability improved
	– Heart rate lowered
	– Stroke volume increased
	– Blood pressure better defended
	– Myocardial compliance improved
Sweating improved	Fluid balance improved
– Earlier onset	– Thirst improved
– Higher rate of redistribution	– Electrolyte loss reduced
– Hidromeiosis resistance	
Skin blood flow improved	Total body water increased
– Earlier onset	
– Higher rate	
Metabolic rate lowered	Plasma volume increased and better defended

body temperature compared to warriors who have not acclimatized. Table 10.4 describes the known physiologic benefits of acclimatization.

In addition to leveraging acclimatization, the MMO needs to be proactive in assessing the environmental stress and implementing appropriate work/rest and hydration strategies. These recommendations are based upon an assessment of the WGBT to determine the heat category. Figure 10.5 details current guidance for ground units published by the the US Army Institute of Environmental Medicine (USARIEM) [6].

Secondary Prevention

Once the warfighter has been exposed to or carries a heat load, their thermoregulatory systems begin to function at a higher rate to maintain homeostasis. While in this state of heat stress, efforts to prevent decompensation into EHI are considered secondary prevention. Proactive strategies for secondary prevention of EHI are also effective for improving performance in the heat. A strategy utilized extensively in the military is "heat dumping," where heat is transferred to the environment using

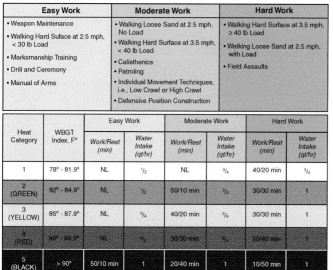

Work/Rest and Water Consumption Table
Applies to average sized, heat-acclimated soldier wearing OCP, hot weather, (See TB 507 for further guidance).

Easy Work	Moderate Work	Hard Work
• Weapon Maintenance • Walking Hard Suface at 2.5 mph, < 30 lb Load • Marksmanship Training • Drill and Ceremony • Manual of Arms	• Walking Loose Sand at 2.5 mph, No Load • Walking Hard Surface at 3.5 mph, < 40 lb Load • Calisthenics • Patroling • Individual Movement Techniques, i.e., Low Crawl or High Crawl • Defensive Position Construction	• Walking Hard Surface at 3.5 mph, ≥ 40 lb Load • Walking Loose Sand at 2.5 mph, with Load • Field Assaults

Heat Category	WBGT Index, F°	Easy Work		Moderate Work		Hard Work	
		Work/Rest (min)	Water Intake (qt/hr)	Work/Rest (min)	Water Intake (qt/hr)	Work/Rest (min)	Water Intake (qt/hr)
1	78° - 81.9°	NL	1/2	NL	3/4	40/20 min	3/4
2 (GREEN)	82° - 84.9°	NL	1/2	50/10 min	3/4	30/30 min	1
3 (YELLOW)	85° - 87.9°	NL	3/4	40/20 min	3/4	30/30 min	1
4 (RED)	88° - 89.9°	NL	3/4	30/30 min	3/4	20/40 min	1
5 (BLACK)	> 90°	50/10 min	1	20/40 min	1	10/50 min	1

• The work/rest times and fluid replacement volumes will sustain performance and hydration for at least 4 hrs of work in the specified heat category. Fluid needs can vary based on individual differences (± 1/4 qt/hr) and exposure to full sun or full shade (± 1/4 qt/hr).

• **NL** = no limit to work time per hr.

• **Rest** = minimal physical activity (sitting or standing) accomplished in shade id possible.

• *CAUTION: Hourly fluid intake should not exceed 1 1/2 qts.*

  Daily fluid intake should not exceed 12 qts.

• If wearing body armor, add **5°F** to WBGT index in humid climates.

• If doing Easy Work wearing NBC (MOPP 4) cloting. add **10°F** to WBGT index.

• If doing Moderate or Hard Work and wearing NBC (Mopp 4) cloting. add **20°F** to WBGT index.

Current guidance for heat injury prevention using work/rest ratios and hydration, as published by the US Army Institute of Environmental Medicine (USARIEM) [6]. Though designed with ground combat units in mind, this guidance is also applicable to other types of military units who conduct outdoor training or operations, and provides appropriate instructions based on varying environmental conditions and workloads.

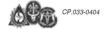

CP.033-0404

Fig. 10.5 Current guidance for ground units published by the US Army Institute of Environmental Medicine (USARIEM) [6]

various techniques. Perhaps the most prevalent are cool mist showers and mist fans. Cooling vests have been increasingly employed by combat units and are now quite prevalent. Cooling vests generally utilize one or a combination of three technologies: (1) embedded packs of phase change materials that absorb large amounts of heat during the transformation from solid ("frozen") to liquid state, effectively maintaining a regulated temperature, (2) advanced evaporative fabrics that stay cool when soaked in water, or (3) pumping chilled water through a network of small-caliber tubing incorporated into the vest adjacent to the skin. Some units also utilize gloves and helmets with similar cooling capabilities. Preliminary studies have shown that evaporative clothing and clothing with embedded phase change materials do provide a cooling effect [22]; however, clinical research on effectiveness for prevention of heat illness remains limited to nil. A novel approach to heat dumping used in the military is the arm immersion cooling system (AICS) (Fig. 10.6).

The AICS takes advantage of the rapid rate of heat transfer from the skin directly into cool water (compared to transfer into evaporative sweat or air) and the large surface area-to-mass ratio of the forearms. Several studies have reported that hand and forearm immersion in cool (50–68 °F or 10–20 °C) water reduces core and skin temperature faster than a non-cooling control, extends tolerance time, and increases total work time [23].

Fig. 10.6 Arm
immersion cooling
system is demonstrated in
the field by a team of
Army troops

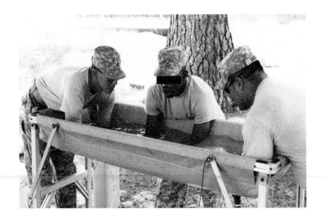

In addition to heat dumping strategies, remote physiologic status monitoring (PSM) technology has enabled improved early detection of heat stress. These systems integrate several wearable or ingestible sensors that transmit various types of data, including core temperature (via ingestible thermistor or telemetry pill that slowly transits the gastrointestinal tract), skin temperature, heart rate, and GPS location. Data is transmitted via radio-frequency or cellular signal to a medic, who is able to remotely monitor the physiologic status and location of a whole team of warfighters. Systems may utilize algorithms to combine physiologic data into a heat strain index that is used to predict whether personnel are beginning to decompensate. PSM systems may enable medics to intervene earlier in the process of heat stress, before the onset of exertional heat stroke.

Other important strategies for secondary prevention include the buddy system, monitoring environmental conditions (usually based on WBGT and stratified into "flag conditions"), and appropriate enforcement of work/rest ratios and hydration policies as discussed above [24].

Tertiary Prevention

When primary and secondary prevention strategies fail and exertional heat stroke ensues, tertiary prevention strategies are employed to minimize risk of morbidity and mortality. Military strategies for tertiary prevention do not differ greatly from civilian methods. Central principles of rapid recognition, core temperature assessment, and on-site whole-body cooling are now written into tri-service policy and widely utilized. However, gaps in practice remain. Implementation within the framework of military training and operations presents multiple challenges, which will be discussed here.

Rapid recognition of EHI is perhaps the most critical of all links in the chain of good care because it carries the greatest potential for delay in cooling, which may be the difference between life and death [25]. Nonmedical personnel are often the first ones to detect altered mental status. When a warfighter begins to display confusion, disorientation, or similar findings while exercising in the heat, the battle buddy, wingman, or shipmate must reach an essential realization that medical help is needed urgently rather than passing it off as simply odd behavior. The ability to recognize a medical emergency such as this requires quality training, which must be disseminated out from the highest to the lowest levels. Training strategies vary by service and region, but highly effective training programs are characterized by simplicity of content, frequent repetition, and leadership buy-in. Hands-on training exercises, such as unannounced "mock heat stroke" scenarios, also provide effective means to identify breakdowns in the emergency action plan. A post-exercise summary report is written by event organizers and signed by leadership, who direct appropriate corrections and ensure preparedness for highly effective response to a real-world EHS.

Core temperature assessment via rectal thermometer is important for diagnosing exertional heat stroke and helping to distinguish from other medical conditions that may have similar presentation. In most military settings, there are no obstacles to obtaining a rectal temperature. Most field medics are well-trained and are familiar with effective means for cooling. However, some field medics may have been trained under outdated curricula and may not have reviewed latest policies, or simply may not be properly equipped with a rectal thermometer. Some field medics may continue in the mistaken practice of checking surface temperatures first (oral, auricular) and reassuring themselves if not significantly elevated. Physician education may also at times present a barrier, as some physicians (both military and civilian) retain their traditional paradigm that "definitive care can only be provided within a hospital or emergency department." When physicians with this paradigm fill leadership positions such as EMS Medical Director, emergency medical teams responding to an exertional heat stroke may be ordered by their Medical Director to "scoop and run," even if effective cooling is available on-site prior to transport. An additional potential barrier to obtaining a core temperature is concern for patient privacy or fear of allegations. In the military training environment, a trainee who files a complaint often triggers an investigation, and many instructors are reluctant to assist medics (e.g., if a combative, disoriented trainee requires restraint in order to obtain a rectal temperature). Finally, the interface between military units and civilian EMS may present a challenge, as some civilian EMS protocols may differ somewhat from military protocols (e.g., may not allow on-site cooling). For example, if a special operations team is training in a remote region of southern Texas and the military field medic identifies a troop with exertional heat stroke, he or she may initiate cooling by cold water immersion and call civilian EMS for evacuation. If the civilian EMS teams arrive and request immediate transport despite persistent hyperthermia, it may be difficult to resolve the conflict in the midst of an ongoing exertional heat stroke response.

Owing to the growing body of evidence, the central role of immediate and aggressive whole-body cooling for victims of exertional heat stroke is largely recognized in the military [6]. At military installations where high-risk or high-volume training occurs, medics are generally well-attuned to the signs of heat illness, and on-site cooling capabilities are generally present. However, the Department of

Defense is very large and diverse with a multitude of units carrying out training in varied conditions across the USA, making the tasks of data collection, communication, and standardization quite difficult. Some units or training locations may lack robust cooling capabilities.

When heat exhaustion or exertional heat stroke is diagnosed, cooling is initiated via whatever means are immediately available [6]. Sometimes this may be dousing in cool water, packing ice around the body (axillae and groin usually preferred if ice quantity limited), and variations of the TACO (tarp-assisted cooling with oscillation) or burrito methods (such as wrapping the body in ice sheets or bed linens soaked in water and frozen). Additional means may be available depending on the circumstances and may include mist fans, cool shower, chilled IV fluids, or helicopter downdraft. While none of these methods cools as rapidly as whole-body cold water immersion (CWI), they are generally adequate for heat exhaustion, and in cases of heat stroke, they can be initiated quickly while transporting the patient to the nearest facility capable of definitive cooling. Data for CWI, specifically referring to whole-body immersion below the neck in ice and water (generally 2–10 °C), have demonstrated superior cooling rates and zero mortality when implemented within the first 10–15 minutes of symptoms. This technique is utilized with success at many DoD installations where high-intensity training occurs.

As important exceptions, physicians at Marine Corps settings, including OCS (Quantico, VA) and the Marine Corps Marathon (MCM; Washington, D.C.), utilize a modified whole-body cooling technique that is arguably better adapted for scenarios when multiple exertional heat strokes are expected to occur simultaneously [26]. This modified technique consists of placing the victim over a tub/pool filled with an ice slurry and dousing the body continuously while simultaneously performing ice massage, giving chilled IV fluids (after checking iSTAT sodium), and directing fans at the victim. Data on efficacy of this modified technique have been published [26], and further reports are being analyzed for publication, but physicians at Quantico describe using it successfully for cooling 297 exertional heat strokes (all confirmed by rectal temperature >104 °F with CNS dysfunction) during calendar years 2016–2018 with zero mortality and extremely low morbidity. In fact, physicians at Quantico report most exertional heat stroke patients return to training approximately 4–5 days later with rare complications. Of note, because exertional heat stroke response infrastructure is so well-trained and robust in these locations, most victims of exertional heat stroke arrive at the "cooling deck" within 5 minutes and rarely delay longer than 15 minutes to initiate definitive cooling, likely contributing to their high success rates [16]. Clinicians who have utilized both CWI and the Quantico/MCM method of ice slurry dousing generally concur that while both are highly effective, pure CWI is optimal and best suited for low numbers of exertional heat strokes, but when large numbers of exertional heat strokes are expected, the Quantico/MCM method has similar cooling efficacy and may be logistically superior for treating multiple heat strokes within a short timeframe.

Return to Duty

Return-to-play/return to duty (RTP/RTD) decisions may be the most challenging component of both athlete and warfighter injury management [27]. Although the final decision is most commonly left to the providing physician, assessments frequently require input from and execution by the athletic trainer, physical therapist, coach, family members, and the athlete. In the military, added input may involve Commanders, noncommissioned officers, and military training guidance. An American College of Sports Medicine (ACSM) guideline on RTP identified several key considerations [28]:

- Status of anatomical and functional healing
- Status of recovery from acute illness and associated sequelae
- Status of chronic injury or illness
- Whether the athlete poses an undue risk to the safety of other participants
- Restoration of sport-specific skills
- Psychosocial readiness
- Ability to perform safely with equipment modification, bracing, and orthoses
- Compliance with applicable federal, state, local, school, and governing body regulations

The RTP/RTD decision-making process requires a fundamental understanding of both the pathophysiology of EHS and how the affected tissues, organs, and/or body systems recover. EHS RTP/RTD is especially challenging because our understanding of the pathophysiological processes involved in the development of and recovery from EHS is incomplete [20]. Current research suggests that most individuals recover completely within a few weeks, especially when patients are treated promptly and cooled aggressively (i.e., cold water immersion) [20, 29]. However, some experience long-term complications that may include multi-system organ (liver, kidney, muscle) and/or neurologic damage and/or reduced exercise capacity and heat intolerance [5, 30, 31]. The most concerning complication facing the MMO is the risk of a recurrent event, with its impact not only on the warfighter but also the military team and mission.

The Risk of a Recurrent Heat Injury

Because warfighters who sustain an EHS may be at higher risk for a subsequent event, the MMO must contemplate the RTD decision carefully, since knowledge of the potential risk for a second event is a critical factor [27]. In one of a number of studies of EHS epidemiology and heat tolerance published by the French military, 15.4% of the 182 military members who were hospitalized after experiencing EHS reported a previous episode of EHS [32]. A few studies in the US military have addressed the issue of heat injury recurrence. This is a cornerstone issue because a history of EHS generally requires a medical waiver, which is a barrier to military enlistment. Phinney et al. evaluated the subsequent risk for re-hospitalization in Marines who suffered EHI during basic training (BT) as outpatients ($n = 872$) or inpatients ($n = 50$) and completed at least 6 months of service [33]. They compared these EHI cases to 1391 non-cases, followed them all for 4 years. EHI cases had about 40% higher subsequent hospitalization rates in military hospitals than non-cases; these differences declined over time, and diagnoses showed little relationship to EHI. Although the authors concluded that hospitalizations for EHI are uncommon during BT, the numbers are too small (five hospitalizations) to provide an accurate comparison.

Nelson et al. recently studied a large cohort of active duty soldiers, observing 238,168 subjects for a total 427,922 person-years of service. Among clinically focused variables, a prior serious EHI event was associated with 4.02 greater odds of experiencing a mild EHI event later, and a mild EHI was associated with a 1.77 greater risk of having a serious EHI event later. These observations strongly confirm the likelihood that a prior EHI event is associated with an increased risk of a subsequent EHI event [34].

Assessment of Recovery

Current civilian and military RTP/RTD guidelines are largely based on anecdotal observations and caution [5, 27, 35]. Although clinicians can utilize basic hematologic parameters and blood chemistries to assess for a return to normal function for renal, hepatic, and coagulation disorders, assessing integrity of the thermoregulatory system remains a gap. Evaluation for potential exercise-heat tolerance deficits, neuropsychological impairments, and/or the altered fitness/acclimatization status are challenging and at this time do not have validated instruments. The absence of clear, evidence-based guidance further complicates decision-making for sports medicine professionals who must guess at the best decision for an individual who has experienced an EHS event. Moreover, the lack of consistency and clinical agreement can negatively affect not only individual athletes and warfighters but also directly influence athletic success and military readiness.

Most guidelines assessing recovery are simply common sense, requiring an asymptomatic state and normal laboratory findings that target end organs (e.g., liver and kidney) coupled with a cautious reintroduction of activity and gradual heat acclimatization. While there are presently no definitive, high level evidence-based guidelines regarding RTP/RTD, the ACSM has published recommendations [5], summarized below.

- Refrain from exercise for at least 7 days after release from medical care.
- Follow-up about 1-week post incident for a physical examination and laboratory testing or diagnostic imaging (biomarkers) of the affected organs. This will address the clinical course of the heat stroke incident.

- When the individual has been cleared for return to activity, he/she should begin exercise in a cool environment and gradually increase the duration, intensity, and heat exposure over 2 weeks to demonstrate heat tolerance and initiate acclimatization.
- If return to vigorous activity is not accomplished within 4 weeks, a laboratory exercise-heat tolerance test should be considered.
- If the athlete proves heat tolerant, he/she may be cleared for full competition between 2 and 4 weeks after the return to full training.

While the ACSM guidance is indisputably useful, many gaps remain. Importantly, the current ACSM process does not address the true risk of recurrence. Although current guidance states that EHS patients may return to practice and competition when they have re-established heat tolerance, clear clinical definitions of heat tolerance/intolerance are distinctly lacking. Suggested recovery periods vary from 7 days to 15 months before EHS victims return to full activity [27, 35]. In addition, both the role of heat tolerance testing and the potential effect of EHS on the thermoregulatory system are areas of scientific question and controversy [36].

What Is Heat Tolerance?

The ability to sustain workloads under conditions of heat stress varies widely across individuals [19, 37]. Under extreme conditions of exertion in the heat, even healthy, well-acclimatized, and physically fit individuals will ultimately be unable to dissipate the excessive heat such that body temperature rises, and a heat injury may ensue. Some individuals may not respond properly to heat stress: their body temperature starts rising earlier and at a higher rate than others under the same conditions. We have defined these individuals as heat intolerant [38]. Heat intolerance is therefore the "inability to efficiently dissipate heat as expected by normal average individuals under similar conditions." The factors that underlie heat intolerance can be categorized as congenital, functional, or acquired (see Table 10.3).

Heat intolerance has been observed in those who experienced an EHS episode from a few weeks to as long as 5 years later; thus heat intolerance may be considered as either temporary or permanent [39, 40]. It has been suggested that heat intolerance may reflect inherent or genetic characteristics and possibly a consequence of a previous EHS event [40, 41]. In a large-scale survey conducted on participants recruited from South African gold mines, 2–4% of the population were found to be heat intolerant yet manifested no apparent disease process [42].

The Role of Heat Tolerance Testing

Heat tolerance testing is currently not a requirement to facilitate the return to duty process for conventional forces in the American military. That being stated, heat tolerance testing is considered in exceptional cases where the return to duty process has been either difficult, prolonged, or a medical evaluation board with potential separation from service is being considered. Heat tolerance testing is additionally considered in unique military settings, such as special operations, where a prior history of exertional heat stroke raises concerns over participation in elite training course participation. Heat tolerance testing is an active area of clinical discussion and controversy and is recognized as one tool in the clinical decision-making process. When heat tolerance testing is used in the clinical setting, currently the most commonly endorsed protocol is that utilized by the Israel Defense Force, which is subsequently described.

For the last few decades, the standard practice in the Israel Defense Force (IDF) Medical Corps has been that all EHI patients undergo a standard exercise HTT about 6 weeks post-event as part of the "return to duty" process [19, 43]. Testing is performed during the early hours of the morning, but for practical reasons time of year and patient acclimatization are not accounted for. However, the test is not performed before complete clinical recovery. The IDF HTT criteria are based primarily on changes in rectal temperature (Trec) and heart rate (HR) during the test. Before testing, subjects undergo a general medical exam and assessment of their baseline core temperature, which should be lower than 37.5 °C (99.5 °F) to be cleared for testing. Subjects are instructed to avoid tobacco and caffeine prior the test, not to perform any exercise or drink any alcohol for at least 24 hours prior to the test, to sleep at least 7 hours during the night, and to drink 0.5 L of water in the hour prior to the test. During the test, the subject wears light clothing: shorts and no shirt for men and shorts and sports bra for women. The HTT is performed in a controlled environmental chamber with the temperature set at 40 °C (104 °F) and a relative humidity of 40%.

Body weight is measured before and after the test. During the test, the subject walks on a treadmill for 120 minutes at 5 km/h (3.1 mph) at a 2% incline, while core body temperature and heart rate are continuously monitored and recorded [38, 44]. Additionally, fluid intake and urine output are measured to compute sweat rate in combination with pre/post body weight. Heat intolerance is defined as a rectal temperature above 38.5 °C, or HR above 150 bpm, or when either does not reach a plateau [40]. A plateau is consistent with a <0.45 °C/hr. increase in core temperature or a Trec/HR ratio (>0.279 °C/bpm). Figure 10.7 presents the Trec dynamics in heat tolerant and heat intolerant individual [41]. Sweat rate is expected to be 0.5–1 L/hr.

Under the IDF protocol, if the thermoregulatory response is abnormal (~5–10% of cases), the soldier is scheduled for a second test that can be performed between 1 and 3 months later, depending on the test results and severity of the prior heat injury. If the second HTT is abnormal according to IDF standards, the subject is defined as heat intolerant and cannot continue service in a combat military unit. After decades of experience and hundreds of cases, the IDF process has yielded almost no indications of heat intolerance after return to duty. A recent study by the IDF military demonstrated that only 6 of 145 subjects (4.1%) who underwent HTT because of a prior EHS experienced recurrent EHI events: 4 (of 35) had been classified as heat intolerant (11.4%) and 2 (of 110) as heat tolerant (1.8%) [44]. Only one of the six

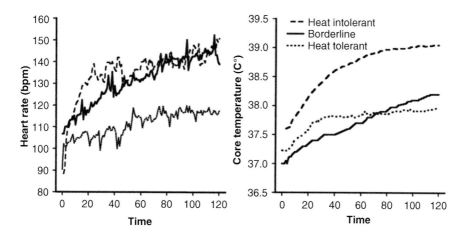

Fig. 10.7 Heat tolerance test output of heart rate and core temperature plotted against time. Examples of heat intolerant, borderline, and heat intolerant individuals are shown. (From O'Connor et al. [41], with permission)

recurrent events was diagnosed as EHS and involved a heat tolerant individual; the other five were diagnosed as heat exhaustions. Based on these data, the sensitivity, specificity, and diagnostic accuracy of the HTT were 66.7%, 77.7%, and 77.2%, respectively.

Current Army Guidance for Return to Duty

The military services do not share consensus recommendations on returning warfighters to duty after sustaining an exertional heat illness [35]. In fact, in many ways, the individual service recommendations are more diverse and varied than those that presently exist in the civilian sector. An ACSM Roundtable was convened at the Uniformed Services University of the Health Sciences (Bethesda, Maryland) from 22–23 October 2008 to address this issue of variability with both military and civilian experts [45]. Specifically, the conference sought to (1) discuss the issue of returning victims (athletes and soldiers) of EHI to either play or duty and (2) develop consensus-based recommendations. The conference results were utilized as a foundation to develop new guidance that is presently used by the Army Medical Department; current exertional heat illness definitions are identified in Table 10.5.

Importantly, the conference recognized the key importance of variability in exertional heat stroke, with the critical importance of the role of timely cooling in both management and recovery. Accordingly, a critical action of the committee was that all warfighters classified as having an exertional heat stroke event would be completely rested for 2 weeks and then reclassified, as follows: EHS without sequelae, all clinical signs and symptoms resolved by 2 weeks following the event; EHS with

Table 10.5 Exertional heat illness as currently defined by the US Army Medical Department

Heat category	Definition
Heat exhaustion	A syndrome of hyperthermia (core temperature at time of event usually ≤40 °C or 104 °F) with collapse or debilitation occurring during or immediately following exertion in the heat, with no more than minor central nervous system dysfunction (headache, dizziness), which resolves rapidly with intervention
Heat injury	Heat exhaustion with clinical evidence of organ (e.g., liver, renal, gut) and/or muscle (e.g., rhabdomyolysis) damage without sufficient neurological symptoms to be exertional heat stroke
Heat stroke	A syndrome of hyperthermia (core temperature at time of event usually ≥40 °C or 104 °F), collapse or debilitation, and encephalopathy (delirium, stupor, coma) occurring during or immediately following exertion or significant heat exposure. Heat stroke can be complicated by organ and/or tissue injury, systemic inflammatory activation, and disseminated intravascular coagulation

sequelae, any evidence of cognitive or behavioral dysfunction, renal impairment, hepatic dysfunction, rhabdomyolysis, or other related pathology that does not completely resolve by 2 weeks following the event; and complex EHS, recurrent or occurring in the presence of a non-modifiable risk factor, either known (e.g., chronic skin condition such as eczema or burn skin graft) or suspected (e.g., sickle cell trait, malignant hyperthermia susceptibility). Following reclassification at the 2-week re-evaluation, the return to duty process is individualized based upon guidance in Table 10.6. Current guidance for return to duty, with a full description of the military profile and medical board system, is detailed in Army Regulation 40–501, Standards for Medical Fitness.

Conclusion

The military tactical athlete is a unique individual subject to stressors that have few parallels in the civilian setting. In addition to environmental challenges that may mitigate performance, the psychosocial stressors that accompany frequent and/or prolonged deployments and the inherent stress associated with combat military operations require significant planning and training on the part of leadership. The MMO is a critical member of the leadership team and uniquely postured to assist the Command to optimize performance and ensure warfighter wellness and safety. This chapter has detailed for the MMO the relevance, past and present, of exertional heat illness as a threat to military operations; discussed military-unique applied physiology, training settings, and risk factors; and detailed primary, secondary, and tertiary strategies currently employed for prevention. Fundamental for the military physician, and as a unique distinction to the care of the civilian athlete, is that the core focus of all training, prevention, and return to duty decision-making is the preservation and accomplishment of the unit's goals and mission. While the MMO has a critical duty to optimize the individual warfighter's safety, in the military, the ultimate focus remains on the team and the mission.

Table 10.6 Profile progression recommendations for the soldier with heat stroke (HS), heat exhaustion (HE), heat injury (HI), and pending medical evaluation board (MEB)

Profile code[a]	Restrictions[b]	EHS without sequelae	EHS with sequelae	Complex EHS or HE/HI pending MEB
T-4 (P)	Complete duty restrictions	2 weeks	2 weeks minimum; advance when clinically resolved	2 weeks minimum; advance when clinically resolved
T-3 (P)	Physical training and running/walking/ swimming/bicycling at own pace and distance not to exceed 60 min per day No maximal effort; no APFT; no wear of IBA; no MOPP gear; no ruck marching No AO	1 month Minimum	2 months Minimum	Pending MEB
T-3 (P)	Gradual acclimatization (TB med 507) No maximal effort; no APFT; no MOPP 4 gear. IBA limited to static range participation May ruck march at own pace/distance with no more than 30 lbs. Nontactical AO permitted	1 month Minimum	2 months Minimum[c]	N/A
T-2 (P)	Continue gradual acclimatization. May participate in unit PT; CBRN training with MOPP gear for up to 30 min; IBA on static and dynamic ranges for up to 45 min; no record APFT. Ruck march at own pace/distance with no more than 30 lbs. up to 2 h Nontactical AO permitted	N/A	Pending completion of 30-day heat exposure requirement, if not accomplished during prior profile[c]	N/A

EHS exertional heat stroke, *APFT* army physical fitness test, *IBA* interceptor body armor, *MOPP* mission-oriented protective posture, *AO* airborne operations

[a]Temporary profile; *Physical capacity P* from *Military Physical Profile Serial System PULHES* (P physical capacity/stamina; U upper extremities; L lower extremities; H hearing/ears; E eyes; S psychiatric)

[b]Soldiers manifesting no heat illness symptomatology or work intolerance after completion of profile restrictions can advance and return to duty without an MEB. Any evidence/manifestation of heat illness symptomatology during the period of the profile requires an MEB referral

[c]Heat stroke with sequelae return to full duty requires a minimum period of heat exposure during environmental stress (heat category 2 during the majority of included days)

References

1. Goldman RF. Introduction to heat-related problems in military operations. In: Wenger CB, editor. Medical aspects of harsh environments, vol. I. Washington, DC: Borden Institute; 2001. p. 3–49.
2. McCallum JE. Military medicine: from ancient times to the 21st century. Santa Barbara, CA: ABC-CLIO, Inc; 2008.

3. Gabriel RA. Between flesh and steel: a history of military medicine from the Middle Ages to the war in Afghanistan. Washington, DC: Potomac Books; 2013.
4. Armed Forces Health Surveillance Branch. Update: Heat illness, active component, U.S. Armed Forces, 2017. MSMR. 2018;25(4):6–12.
5. Armstrong LE, Casa DJ, Millard-Stafford M, Moran DS, Pyne SW, Roberts WO. American College of Sports Medicine position stand. Exertional heat illness during training and competition. Med Sci Sports Exerc. 2007;39(3):556–72.
6. TB MED 507/Air Force Pamphlet 48-152, Heat Stress Control and Heat Casualty Management. 7 Mar 2003. Washington DC: Headquarters Department of the Army and Air Force.
7. Ely BR, Ely MR, Cheuvront SN, Kenefick RW, Degroot DW, Montain SJ. Evidence against a 40 degrees C core temperature threshold for fatigue in humans. J Appl Physiol (1985). 2009;107(5):1519–25.
8. Leon LR, Bouchama A. Heat stroke. Compr Physiol. 2015;5(2):611–47.
9. Roux-Buisson N, Monnier N, Sagui E, Abriat A, Brosset C, Bendahan D, et al. Identification of variants of the ryanodine receptor type 1 in patients with exertional heat stroke and positive response to the malignant hyperthermia in vitro contracture test. Br J Anaesth. 2016;116(4):566–8.
10. Kim JH, Jarvik GP, Browning BL, Rajagopalan R, Gordon AS, Rieder MJ, et al. Exome sequencing reveals novel rare variants in the ryanodine receptor and calcium channel genes in malignant hyperthermia families. Anesthesiology. 2013;119(5):1054–65.
11. United States Air Force Academy. The Application Process. https://www.academyadmissions. com/admissions/the-application-process/fitness-assessment/. Accessed 20 Jun 2019.
12. United States Military Academy West Point. Admissions. Steps to Admission. https://www. usma.edu/admissions/steps-to-admission. Accessed 20 Jun 2019.
13. U.S. Naval Academy. Application Instructions. https://www.usna.edu/Admissions/Candidate-Fitness-Assessment.php. Accessed 20 Jun 2019.
14. Schogol J. Marines roll out tougher initial strength test for poolees. Marine Corps Times. 23 Feb 2016. https://www.marinecorpstimes.com/news/your-marine-corps/2016/02/24/marines-roll-out-tougher-initial-strength-test-for-poolees/. Accessed 20 Jun 2019.
15. Vergun D. Army implements new fitness standards for recruits and MOS transfers. U.S. Army Website. 3 Jan 2017. https://www.army.mil/article/180199/army_implements_new_fitness_standards_for_recruits_and_mos_transfers. Accessed 20 Jun 2019.
16. Personal communication. LCDR Clifford Madsen: Description of heat illness rates, risk factors, and response procedures in Marine Corps Officer Candidate School, 2016–2018.
17. Deuster PA, Lieberman HR. Protecting military personnel from high risk dietary supplements. Drug Test Anal. 2016;8(3–4):431–3.
18. Risk management. Army Techniques Publication 5–19. Risk Management. April 2014. Washington, DC: Headquarters, Department of the Army.
19. Epstein Y. Heat intolerance: predisposing factor or residual injury? Med Sci Sports Exerc. 1990;22(1):29–35.
20. Casa DJ, Armstrong LE, Ganio MS, Yeargin SW. Exertional heat stroke in competitive athletes. Curr Sports Med Rep. 2005;4(6):309–17.
21. Glaser EM. Acclimatization to heat and cold. J Physiol. 1949;110(3–4):330–7.
22. Wang F, Song W. An investigation of thermophysiological responses of human while using four personal cooling strategies during heatwaves. J Therm Biol. 2017;70.(Pt A:37–44.
23. DeGroot DW, Kenefick RW, Sawka MN. Impact of arm immersion cooling during ranger training on exertional heat illness and treatment costs. Mil Med. 2015;180(11):1178–83.
24. Epstein Y, Druyan A, Heled Y. Heat injury prevention—a military perspective. J Strength Cond Res. 2012;26(Suppl 2):S82–6.
25. Costrini A. Emergency treatment of exertional heatstroke and comparison of whole body cooling techniques. Med Sci Sports Exerc. 1990;22(1):15–8.
26. McDermott BP, Casa DJ, O'Connor FG, Adams WB, Armstrong LE, Brennan AH, et al. Cold-water dousing with ice massage to treat exertional heat stroke: a case series. Aviat Space Environ Med. 2009;80(8):720–2.

27. Asplund CA, O'Connor FG. Challenging return to play decisions: heat stroke, exertional rhabdomyolysis, and exertional collapse associated with sickle cell trait. Sports Health. 2016;8(2):117–25.

28. American College of Sports Medicine. The team physician and return-to-play issues: a consensus statement. Med Sci Sports Exerc. 2002;34(7):1212–4.

29. McDermott BP, Casa DJ, Yeargin SW, Ganio MS, Armstrong LE, Maresh CM. Recovery and return to activity following exertional heat stroke: considerations for the sports medicine staff. J Sport Rehabil. 2007;16(3):163–81.

30. Mehta AC, Baker RN. Persistent neurological deficits in heat stroke. Neurology. 1970;20(4):336–40.

31. Royburt M, Epstein Y, Solomon Z, Shemer J. Long-term psychological and physiological effects of heat stroke. Physiol Behav. 1993;54(2):265–7.

32. Abriat A, Brosset C, Brégigeon M, Sagui E. Report of 182 cases of exertional heatstroke in the French Armed Forces. Mil Med. 2014;179(3):309–14.

33. Phinney LT, Gardner JW, Kark JA, Wenger CB. Long-term follow-up after exertional heat illness during recruit training. Med Sci Sports Exerc. 2001;33(9):1443–8.

34. Nelson DA, Deuster PA, O'Connor FG, Kurina LM. Timing and Predictors of Mild and Severe Heat Illness among New Military Enlistees. Med Sci Sports Exerc. 2018;50(8):1603–12.

35. O'Connor FG, Williams AD, Blivin S, Heled Y, Deuster P, Flinn SD. Guidelines for return to duty (play) after heat illness: a military perspective. J Sport Rehabil. 2007;16(3):227–37.

36. Kazman JB, Heled Y, Lisman PJ, Druyan A, Deuster PA, O'Connor FG. Exertional heat illness: the role of heat tolerance testing. Curr Sports Med Rep. 2013;12(2):101–5.

37. Kazman JB, Purvis DL, Heled Y, Lisman P, Atias D, Van Arsdale S, Deuster PA. Women and exertional heat illness: identification of gender specific risk factors. US Army Med Dep J. 2015:58–66.

38. Druyan A, Ketko I, Yanovich R, Epstein Y, Heled Y. Refining the distinction between heat tolerant and intolerant individuals during a heat tolerance test. J Therm Biol. 2013;38(8):539–42.

39. Keren G, Epstein Y, Magazanik A. Temporary heat intolerance in a heatstroke patient. Aviat Space Environ Med. 1981;52(2):116–7.

40. Hosokawa Y, Stearns RL, Casa DJ. Is heat intolerance state or trait? Sports Med. 2019;49(3):365–70.

41. O'Connor FG, Heled Y, Deuster PA. Exertional heat stroke, the return to play decision, and the role of heat tolerance testing: a clinician's dilemma. Curr Sports Med Rep. 2018;17(7):244–8.

42. Strydom NB. Acclimatization practices in the South African gold mining industry. J Occup Med. 1970;12(3):66–9.

43. Moran DS, Erlich T, Epstein Y. The heat tolerance test: an efficient screening tool for evaluating susceptibility to heat. J Sport Rehabil. 2007;16(3):215–21.

44. Schermann H, Heled Y, Fleischmann C, Ketko I, Schiffmann N, Epstein Y, Yanovich R. The validity of the heat tolerance test in prediction of recurrent exertional heat illness events. J Sci Med Sport. 2018;21(6):549–52.

45. O'Connor FG, Casa DJ, Bergeron MF, Carter R, et al. American College of Sports Medicine Roundtable on exertional heat stroke—return to duty/return to play: conference proceedings. Curr Sports Med Rep. 2010;9(5):314–21.

Chapter 11
Considerations for Road Race Medical Staff

John F. Jardine and William O. Roberts

There are approximately 38,400 road races from 5 K through marathon and beyond, in the United States each year [1]. In 2017, more than 18.3 million runners registered to participate in road races, with ages ranging from young children to 65-plus years old [1].

People run for general health and fitness reasons and benefit from lower blood pressure and body weight. Despite the health benefits of running, there are risks for injuries and medical conditions that may require medical intervention during and after road races. 86% of running races are commonly held in the spring, summer, and fall to encourage maximum participation, with novice runners and elite level athletes competing in the same race [1]. It is during these warm weather events that runners are at risk for exertional heat stroke and other problems of exercise in hot weather, especially during unexpectedly hot conditions.

While there is no formal governing body to mandate medical care for these events, on-site medical care should be considered for events with more than 1000 participants or smaller events when there is a known high number of medical encounters that could interrupt community access to the emergency medical system [2]. This chapter will discuss the organization of the medical team, staffing needs, specific protocols and procedures, adverse conditions, runner education, and the supplies needed for on-site health care at mass participation events.

J. F. Jardine (✉)
Korey Stringer Institute, University of Connecticut, Storrs, CT, USA

W. O. Roberts
Sports Medicine Program, Department of Family Medicine and Community Health, University of Minnesota, Minneapolis, MN, USA

© Springer Nature Switzerland AG 2020
W. M. Adams, J. F. Jardine (eds.), *Exertional Heat Illness*,
https://doi.org/10.1007/978-3-030-27805-2_11

Organization

Organizing a medical plan for an event requires a multidisciplinary team effort that includes the race administration, medical experts, community emergency medical services (EMS), and public safety personnel. The medical plan should address the health and safety of the athletes, spectators, and event staff on race day. Planning should focus on the common injuries and medical conditions that affect runners during distance running races. It is best to leave the multitude of medical emergencies typical in the general population that may occur during the race to the community emergency medicine services.

The team should be led by a medical director or directors, ideally a physician with an interest in road race and event medicine. The medical director should understand exercise physiology, interpretation and application of meteorological data, heat and cold illness reduction strategies, liability issues, and the evaluation and management of medical problems associated with endurance events in varying environments [3].

The duties of the medical director(s) include but are not limited to:

1. Recruit and supervise the medical personnel
2. Develop medical protocols for the common conditions expected for the event
3. Coordinate services with the local health-care provider(s), emergency medical services, and local public safety personnel
4. Ensure the supplies and equipment are available for all medical care areas (Table 11.1)
5. Prepare a medical informational manual for the medical team
6. Prepare a medical training program available to the medical team
7. Ensure the correct accreditation and/or licensure of the medical staff
8. Assist the event director in developing a budget for any medical needs
9. Compile all medical records created at the event
10. Prepare an after-event report for the event director [4]

Medical teams can be volunteer or paid; however, there are very few paid medical teams in road racing. The medical team is best organized in a unified command structure [5]. A chain of command establishes the responsibilities of the personnel involved and connects the medical personnel with the public safety assets in the community. The medical team should work closely with local emergency medical services (EMS) and health-care facilities to integrate within the community and reduce the impact on the community health care. Some events will reach the level of prominence that requires heightened security for participants, spectators, and staff, which may involve personnel from federal and state agencies as part of the health and safety plan for the event.

A communications system is a critical part of the race command structure and the medical team. The medical team must have communication with personnel along the course and in the finish area, as well as race officials, local EMS, and health-care facilities. A redundant system with mobile phones, hand held radios, and ham radios will reduce the risk of communications failure. Security services are critical for medical care areas, equipment storage, and supplies to avoid theft and tampering. Security on race day is essential to reduce unnecessary traffic through the medical area and to preserve runner confidentiality. A diagram depicting a recommended medical team structure is shown in Fig. 11.1 [6].

Table 11.1 Equipment required for medical care area

Patient transport	Stretchers
	Wheelchairs
Triage	Cots
	Thermometers (rectal)
	Blood pressure cuffs
	Stethoscopes
	Pulse oximeters
	Disposable gloves
Heat emergencies	Ice
	Immersion tubs
	Water
	Fans
	Towels
Hydration	Oral fluids
	Cups
	Intravenous (IV) fluids with IV start kits (catheters, etc.)
	Sharps container for needle disposal
	Handheld blood gas and electrolyte analyzer (e.g., i-STAT system; Abbott, Princeton NJ, USA)
	Salt/bouillon cubes
Sudden cardiac events	Automated external defibrillator (AED)
	Electrocardiogram (ECG) monitors
	Oxygen tanks/masks/cannulas
Musculoskeletal injuries	Elastic bandages
	Splints
	Plastic bags/ice packs
Wound care	Gauze bandages
	Tape
Medications	Benzodiazepine (midazolam, diazepam) for seizures
	Allergy kit (diphenhydramine) (EpiPen; Meridian Medical Technologies, Columbia, MD, USA)
	Metered-dose inhalers (MDIs) for asthma
	Advanced Cardiac Life Support (ACLS) medications
	Clipboards
	Pen

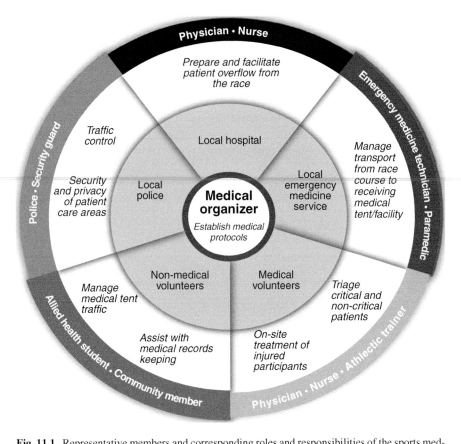

Fig. 11.1 Representative members and corresponding roles and responsibilities of the sports medicine team that are recommended to be included when organizing and executing a medical program at a mass participation event. (From Adams et al. [6], with permission)

The medical team should be easily identified on race day with T-shirts, jackets, vests, bibs, or caps. Credentials with the individual's name, level of training, and role should be worn by all volunteers. Medical care sites should be clearly identified and easily accessible to the runners.

The location of medical care areas along the racecourse is often determined by the geography of the course, the anticipated environmental conditions, and the number of participants involved. The Falmouth Road Race (11.4 km) that takes place every year in Falmouth (Cape Cod), Massachusetts, USA, in August, (https://falmouthroadrace.com/), with 12,000 runners, has 2 runners with exertional heat stroke (EHS) per 1000 participants that occur at or near the finish line [7]. The medical care areas must prepare to triage runners to find and accommodate at least 2 runners per 1000 participants who will have EHS (Fig. 11.2). There is often a constant flow of runners that cross the finish line, requiring the medical team to manage many patients simultaneously. (Observations over a 3-year period at this race show a rather predictable pattern of activity at the finish line medical tent (Fig. 11.3) [8]).

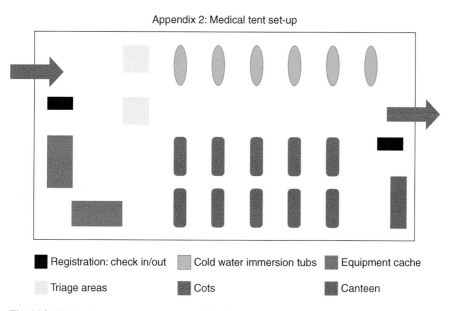

Appendix 2: Medical tent set-up

- ■ Registration: check in/out   ▢ Cold water immersion tubs   ▨ Equipment cache
- ▢ Triage areas   ▨ Cots   ▨ Canteen

Fig. 11.2 Medical tent setup at a mass participation sports event

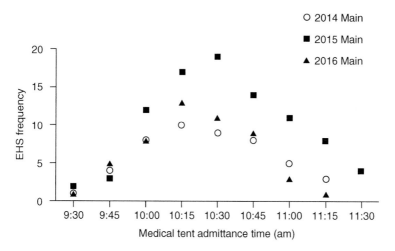

Fig. 11.3 Admittance of exertional heat stroke (EHS) patients to the medical tent and the number of cooling stations needed to effectively treat each patient, assuming that each patient required at least 20 min of cooling treatment and medical attention. The race started at 9:00 am (zero point in the *x* axis). (From Hosokawa et al. [8], with permission)

Longer-distance races will usually have medical care areas dispersed along the route. In very large mass participation events, a medical care area may be necessary at the start area with the entire field of runners confined to a relatively small area. Along the course, teams of at least two providers can be stationed at intervals along the route equipped with an AED, basic first-aid supplies, and a radio for communication with the course unified command center for dispatch of more advanced care. On course, teams may be stationary and on-foot or use bicycles, golf carts, or Gators to be mobile.

The major medical areas are placed at sites with the most medical encounters. For most road races, the demand for medical care will likely be at or near the finish line. The finish line medical care area is usually located downstream from the finish line at a geographically convenient site that has ambulance access. It is reasonable to allow a space of 50–100 m to allow runners to "catch their breath," but not so that it is difficult to transport collapsed runners to the medical tent [9].

Designated medical care areas along the course or at the finish area can be fixed or temporary structures depending on the location of the racecourse. Races that finish in a stadium or near a civic center or other large public building may utilize these fixed structures as medical care areas [10]. Otherwise, temporary structures such as tents or trailers may be used.

The geography of the course must be taken into consideration. It is important to have access to the runners and to have a clear egress for collapsed runner requiring transport to advanced medical care at the hospital. Long bridges, parkways, and limited access neighborhoods may present access challenges to the medical team. Train schedules may have to be altered to accommodate the course and can interfere with EMS response if roads are closed by trains passing through the race area. The Boston Marathon and Marine Corps Marathon in Washington, D.C., cross town and state borders, respectively, and require integrating several EMS jurisdictions into the medical plan. Determining mutual aid contingencies to assure continuous care between different jurisdictions is critical to runner safety. The central command model with integrated race protocols developed in advance of race day will allow the transition of care between regional EMS systems. Geographically isolated races may need to consider other evacuation methods such as watercraft or by air, but these methods can easily be limited by weather conditions and will need to be integrated into race cancelation protocols.

For all race venues, the majority of work for a safe and successful event is in the preparation phase leading up to the event. Planning for the medical coverage of a large-scale event should start months in advance. The medical director typically assembles a race medical operations committee to initiate pre-race planning. The medical personnel must be recruited and educated prior to the event. Volunteers not familiar with race medicine will need specific instruction to care for the common race maladies. The supplies and equipment needed to provide event-specific care must be obtained (see Table 11.1). The medical director(s) and medical operations team leads should work with the event coordinators to develop a budget that is sufficient to obtain the essential supplies and training for runner safety. The medical operations committee is responsible for developing a medical manual with protocols addressing common race medical problems for the medical team to review in advance of the race. A medical record is critical for accurate record keeping on race day; this forms the database that informs future races and is the legal record of care provided during the race. Local EMS, hospitals, and other health-care facilities should be aware of the event and the likely patient problems that may present from the event. It may be necessary for emergency departments to "staff up" so the potential influx of patients does not overload the emergency department (ED) and affect the care available to the community. Pre-planning in the unified command model involves the local EMS and public safety personnel, which ensures that routes to the local EDs affected by road closures or other detours are known in advance of the event.

Staffing

Staffing of on-site medical teams should include the personnel needed to care for the anticipated medical problems associated with the event. A combination of physicians, nurses, paramedics, emergency medical technicians (EMT), athletic trainers (AT), and physical therapists can address the usual medical problems. Nonmedically trained personnel are helpful as assistants for transporting runners, retrieving clothing, distributing food and drink, setting up and tearing down of the medical area, and recording patient information.

The number of participants and environmental conditions will determine the number of anticipated medical encounters, which in turn dictates the number of medical personnel needed for an event. The International Association of Athletics Federations (IAAF) has published competition medical guidelines with staffing recommendations that are useful for a new event, but the event historical data will drive the numbers for future races [11]:

Physicians	2–3 per 1000 runners
Nurses	4–6 per 1000 runners
Other professionals (EMT, AT, etc.)	4–6 per 1000 runners
Nonmedical (fetchers, scribes, etc.)	4–6 per 1000 runners

The fitness level of the participants may further influence staffing needs. An exclusively elite competition will utilize different resources than an event that has a mix of competitors from all ability levels, including first-time participants [5].

For warm weather events, the staffing and supply needs increase as the wet-bulb globe temperature reaches higher levels and both the number of medical encounters and race dropouts increase [12, 13]. A study done at the Falmouth Road Race found a clear relationship between the ambient temperature and humidity and the occurrence of EHS [14]. Weather conditions most accurately predict staffing needs, and the staff needed is better predicted when conditions and the number of runners are relatively stable from year to year. Staffing needs are most difficult to predict in spring and fall races where there can be wide swings in temperature and relative humidity. Medical encounters will usually be in the 2–3% of total participant range with this level rising to 5–8% when environmental conditions become more extreme [15]. It is best to staff for the worst-case scenario to best address runner safety in all conditions.

Protocols/Procedures

The medical problems that occur during road races are from three basic categories: life-threatening, self-limiting musculoskeletal, and skin-related conditions. Protocols for running races should address each area with an emphasis on recognizing and managing life-threatening conditions as the basis of an emergency action plan [15]. The type of medical care offered on-site is largely dependent on the resources and assets of the community. The life-threatening problems like sudden cardiac arrest can occur at any distance but tend to be more prevalent when the race field is older and male [16, 17]. Some problems like exercise associated hyponatremia are more common in longer distance and duration events, and exertional heat stroke is more common in unexpectedly hot conditions but can occur in cool conditions [18, 19]. Furthermore, the latter is usually most often seen in shorter races (10 k to half marathon distance), where metabolic heat production is typically greater due to the greater exercise intensity given the shorter distance covered. Most runner collapse in longer-distance races is easily managed with leg elevation and rest or active walking to keep the muscle pump of the lower extremity returning blood to the heart [20, 21]. This section will stress the recognition and management of conditions typically associated with warm weather events and the medical care for exertional heat illnesses.

A study by Rav Acha et al. reviewed six fatal cases of exertional heat stroke in the Israeli Defense Forces and found two factors that contributed to all six deaths [22]. The first was the absence of proper medical triage and clearly endorses the need for on-site medical care at high-risk road races. Runners suffering from exertional heat stroke must be rapidly identified and rapidly treated to prevent fatalities. The second factor was a physical effort that was not matched to physical fitness, which is synonymous with novice runners competing at a pace or intensity beyond their ability or attempting a personal best in hot conditions. Pre-planning is important to protect competitors at all levels.

When an athlete collapses or needs medical attention during or following a road race, rapid assessment for life-threatening conditions is critical, as life-threatening conditions require rapid intervention to preserve tissue. A triage system should be set up at the finish area and at each medical treatment area. Triage is typically done by experienced providers who are able to distinguish runners who need evaluation for life-threatening condition from runners who are fatigued from the run. Patients requiring acute medical care should be moved to the appropriate level of care. There is often a second level of triage in the medical care area that includes measuring vital signs, including a core temperature estimate, to determine the severity of illness. Core temperature is best estimated in field conditions by rectal thermometry, as other temperature measures to do not correlate well with core temperature in the field [23–25].

Patients presenting with hyperthermia, i.e., rectal temperature >40 °C (104 °F), must be assessed for exertional heat stroke (EHS). EHS is defined as central nervous system (CNS) changes with hyperthermia (>40 °C). CNS changes are often changes in mental status (e.g., confusion, disorientation, aggressive behavior, irritability, etc.) that can be missed if not carefully assessed. Any runner with a presumptive diagnosis of EHS requires rapid cooling. The gold standard for treating patients with EHS is cold-water immersion (CWI) [26]. Warm weather races with a potential for runners presenting with EHS should be prepared to treat EHS with CWI.

The medical plan should include the personnel (nurses, EMTs, ATs) for the cooling teams and have the equipment needed to immerse hyperthermic runners in tubs with ice and water mixture. The Falmouth Road Race and Boston Marathon currently use 50-gallon polyurethane stock tanks (Rubbermaid Mfr #: FG424300BLA, Agrimaster Mfr # 52110067GS; Rubbermaid Commercial Products/DB Industrial Supply, Saratoga Springs, NY, USA). Plastic kiddy pools are less expensive, but are less durable. The aforementioned tanks can adequately immerse the patient's torso, while keeping the head safely out of the water. Tanks filled with 30–40 gallons of water with 10 pounds of ice provide a cooling rate in the range of 0.22 °C/minute [26].

Reducing core body temperature in EHS patients is critical to survival. Although cold-water immersion is considered best practice for rapid cooling in EHS, there will be situations where stationary tubs for cold-water immersion are not available. Any cooling method should be initiated when tubs are not available. Rotating towels, tarp cooling, and cold-water dousing are acceptable field methods that provide satisfactory cooling rates and can be initiated at the site of collapse.

Rapidly rotated ice water-soaked towels applied sequentially to the extremities, trunk, and head can produce cooling rates similar to immersion [27]. A portable cooler with ice, water, and 6–8 towels may provide treatment to a hyperthermic runner within seconds of collapse. Rotating cold, wet towels every 2–3 minutes will begin the cooling process and may be adequate to reduce core temperature to safe levels. If cooling is not successful, immersion-cooling modality may be used if it is available.

Tarp-assisted cooling is another acceptable alternative that does not require a stationary location [28]. This requires a large sheet of waterproof fabric, water, and ice. Three or more persons hold the tarp to form a portable vessel into which is poured 20 gallons of water with 10 gallons of ice. The patient is immersed in the ice water with the persons holding the tarp oscillating the water to continually circulate the cold water.

Cold-water dousing, a modification of cold-water immersion, is another stationary method of cooling. The patient is placed on a porous stretcher over a large tub filled with ice water, and the cold water from the tub is continuously poured over the patient. This method is used at the Marine Corps Marathon and successfully cools runners with EHS [29].

The Falmouth Road Race Protocol

A specific protocol should be developed to direct the care and cooling strategy for runners with EHS at each event. The Falmouth Road Race protocol defines EHS as a rectal temperature >40 °C (104 °F) with CNS changes, which clearly identifies runners requiring CWI for rapid cooling. Runners are cooled to a safer temperature of 38.9 °C (102 °F) before being removed from the cooling tub (Figs. 11.4 and 11.5). Thermistors with flexible rectal probes (Fig. 11.6) are especially helpful to continuously record rectal temperatures and observe the active cooling rates. If thermistors are not available, patients can be cooled until they "wake up" and then repeat the rectal temperature measurement or have repeated rectal temperatures every 10 minutes until the target cooling temperature is reached. In some instances, some runners' rectal temperatures continue to drop following removal from cooling (i.e., hypothermic after drop); thus, it is essential that rectal temperature is continually monitored along with their cognitive function to determine if rewarming methods (e.g., bare hugger, blankets, moving runner out of the tent into the sun) are needed. Normothermic runners with clear cognitive function can be offered hydration and/or other nutrition by mouth. Runners who have been cooled and exhibit normal cognitive function with stable vital signs may be discharged to family and home. If there are questions regarding medical sequelae, the runner can be transported to the nearest emergency department (ED) for further evaluation. Runners with EHS should follow up with their personal physician within 2 days to monitor liver and kidney function.

Patients suffering from mild hyperthermia or hyperthermia without CNS changes may be identified by the triage process. Immersion is not indicated for these patients, but they should be provided with a cool area (shade, air-conditioned, etc.) for their care. These patients should be provided with fluids, usually by mouth, or intravenously if necessary. Physical therapists may be helpful in the care of these patients, especially with regards to painful muscle cramps. Protocols should be developed for these patients including disposition decisions.

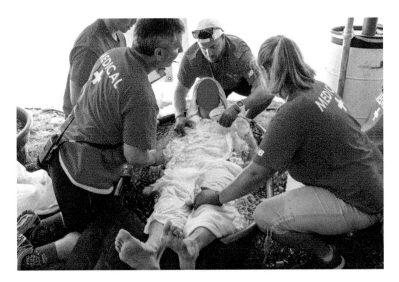

Fig. 11.4 A patient in the immersion tub at the Falmouth Road Race

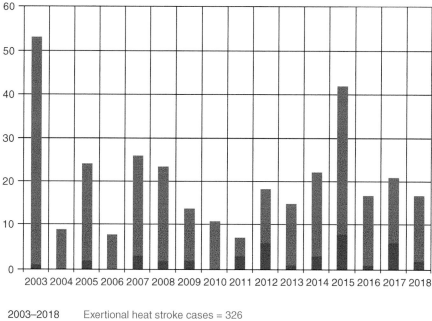

Exertional heat stroke at the falmouth road race

2003–2018 Exertional heat stroke cases = 326
EHS transported to the ED = 40

88% of EHS cases discharged from site

Fig. 11.5 Exertional heat stroke (EHS) in the Falmouth Road Race (2003–2018). EHS cases = 326; EHS transported to the local emergency department = 40. 88% of EHS cases discharged from site

Fig. 11.6 Small, light, transportable body temperature monitoring. (DataTherm II®; Geratherm Medical AG, Geschwenda, Germany)

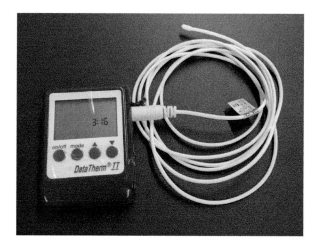

EHS protocols specific to each road race should be developed in conjunction with local EMS agencies to be sure there is agreement on the care protocol. It is critical that on-site cooling be completed before transferring an EHS victim unless the runner is unstable for other reasons. The "cool first, transport second" protocol [30] may not be in many local EMS protocols. EHS survival requires rapid cooling, and the road race EHS protocol may supersede the usual local EMS protocols on race day in the medical tent. It may be prudent to transfer a collapsed runner to a race medical care area equipped with CWI tubs in lieu of the local ED. In turn, the local ED(s) should be aware of this protocol but, at the same time, be prepared to receive EHS patients that may require rapid cooling. It is recommended, where possible, that EDs expecting to receive patients from a road race have CWI equipment available, and this should be communicated well in advance of race day.

Adverse Conditions

Weather patterns and trends in temperatures may help predict conditions on race day. Wet-bulb globe temperatures (WBGT) reflects the heat stress imposed on the participating athletes and should be measured along the course to help race administrators and participants with pace and competition decisions. WBGT should be used to guide the decision to start or continue the race [12]. Increasing WBGT is associated with increased EHS risk, especially if the participants are not acclimatized to the conditions [12]. Charts are available to guide decision-making with temperature ranges, but the ranges vary with the geographical location of the race and reflect the acclimatization of living in a specific region (Fig. 11.7).

The medical director(s) and the event director should determine the race cancelation parameters in advance of the event based on race data when available. Canceling a race before it starts is safer than canceling midrace as participants already on the course continue to run and may overload the race and community medical system [12].

Guidance for athletic trainers			
WBGT	Flag color	Level of risk	Comments
<18°C (<65°F)	Green	Low	Risk low but still exists on the basis or risk factors.
18–23°C (65–73°F)	Yellow	Moderate	Risk level increases as event progresses through the day.
23–28°C (73–82°F)	Red	High	Everyone should be aware of injury potential: individuals at risk should not compete.
>28°C (82°F)	Black	Extreme or hazardous	Consider rescheduling or delaying the event until safer conditions prevail: if the event must take place. be on high alert.

Fig. 11.7 Example of guidance for athletic trainers. WBGT (wet-bulb globe temperature)

Races may employ a flag system or electronic sign boards positioned along the course to warn runners of dangerously high WBGT readings and increasing heat stress.

Education of Runners

Pre-race runner education is an underutilized modality to reduce heat illness associated with warm weather events. Runners should be informed of heat stress precautions and race protocols including the process of race day weather data distribution in their race registration materials. Lack of heat acclimatization may predispose runners to EHS and heat acclimatization recommendations should be included with the educational materials. This is especially important for competitors coming from cooler climates to compete in locations with higher ambient temperature or relative humidity than where they reside [5]. Acclimatization challenges may still occur when there are unusually hot conditions on race day. This is especially true in Spring (Boston), and Fall (Chicago) marathons that are typically preceded by several weeks of cooler weather [12].

Informational videos may be used to educate runners about heat illness. Falmouth Road Race, for example, has produced a heat education video that is used for race entrants. A study of this video had runners take a pre-video survey to assess their knowledge of heat acclimatization, hydration, and heat illnesses. After watching the 5-minutes video on heat safety and hydration strategies to optimize running performance and safety in the heat, the runners' post-video surveys showed an increased understanding of these principles [31]. Embedding this video into the registration process would expose all runners to the concepts of heat safety and potentially prevent a severe medical emergency.

References

1. Running USA. 2018 National Runner Survey. https://www.runningusa.org/.
2. De Lorenzo RA. Mass gathering medicine: a review. Prehosp Disaster Med. 1997;12(1):68–72.
3. Armstrong LE, Epstein Y, Greenleaf JE, Haymes EM, Hubbard RW, Roberts WO, Thompson PD. American College of Sports Medicine position stand. Heat and cold illnesses during distance running. Med Sci Sports Exerc. 1996;28(12):i–x. Review.
4. American College of Sports Medicine. Mass participation event management for the team physician: a consensus statement. Med Sci Sports Exerc. 2004;36(11):2004–8.
5. Yao KV, Troyanos C, D'Hemecourt P, Roberts WO. Optimizing marathon race safety using an incident command post strategy. Curr Sports Med Rep. 2017;16(3):144–9.
6. Adams WM, Hosokawa Y, Troyanos C, Jardine JF. Organization and execution of on-site health care during a mass participation event. Athl Train Sports Health Care. 2018;10(3):101–4.
7. DeMartini JK, Casa DJ, et al. Effectiveness of cold water immersion in the treatment of exertional heat stroke at the Falmouth Road Race. Med Sci Sports Exerc. 2014;47(2):240–5.
8. Hosokawa Y, Adams WM, Belval LN, Davis RJ, Huggins RA, Jardine JF, et al. Exertional heat illness incidence and on-site medical team preparedness in warm weather. Int J Biometeorol. 2018;62(7):1147–53.
9. Roberts WO. Management of mass participation events. In: Madden C, Putukian M, McCarty E, Young C, editors. Netter's sports medicine: the team physician's handbook. 2nd ed. Philadelphia PA: Elsevier; 2017. p. 736–43.

10. Cianca JC, Roberts WO. Distance running events: medical coverage. In: Wilder RP, O'Connor FG, Magrum EM, editors. Running medicine. 2nd ed. Monterey, CA: Healthy Learning; 2014.
11. International Association of Athletics Federations. IAAF Competition Medical Guidelines: A practical guide. Jan 2013. Monaco: IAAF. https://www.friidrett.no/globalassets/aktivitet/dommer/annet-materiell/iaaf-competition-medical-guidelines.pdf. Accessed 8 Jun 2019.
12. Roberts WO. Determining a "do not start" temperature for a marathon on the basis of adverse outcomes. Med Sci Sports Exerc. 2010;42(2):226–32.
13. Roberts WO. Heat and cold: what does the environment do to marathon injury? Sports Med. 2007;37(4–5):400–3.
14. DeMartini JK, Casa DJ, Belval LN, Crago A, Davis RJ, Jardine JJ, Stearns RL. Environmental conditions and the occurrence of exertional heat illnesses and exertional heat stroke at the Falmouth Road Race. J Athl Train. 2014;49(4):478–85.
15. Nguyen RB, Milsten AM, Cushman JT. Injury patterns and levels of care at a marathon. Prehosp Disaster Med. 2008;23(6):519–25.
16. Drezner J, Courson R, Roberts WO, Mosesso V, Link M, Maron B. Inter-Association Task Force recommendations on emergency preparedness and management of sudden cardiac arrest in high school and college athletic programs: a consensus statement. J Athl Train. 2007;42(1):143–58.
17. Kim JH, Malhotra R, Chiampas G, d'Hemecourt P, Troyanos C, Cianca J, et al.; Race Associated Cardiac Arrest Event Registry (RACER) Study Group. Cardiac arrest during long-distance running races. N Engl J Med. 2012;366(2):130–40.
18. Roberts WO, Roberts DM, Lunos S. Marathon related cardiac arrest risk differences in men and women. Br J Sports Med. 2013;47(3):168–71.
19. Roberts WO. Exertional heat stroke during a cool weather marathon: a case study. Med Sci Sports Exerc. 2006;38(7):1197–202.
20. Roberts WO. Exercise-associated collapse care matrix in the marathon. Sports Med. 2007;37(4–5):431–3.
21. Asplund CA, O'Connor FG, Noakes TD. Exercise-associated collapse: an evidence-based review and primer for clinicians. Br J Sports Med. 2011;45(14):1157–62.
22. Rav-Acha M, Hadad E, Epstein Y, et al. Fatal exertional heat stroke: a case series. Am J Med Sci. 2004;328(2):84–7.
23. Ronneberg K, Roberts WO, McBean AD, Center BA. Temporal artery and rectal temperature measurements in collapsed marathon runners. Med Sci Sports Exerc. 2008;40(8):1373–5.
24. Armstrong LE, Maresh CM, Crago AE, Adams R, Roberts WO. Interpretation of aural temperatures during exercise, hyperthermia, and cooling therapy. Med Exerc Nut Health. 1994;3(1):9–16.
25. Roberts WO. Assessing core temperature in collapsed athletes: choosing the best method. Physician Sportsmed. 1994;22(8):49–59.
26. Casa DJ, McDermott BP, Lee EC, Yeargin SW, Armstrong LE, Maresh CM. Cold water immersion: the gold standard for exertional heat stroke treatment. Exerc Sport Sci Rev. 2007;35(3):141–9. Review.
27. McDermott BP, Casa DJ, Ganio MS, Lopez RM, Yeargin SW, Armstrong LE, Maresh CM. Acute whole-body cooling for exercise-induced hyperthermia: a systematic review. J Athl Train. 2009;44(1):84–93.
28. Hosokawa Y, Adams WM, Belval LN, Vandermark LW, Casa DJ. Tarp-assisted cooling as a method of whole-body cooling in hyperthermic individuals. Ann Emerg Med. 2017;69(3):347–52.
29. McDermott BP, Casa DJ, O'Connor FG, Adams WB, Armstrong LE, Brennan AH, et al. Cold-water dousing with ice massage to treat exertional heat stroke: a case series. Aviat Space Environ Med. 2009;80(8):720–2.
30. Casa DJ, Armstrong LE, Kenny GP, O'Connor FG, Huggins RA. Exertional heat stroke: new concepts regarding cause and care. Curr Sports Med Rep. 2012;11(3):115–23. Review.
31. Hosokawa Y, Johnson EN, Jardine JF, Stearns RL, Casa DJ. Knowledge and belief toward heat safety and hydration strategies among runners: a preliminary evaluation. J Athl Train. 2019;54(5):541–9. https://doi.org/10.4085/1062-6050-520-17.

Chapter 12
Climate Change and Heat Exposure: Impact on Health in Occupational and General Populations

Glen P. Kenny, Sean R. Notley, Andreas D. Flouris, and Andrew Grundstein

Introduction

While human health has always been affected by climate and weather, the rise in global temperature caused by climate change is considered the greatest threat to health of the twenty-first century. Recently, the United Nation's Intergovernmental Panel on Climate Change (IPCC) warned that the earth is already 1 °C warmer than preindustrial levels and is in danger of reaching or exceeding an increase of 1.5 °C in the coming years [1]. Of greatest concern is that even small elevations from summer average temperatures can result in illness and death and every fraction of additional warming beyond current levels would dramatically worsen these effects. Indeed, days hotter than the seasonal average can reduce functional ability [2, 3], quality of life (including sleep quality) [4, 5], mental fatigue [5], and thermal comfort [5–7] and even result in death. However, since dynamic interactions between extreme heat events and population vulnerability occur, it can be difficult to quantify the complete effects of extreme heat on human health.

Countries around the world are entering unchartered territory as the periods of extreme heat are predicted to be more frequent and five times more deadly in the

G. P. Kenny (✉) · S. R. Notley
Human and Environmental Physiology Research Unit, School of Human Kinetics, University of Ottawa, Ottawa, ON, Canada
e-mail: gkenny@uottawa.ca

A. D. Flouris
FAME Laboratory, Department of Exercise Science, University of Thessaly, Karies, Trikala, Greece

A. Grundstein
Department of Geography, University of Georgia, Athens, GA, USA

© Springer Nature Switzerland AG 2020
W. M. Adams, J. F. Jardine (eds.), *Exertional Heat Illness*,
https://doi.org/10.1007/978-3-030-27805-2_12

next decade [8]. It is an ominous sign of what increasing temperatures portend for the most vulnerable – children, older adults, those who are chronically ill, the socially disadvantaged, and workers in various occupational settings. In parallel, most industrialized countries are faced with an aging population [9] and work-force [10], which is coupled with a concurrent rise in the prevalence of chronic health conditions linked to heat vulnerability [9, 11]. The reasons for concern are plenty as extreme heat causes some of the highest death tolls among all natural weather hazards [12, 13] dramatically increasing short-term mortality in vulnerable populations [14, 15].

Extreme heat is a "silent" killer because it's not a visible threat. Heat stress is created by the combined heat load from the environment (higher ambient temperatures increase the requirements for the body to dissipate heat, while increased ambient humidity restricts heat loss via sweat evaporation), clothing (restricts heat loss), and heat generated from metabolic processes (increases in metabolic rate augments the heat produced by the body and thus rate that heat must be dissipated) [16, 17]. The resulting physiological, psychophysical, and performance effects characterize the heat strain response. Excessive heat stress can result in performance decrements and multiple physiological adjustments that can lead to a range of deleterious health effects, including heat stroke, heat exhaustion, dehydration and chronic kidney diseases, and, if left unchecked, death [18]. Moreover, it can lead to a worsening of cardiovascular [19, 20] and respiratory diseases, diabetes-related conditions, mental health degradation, and cognitive impairment [21, 22] as well as a reduction in well-being [23, 24]. Prolonged exposure to hot environments is associated with increased hospital admissions for cardiovascular, kidney, and respiratory disorders. Exposures to high minimum temperatures may also reduce the ability of the human body to recover from high daily maximum temperatures further complicating heat-related health problems [5].

In addition to the dramatic effects on population morbidity and mortality, heat-related health effects have economic consequences through incurred medical treatment and healthcare costs and loss of work productivity [25]. While the economic impacts of heat on human health are significant, they are difficult to accurately quantify [26]. Conservative estimates indicate that countries will face billions in additional healthcare costs and may place an unsurmountable strain on healthcare systems worldwide [26–28]. This is because the excess morbidity and mortality caused by extreme heat events are associated with increased ambulance call-outs, emergency department visits, and hospitalizations [29]. Between 2000 and 2009, extreme heat events resulted in nearly US$5.4 billion in additional healthcare costs in the United States [27] (representing 37% of the $14 billion in healthcare costs associated with climate change-related events including infectious disease outbreaks, hurricanes, wildfire, floods, etc.). The total health cost associated with a single 2-week (July 15–August 1, 2006) heat wave in California was estimated at US$5.4 billion [29]. In Canada, it is estimated that the impact on provincial healthcare systems and society in general would exceed CDN$33 billion over the next 50 years with an estimated associated additional 20,000 deaths due to rising temperatures [28]. For industry, persistently reduced labor productivity may be one of the largest economic impacts of rising temperatures (2.6% productivity loss per extra degree above 25 °C [30], 2–3% decrease in income per capita per °C above average yearly temperatures [31, 32]). The first quantitative estimates of the economic cost of excessive heat at work, reducing labor productivity, would be approximately US$2 trillion globally in 2030 [30]. With the predicted increase in global temperatures, a concomitant rise in adverse health outcomes can be expected which may subsequently burden the already overloaded and budget-constrained healthcare system [33]. Taken together, these outcomes underline a critical role for ambitious adaptation.

International experience suggests appropriate public health programs (e.g., heat-health warnings and heat action plans) can protect the health and well-being of individuals and greatly limit heat-related mortality [34–36] and can translate to substantial economic savings especially for large metropolitan cities [37]. However, their success requires that policy makers, frontline clinical staff, health managers, and others have comprehensive knowledge of factors affecting heat-vulnerable populations [34], which is currently lacking. Moreover, existing guidelines adopted and recommended for use by government agencies worldwide (e.g., WHO, CDC, others) to protect the public and workers also assumes a "one size fits all" approach to protect human health. These guidelines generally prescribe protective measures (e.g., heat advisories, exposure limits) using models defined by the assessment of heat strain in young and or relatively healthy adults. They fail to consider key factors such as sex, age, health status, and other factors, which can markedly alter a person's tolerance to heat, thereby leaving a large segment of the population under-protected (see section "Basic Overview of Temperature Regulation" for detailed information). For instance, recent studies show that the body's response to heat is impaired in healthy adults as young as 40 years [38]. This impairment is worse in women [39–43] and in older adults [44–48], especially in those with health conditions [49]. In these individuals, heat tolerance is reduced as the body is unable to cool itself via the evaporation of sweat, placing them at increased risk of heat-induced illnesses or death. Furthermore, in their current form, protective measures are primarily defined by heat-related mortality data and/or sociodemographic, environmental (ambient temperature), and territorial (neighborhood building density, dwelling type, location, others) data. They do not however consider the level of heat stress where physiologic vulnerability may occur which represents a critical shortcoming.

A warmer future is projected to lead to marked increases in future mortality worldwide. Currently, about 30% of the world's population currently experiences at least 20 days per year of extreme heat conditions that can be considered deadly [50], and it is expected that by the year 2100, three out of four people could be subject to this same threat. Consequently, the need to define appropriate heat action plans to protect human health is therefore paramount. To increase our readiness and ability to protect people during extreme heat events, we must continue building our understanding of the physiological factors that contribute to increased heat vulnerability. In this review, we examine the consequence of the anthropogenic rise in global temperatures on human health. This includes an evaluation of the cause-and-effect relationships between the thermal environment and the body's physiological capacity to dissipate heat. Additionally, we assess how physiological adaptations, behavioral adjustments, and the implementation of heat management (e.g., work exposure limits, others) and monitoring strategies can play a role in mediating an individual's susceptibility to heat stress. Finally, we discuss current initiatives and approaches to create communities and industries resilient to climate change and protect the public and workers against the projected rise in temperatures.

Climate Change and Rising Temperatures

There is strong undisputable evidence that human activities, especially the emission of greenhouse gases, are changing the climate [1]. Variations in environmental factors such as temperature or humidity affect heat stress and have important consequences for human health, safety, and productivity. The following section will discuss observed changes in climate that may affect heat stress as well as forecasts of climate in the mid to late twenty-first century.

Environmental Factors Influencing Heat Stress

Four environmental factors influence heat stress in humans – air temperature, radiant heat, humidity, and air movement [51]. Based on these environmental factors, a number of indices have been developed to estimate the thermal stress faced by an individual [51]. The indices can range from direct measures of environmental variables such as the wet-bulb globe temperature [52] to those that are based on the heat balance equation such as the apparent temperature/heat index or Universal Thermal Climate Index (UTCI) [53, 54]. A common feature among all the indices is the use of ambient air temperature and humidity as input parameters [50]. This is particularly relevant given that temperature and humidity are the most critical weather variables for predicting lethal heat events [50]. Sherwood and Huber [55] developed a physiological upper limit for humans using the wet-bulb temperature, which incorporates humidity and air temperature. They showed that values in excess of 35 °C for prolonged periods of time would make it physiologically impossible for humans to maintain heat balance.

Observed Changes in Climate Related to Heat Stress

Climate change is contributing to more frequent, severe, and more prolonged temperature extremes paralleled by elevated minimum (nighttime) temperatures. Global average temperatures have increased by approximately 1.0 °C over the 1901–2016 period, and 20 of the warmest years on record occur over the past 22 years [1]. Not only are mean temperatures increasing but extreme temperature events are becoming more common. Already, successive days of extreme heat have increased in frequency, length, and intensity in large parts of Europe, Asia, and Australia [56]. In Western Europe, for example, the length of intense heat waves has doubled between 1880 and 2003 and is paralleled by a 40% increase in heat wave frequency [57]. A study of 217 urban areas across the globe showed that almost half have experienced significant increases in the number of extreme hot days (above 99th percentile) and almost two-thirds of the cities had significant increases in peak nighttime temperatures over the 1973–2012 period [58].

The effects of the most lethal heat waves are due to not only high temperatures but also the effects of humidity [50]. The co-occurrence of consecutive hot and humid days during a heat wave can strongly affect human health. Normally, the body can cool itself through sweating, but when humidity is high, heat loss via the evaporation of sweat is restricted, potentially leading to heat exhaustion or heat stroke and, if left unchecked, death. While the effect of anthropogenic climate change on humidity is more complex than it is on temperature, climate model projections suggest that the effect of humidity at a 1.5 °C global warming will amplify the effect of extreme heat events [59].

Many studies have examined the integrated effect of temperature and humidity on heat stress using indices such as the apparent temperature/heat index or wet-bulb globe temperature [52, 53]. While there are differences in the computation of these indices, they all behave in a similar manner for combinations of high air temperature and humidity [60]. Regional studies, such as those in the United States, Australia, and India, show increasing trends in measures that incorporate temperature and humidity (e.g., apparent temperature/heat index, equivalent temperature) over time [61–65]. More broadly, positive trends in wet-bulb globe temperature (WBGT) [66, 67] and heat index [68] have been observed across most, although not all, regions of the world.

Future Climate Scenarios and Heat Stress

Climate model projections of future temperature extremes can be combined with the estimated relationships between temperatures and health in order to assess how deaths and illnesses resulting from extreme heat events can change in the future [69]. The projections are typically presented as a range of possible scenarios to capture the uncertainty of human activities in greenhouse gas emissions. For instance, one scenario might assume no attempts to limit greenhouse gas emissions and very high greenhouse gas concentrations in the future, while others assume lower greenhouse gas levels in response to active mitigation measures. Projections are also typically made for multi-decadal periods in the middle twenty-first century (e.g., 2040–2079) or late twenty-first century (e.g., 2070–2099).

Global surface mean temperatures are predicted to increase relative to the 1986–2005 period between 0.3 °C and 0.7 °C in the middle of the twenty-first century and from as low as 0.3 °C up to 4.8 °C in the late twenty-first century, with larger temperature increases for scenarios assuming greater greenhouse gas accumulations [1]. The warming is not uniform across global land surface areas, however, with greater warming in arctic regions [1]. A continuation of the trend toward more frequent, longer, and more intense extreme heat events is expected across the globe in the twenty-first century [70, 71].

Beyond temperature, several studies have identified integrated variables that affect the human comfort, health, and productivity/performance. Mora et al. [50] determined thresholds in temperature and humidity that historically led to increased mortality and examined them in the context of low, moderate, and high greenhouse gas emission scenarios (i.e., representative concentration pathway (RCP) 2.6, 4.5, 8.5) by 2100. Between 48% and 74% of human population as currently distributed will be exposed to ≥20 days in excess of the lethal threshold, depending on the scenario. Further, higher latitudes will undergo more warming than tropical regions, but the humid tropical areas will be disproportionally exposed to more days with deadly climatic conditions. This is because humid tropical areas have year-round warmer temperatures and higher humidity, thus requiring less warming to exceed the deadly threshold. Taking this one step further, Sherwood and Huber [55] identified how climate change may push many areas toward the physiological limit of environmental conditions (wet-bulb temperature ≥35 °C). They note a 7 °C warming, a high-end scenario by 2100, would create small zones that would be uninhabitable and a 11–12 °C warming which may be possible by 2300 would expand these areas to encompass the majority of human population as it is currently distributed.

It is without question that climate change will increase heat stress across the globe, affecting public health, labor productivity, and leisure activities such as sports. The future impacts on people will be determined by human attempts to mitigate greenhouse gas emissions and adaptive behaviors. Greater mitigation of greenhouse gas emissions will reduce future warming and therefore heat stress. In addition, factors such as physiological adaptation to heat, relocation to cooler environments, and changes in labor intensities will all modulate the influence of increased warming upon humans.

Basic Overview of Temperature Regulation

To maintain the *milieu intérieur* (a stable internal environment), humans strive to regulate body temperature within a narrow range. This requires a balance between the heat produced from metabolic processes and the heat exchanged between the body and surrounding environment. Those heat exchanges occur passively and are actively driven by behavioral (e.g., application or removal of clothing) and autonomic effector mechanisms (vasomotion, sudomotion, and thermogenesis). In this section, attention will be directed to the challenges associated with body temperature regulation during rest and physical activity in the heat, with specific emphasis on the inter- and intraindividual factors that can influence autonomic effector function, and, thus, one's physiological capacity to dissipate heat.

Thermoregulation During Rest and Physical Activity in Hot Environments

As dictated by the *First Law of Thermodynamics*, the thermal energy within any open system, including the body, will remain constant only when the energy (heat) entering and exiting that system is equal. Therefore, for body temperature to be stable, body heat storage must be zero. This requires a balance between metabolic heat production, which represents the difference between the heat produced from metabolic processes (i.e., metabolic rate) and the heat released during external work, and the dry (convection, radiation, conduction) and evaporative heat exchanges occurring between the body and surrounding environment [17]. Those heat exchanges obey the *Second Law of Thermodynamics*, whereby heat transfer occurs as a function of the thermal- (dry) and water-vapor pressure gradients (evaporative) between the skin and surroundings environment. Dry-heat exchange is therefore bidirectional, with dry-heat loss occurring when a positive thermal gradient exists between the skin surface and surrounding environment, while dry-heat gain takes place when there is a negative thermal gradient. It follows that the heat released (~2.426 kJ) [72] during the evaporation of sweat forms the primary avenue for heat dissipation when the ambient temperature exceeds that of the skin (i.e., promoting dry-heat gain) [73], with the rate of sweat evaporation being determined by the water-vapor pressure gradient between the skin and the ambient air, as well as the skin temperature and airflow across the skin. While convective and evaporative heat losses can also occur from the respiratory tract, those heat exchanges contribute minimally to human heat balance during physical activity in the heat [74]. As such, the total (net) rate of heat loss may be quantified in such conditions as the sum of dry and evaporative heat exchange.

During resting heat exposure or when performing physical activity in hot environments, the combined metabolic (i.e., metabolic heat production) and environmental heat load (i.e., dry-heat gain occurring when the ambient temperature is greater than that of the skin) initially exceeds that of total heat loss. This causes a positive change in body heat storage and a subsequent rise in body temperature [17]. Thermoreceptors, which are located in the skin, muscle and throughout deeper-body structures [75, 76], contain a high density of thermally sensitive neurons that detect these temperature changes [77]. Thermoafferent feedback from these receptors is integrated in the central nervous system (preoptic anterior hypothalamus), triggering one or more effector mechanisms to restore heat balance [78]. The most powerful of those thermoeffectors is of behavioral origin [79], including moving to a cooler location, pacing work effort, removal of clothing, etc. However, since we are either unwilling or unable to make such behavioral adjustments (e.g., during competition, work, etc.), in many instances, we rely upon autonomic thermoeffector responses of cutaneous vasodilation (vasomotion) and eccrine sweating (sudomotion) to facilitate heat loss. The resulting elevations in cutaneous blood flow facilitate the convective heat transfer from deep-body structures to the skin surface to buffer dry-heat gain and increase the cutaneous water-vapor pressure gradient for evaporation when the surrounding environment is hotter than the skin surface [80], while increases in sweat secretion promote evaporative cooling.

Under thermally compensable conditions, where changes in cutaneous blood flow and sweating can facilitate the total heat loss (dry ± evaporative heat exchange) required to attain heat balance, heat storage will return to zero and body temperature will stabilize following ~30–60 min of continuous heat exposure or physical activity [48, 73]. However, during exposure to more extreme heat or when performing more intense physical activity, the rate of total heat loss required to maintain heat balance often cannot be achieved, due either to limitations in the body's physiological capacity to dissipate heat and/or due restrictions in the maximal rate of heat loss that may be achieved (e.g., humid environments that prevent sweat evaporation) [81]. In these uncompensable states, heat storage and body temperature will continue to rise as heat exposure or exercise continues, leading to heat-related illnesses and even death [82]. This is often the case for workers employed in physically demanding occupations (e.g., construction, firefighting, agriculture, electrical utilities), who commonly operate in hot, humid environments with substantial solar/radiation load [23, 83–85]. Further, to protect from other exogenous heat sources (e.g., fire, hot machinery) and noxious gases or materials, many occupations necessitate the use of heavy and often impermeable and/or highly insulated protective clothing systems. Such clothing can exacerbate heat strain and cause more rapid rises in body temperature by (i) causing movement restriction that increases the metabolic demands of manual work [86–88] and (ii) creating a hot, humid microclimate around the worker that increases dry-heat gain and impedes sweat evaporation [89–91].

Heat exposure and work and/or physical activity in the heat represent a challenge not only to thermoregulation but also to blood pressure and body fluid regulation. In such conditions, cardiac output often exceeds metabolic demand to support thermoregulatory increases in cutaneous blood flow [92, 93]. The resulting elevations in cutaneous blood flow cause increases in venous volume that reduce cardiac filling pressure and cardiopulmonary (low pressure) baroreceptor unloading. To maintain mean arterial pressure, compensatory elevations in sympathetic activity occur to increase cardiac contractility and heart rate, while blood volume from inactive skeletal muscle and visceral structures (e.g., liver and splanchnic regions) is redistributed centrally [94]. That cardiovascular strain can be exacerbated when sweat losses cannot be matched by fluid intake during prolonged heat stress, and dehydration-induced reductions in plasma volume (hemoconcentration) cause plasma hypertonicity (hypertonic, hypovolemia), which further reduces central venous and mean arterial pressures [95]. Progressive dehydration has also been shown to attenuate sweat secretion [96] and elicit a 0.2–0.4 °C increase in body core temperature for every 1% of body mass lost from fluid [97, 98]. Unsurprisingly, dehydration is a key factor predisposing workers and the general population to heat-related illness [82].

Inter- and Intraindividual Determinants of Heat Strain

As with many physiological processes, there is extensive individual variability in one's heat strain response to a given heat stress. This is due, in large part, to the numerous interindividual factors (e.g., age, sex, chronic disease, others) and intraindividual factors both within (e.g., alcohol and medication use, fitness, acclimation and hydration state, others) and beyond an individual's control (e.g., exposure duration, illness, others), which can modulate heat exchange and, thus, influence heat strain [18, 99]. Some individuals may therefore better tolerate heat stress, while others may develop heat-related illness even in temperate conditions. For this reason, it is fundamentally important to understand how these individual factors and their interactive effects may modulate heat strain.

Perhaps the largest source of individual variation in thermoregulatory function arises from characteristics that differ among individuals. Over the past two decades, we have made significant advancements in our understanding of the interindividual factors that can modulate whole-body heat exchange during both rest and physical activity in the heat. Specific efforts have been made to isolate the effects of the interindividual factor in question by accounting for secondary factors known to modulate heat exchange that also differ among the individuals being studied. This is performed either using statistical procedures or by studying homogeneous subject groups who differ primarily in the factor of interest. Using these approaches, we now know that multiple interindividual factors (e.g., age, sex, body morphology, aerobic fitness, and chronic disease, among others) can independently influence whole-body heat exchange during rest and physical activity in the heat [38, 41, 42, 44, 45, 47–49, 100–104]. Further, those studies have revealed that the effects of many of such factors display a heat-load dependency, modulating heat exchange to a greater extent at higher exercise-induced heat loads. While a detailed discussion of each of these interindividual factors is beyond the scope of this communication and can be found in other reports [99], our current state of knowledge on the interindividual factors that can modulate heat exchange and the exercise-induced heat load at which those differences occur is summarized in Fig. 12.1.

In addition to these interindividual factors, individual variation in thermoregulatory function during heat stress can arise from day-to-day and within-day variation changes both within (e.g., including acclimation and hydration state and caffeine, alcohol, and medication use, among others) and beyond a person's control (e.g., heat exposure duration, acute illness, consecutive work shifts, shift duration, and illness, among others). For instance, it is well established that repeated heat exposure or exercise in hot environments can confer thermoregulatory adaptations [105], with these changes being recently shown to enhance whole-body evaporative heat loss as a function of the exercise-induced heat load, and thus, markedly reduce body heat storage during exercise in the heat [106, 107]. Conversely, during exercise-heat stress, fluid consumption that is insufficient to offset sweat losses can result in hypohydration, which can exacerbate body heat storage by attenuating sweat production, and thus, whole-body evaporative heat loss [108]. Further, workers in many industries (e.g., mining, electric utilities, others) often perform consecutive days of prolonged (~10–12 hours), strenuous work in the heat. These conditions cause

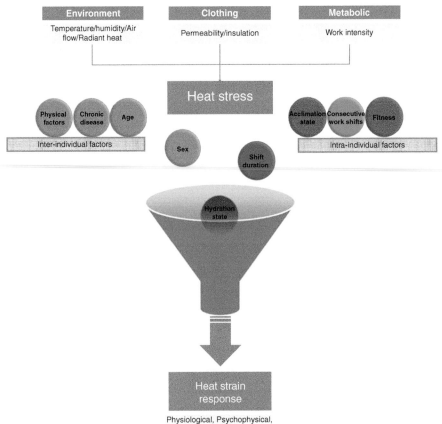

Fig. 12.1 A summary of the potential sources of heat stress, the resulting effects of that heat stress (i.e., heat strain) and the interindividual factors (*green circles*) and intraindividual factors both within (*red circles*) and beyond (*blue circles*) the individual's control that may modify an individual's response to a given level of heat stress. Heat stress represents the combined heat load from the environment, clothing, and heat generated from metabolic processes, while the resulting physiological, psychophysical, and performance effects characterize the heat strain response. Excessive and/or prolonged heat strain can progress to heat-related illness or death without appropriate monitoring

considerable heat strain [84], which can cause carry-over effects that impair whole-body heat loss, and, thus, exacerbate body heat storage and the resulting changes in heat strain in older adults on the next work day [109], with those effects potentially worsening over two or more work days [110]. However, while we have markedly improved our understanding of these intraindividual factors over recent years, we know relatively little about the independent effects of other common factors during heat exposure or physical activity in the heat, including sleep deprivation and alcohol and medication use, among others. Given that many of those factors have been shown to modulate local heat loss responses of skin blood flow and sweating [111–113], examining the integrated effects of these changes on whole-body heat exchange and body heat storage represents an important area of future research.

Up until this point, emphasis has been directed to the inter- and intraindividual factors known to independently modulate whole-body heat exchange when examined in isolation. While that research has improved our understanding of the independent effects of those factors, we possess only limited knowledge of the interactive effects of multiple inter- and/or intraindividual factors. Such interactions may exert an additive effect on heat strain, while others may reduce the additional heat strain associated with a given factor. For instance, it is known that sedentary middle-aged adults display age-related reductions in whole-body evaporative heat loss relative to young adults, whereas aerobically trained middle-aged adults display a similar capacity to dissipate heat compared to their young counterparts [44]. As another example, recent work has demonstrated that sweat-induced hypohydration (~4% body mass loss) causes marked reductions in evaporative heat dissipation (via sweating), likely to conserve fluid to support blood pressure regulation [114], which exacerbate body heat storage during exercise-induced heat stress in in young, but not older adults [108]. Since both the general and working population are heterogeneous for multiple interindividual factors, improving our understanding of the interactive effects of these intraindividual factors is critical for explaining individual variation in heat exchange and the resulting changes in heat strain during heat exposure and physical activity in the heat.

Heat and Impact on Population Health

High ambient heat has been associated with adverse impacts on health which include a worsening of preexisting health conditions (e.g., cardiovascular, respiratory, and renal illnesses; diabetes; mental health issues). Due to an insufficient ability to thermoregulate, children are particularly vulnerable during extreme heat events. The degree to which people are negatively affected by an extreme heat event is to a large extent dependent on the frequency and duration of heat of the event. Moreover, the severity and extent of health effects associated with extreme heat events are unique to the human, societal, and environmental circumstances at the time and location where the heat event occurs. This complex set of factors can moderate or exacerbate health outcomes and vulnerability in the affected people and communities.

Having strong adaptive capacity contributes to heat-resilient people and communities—the ability to prepare and plan for, absorb, recover from, and more successfully adapt to adverse events. During extreme heat events, heat-related morbidity and mortality is especially elevated in people with low adaptive capacity and that have difficulty responding or relocating when necessary. As discussed in the following section, heat-health relationships are complex, and vulnerability to heat varies as a function of nonphysiological (e.g., geographical location, urban density, building design) and physiological (e.g., natural aging, state of health) factors.

Heat and Human Health

A recent report concluded that the threat to human life from excess heat now is inevitable [50]. Extreme heat causes some of the highest death tolls among all natural weather hazards [12, 13] dramatically increasing short-term mortality in vulnerable populations (i.e., children, the elderly, the physically challenged or the sick, deprived individuals, others) [14, 15]. Change of 0.7–3.6% in all-cause mortality has been reported for a 1 °C increase in average daily temperature during hot weather [115]. In addition to the above groups, people living at home alone as well as deprived individuals show increased mortality rates during heat waves [14, 116–124], which highlights the key roles of isolation and socioeconomic factors on the vulnerability to heat waves [119].

The dramatic effect of heat on human health was revealed during a major heat wave in Chicago in 1995. Record high temperatures of 41 °C resulted in 739 heat-related deaths over a 5-day period primarily in the elderly, especially those without air conditioning or those who were unable to open their windows due to fear as a result of the unprecedented increase in crime [125]. Additionally, thousands of people, including the young, were hospitalized with heat-related illnesses. In 2003, a large-scale catastrophic effect of extreme heat on population health occurred when between 30,000 and 70,000 premature deaths were recorded in Europe during a 2-month heat wave (average temperature ≥30 °C; peak temperatures >40 °C) [126]. As in the case of the Chicago heat wave, overheating in homes caused wide-scale fatalities in the 2003 European heat wave [126]. There were 55,000 excess deaths during a heat wave in Russia in 2010 [127].

The Temperature-Mortality Relationship

Variations in both morbidity and mortality rates with temperature are non-linear [128]. Most commonly, these relationships are expressed as U-, V-, or J-shaped curves with minimum morbidity/mortality at some temperature threshold [129, 130] (Fig. 12.2). The temperature-mortality relationship, however, is not constant and may vary geographically, temporally, and even by disease. The impact on human health of a given heat event is dependent on where and when it occurs. The evidence also shows hospital admission rates and excess mortality during extreme heat events are greater in cities where temperatures are typically cooler as compared with warmer cities. Several studies note that cities with milder climates have lower minimum mortality thresholds than those in warmer climates due to some combination of acclimatization to the hotter weather and behavioral adaptations such as the prevalence of air conditioning [130, 131]. This can be similarly shown with morbidity to specific diseases. In New York, for instance, hospital admissions for respiratory diseases increased for temperatures >28.9 °C but at 23 °C in London, which has milder summers [132]. Sensitivity to heat may vary over different time horizons.

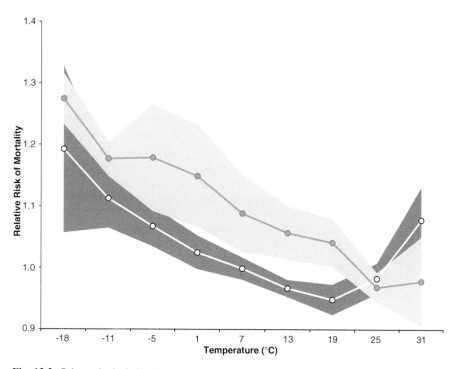

Fig. 12.2 Schematic depicting the relationship between outdoor temperature and human health. Assessment of the thermal environment on temperature-attributable mortality serves as a valuable tool to assess the acute health effects of heat exposure that fluctuate over time. As exemplified by the white and orange tracing, the temperature-mortality relationship is not constant and can vary as function of geographical location, climate type, seasonal influences, as well as population groups (e.g., older adults, individuals with chronic disease, others) (adapted from 130)

Some studies indicate greater health impacts early in the season when people are less acclimatized [133–135]. Other studies show that mortality has decreased over time in response to greater awareness of heat hazards due to improved heat watch warning systems or increased prevalence of air conditioning [136, 137]. Finally, thresholds for morbidity may vary by disease. As an example, hospital admissions in London increased for respiratory diseases at >23 °C but at a lower threshold of >18 °C for renal diseases [138].

Heat Health and Aging

As mentioned in the subsection above (*Inter- and Intraindividual Determinants of Heat Strain*), vulnerability to heat depends on climate factors such as the frequency of heat waves, but it is also dependent on individual risk factors (e.g., age, sex, health status, etc.; see Fig. 12.1) [139, 140]. The impacts of heat are disproportionately borne by older adults and individuals with type 2 diabetes [123, 141, 142], especially those with associated comorbidities such as obesity [143, 144] and/or cardiovascular disease [120, 123, 142]. The issue of aging and its implications on heat tolerance and thermal comfort has become an important concern especially with our aging population and climate change. A growing body of evidence indicates that the ability of humans to manage heat stress progressively decreases with age [38, 40]. Individuals over the age of 65 years are among those most at risk for adverse heat-related events [14], as evidenced by an increased risk for hospital/ emergency department admissions [29, 138, 142] and death [118, 121, 123, 145] during extreme heat events compared with younger populations. These findings are attributed to social and community factors [119], as well as to marked reductions in the ability of older individuals to dissipate heat [39, 40, 44, 48]. Recent evidence even suggests that this impairment in thermoregulation can be detected as early as 40 years of age [38] and, by the age of 55 years, it leads to a substantially increased risk for hyperthermia when working or exercising in the heat [140]. The impact of this decrement in heat loss capacity also appears to be dependent upon the heat load such that the magnitude of difference in heat loss as a function of age increases progressively along with increasing levels of heat stress [39, 44].

Heat Health and Chronic Disease

Chronic health conditions commonly associated with aging such as obesity, diabetes, hypertension, and cardiovascular disease have also been shown to independently diminish one's capacity to regulate core temperature during heat stress. Obesity was a comorbidity in the 2003 European heat wave [146], which supports previous findings showing that fatal heat strokes occur at a rate of 3.5 times higher in those who are obese or overweight than in those of normal weight [147]. Furthermore, those who have diabetes suffer disproportionately during extreme heat events compared with the general population [14, 148]. Type 2 diabetes has been linked to impairments in sweating and skin perfusion [148]. As a consequence individuals with type 2 diabetes have a reduced capacity to dissipate heat and therefore a compromised ability to regulate core temperature during heat stress [49]. Moreover, the magnitude of those impairments is exacerbated by complications from diabetes (e.g., peripheral and autonomic neuropathies, poor glucose control, others) [148].

While there remains a paucity of information regarding the extent to which individuals with cardiovascular disease may have an impaired capacity to dissipate heat, some links have been found between increased mortality during heat waves and the presence of cardiovascular diseases [14, 125, 149]. For example, mortality in those who had cardiovascular diseases was 30% higher during the 2003 European heat wave than during other "normal" heat days [149]. Cardiovascular disease was also prominent among health conditions ascribed to the excess mortality recorded during the 1995 Chicago heat wave [125]. Additionally, hypertension was a common comorbidity factor in those who died from heat effects during the Chicago 1995 heat wave [150].

Heat Health and Children

Children are regarded as a population group that is especially vulnerable to the effects of heat and extreme heat events. Children are usually defined as humans under 18 years of age [151]. There are several physiologic differences between children and adults (e.g., higher surface area-to-mass ratio, lower sweat rate, smaller blood volume, others) that could explain a higher vulnerability to heat [152]. Surprisingly, only a few studies have examined the association of heat and mortality among young children [153]. Using different age ranges, some studies have found a relationship [153–155], while others have observed no association [156, 157]. According to the most conservative estimates, children under 14 have a 1.5-fold greater risk of experiencing a heat-related fatality as compared to young healthy adults [158].

Despite the growing evidence that heat-related morbidity and mortality is elevated in children, relatively little is known about the physiologic responses of children exposed to heat stress conditions. Inbar and colleagues were among the first to suggest that children's thermoregulation differed markedly from that of adults. This was evidenced by their observation that children demonstrate a reduced tolerance to heat [159]. A number of other studies showed similar reductions in heat tolerance in children [160, 161] albeit responses have been variable [161–163]. It was also demonstrated that the process of maturation, and not only physical growth, may modulate thermoregulatory function in children [164–166], although the mechanism(s) underpinning this response has yet to be elucidated. This is likely associated with multiple factors related to morphologic, metabolic, and cardiovascular differences [167].

Heat Health: Social and Community Determinants

Epidemiological studies examining trends in heat-related mortality have noted in several instances that there is an unequal distribution of morbidity and mortality among the various socioeconomic groups [118, 141, 168–170]. Studies show a greater risk of mortality was associated with lower levels of education [168, 171] and lower income (includes living in poverty and poor housing) [121, 130, 170]. A direct inverse correlation has been found between income and education and the rates of obesity, hypertension, cardiovascular disease, and type 2 diabetes [172–178]. Those with higher income and education are also more likely to be physically active [179–181], adding an element of protection against heat injury and illness. In addition, those in lower socioeconomic strata are often at a disadvantage in terms of self-care due to the costs of monitoring and treatment that may not be covered by health insurance. As a result, the socioeconomically disadvantaged often have lower treatment compliance rates and higher rates of long-term disease-related complications [182–184]. This, in turn, would make them even more susceptible to heat-related injury and illness when exposed to hot weather.

Lack of social contact is considered an important risk factor for heat-related mortality. It is estimated that people, especially the most vulnerable, spend the majority (80–90%) of their time indoors [185, 186]. Living alone has generally been shown to be one of main risk factors for mortality [121, 123, 125, 187], although some studies observed no greater risk which may be linked to differences in geographical location [188, 189]. Involvement in group activities, maintaining friendships, or even having a pet in the household have been shown to provide some measure of protection [121, 123]. While living alone should not be equated with social isolation, changes in the social and built environments may have led to an increase in the number of people living alone, who are also socially isolated. It is noteworthy that there has been an increase in recent years in the number of individuals, especially seniors, who live alone [190]. There has also been a trend toward the decreasing availability of safe public spaces and supported housing arrangements, thereby decreasing the availability of social contact for many vulnerable individuals (e.g., senior citizens, individuals with mental illness) [125].

The direct relationship between heat-related mortality and race/ethnicity is less obvious, possibly due to the complex interplay of many factors that may influence vulnerability [191]. While some report a higher risk of heat-related morbidity and mortality in individuals of nonwhite origin [141, 168, 169], and in particular African Americans compared with Caucasians [142, 191, 192], others have reported no differences [193, 194].

Heat Health and Geographical Location

Many studies have documented the importance of geographic location in heat-health relationships. Populations adapt to local climate conditions physiologically and through cultural and behavioral practices [195]. As noted earlier, minimum mortality thresholds increase in warmer climates. This is well illustrated by McMichael et al. and colleagues [195] who evaluated 12 cities across the globe, spanning tropical (12°N) to mid-latitude regions (46°N). They observed that minimum mortality thresholds varied from 16 °C to 31 °C, generally increasing in warmer climates. Irrespective of geographical locations, global average surface temperatures are predicted to rise, and heat waves are expected to increase in intensity, frequency, and duration; dense urban environments will be most impacted because of the urban heat island effect [129, 196–198].

Heat islands can form over any built-up area, but especially occur over large cities where surfaces absorb large quantities of solar radiation during the day and radiate it during the night, sustaining higher temperatures than surrounding rural areas and intensifying the effects of heat waves [12, 199]. The magnitude other urban heat island effect varies through the day, by season, and geographically. While green spaces are associated with decreased heat-related morbidity and mortality in urban areas [200], these spaces are increasingly limited in large metropolitan cities. The hottest areas tend to have high density of buildings or roadways, little greenspace, intense generation of anthropogenic heat such as by factories, and low air circulation caused by a very dense cluster of building and narrow streets [201]. While urban density is a major factor contributing to the urban heat island effect, studies indicate that surface temperatures in lower-density land use caused by urban sprawl in large cities [202] are also on the rise. Urban sprawl has been shown to increase the probability and intensity of heat waves [203] increasing the likelihood of high indoor temperatures that can pose a danger to a person's health and well-being.

Even within the same city, heat exposure may differ among neighborhoods based on land-use patterns and land cover [204]. In this context, individuals are not uniformly exposed to similar levels of heat stress during extreme heat events. A report by Hondula and co-workers showed significant fine-scale spatial variability in heat-related mortality within Philadelphia such that heat-related mortality across different sectors of the city varied by as much as 50% [197]. Several studies have incorporate multiple variables such as those associated with environmental (e.g. land-use type or greenspace), sociodemographic (e.g., education, income, age, ethnicity), living conditions (e.g., access to air conditioning), and health (e.g., diabetes) determinants to develop heat vulnerability indices [205] or heat maps [206] that are useful for identifying geographic patterns of sensitivity to heat. These measures have been shown to be effective indicators of geographic vulnerability to heat-related mortality and morbidity within cities and can assist health officials develop action plans for extreme heat events including resource allocation needed to support increased hospital admissions, ambulance transport needs, public cooling centers, and others [206, 207].

As outlined above, there are a number of factors that can affect temperature and therefore human health during an extreme heat event. However, the challenge remains in quantifying a person's level of heat exposure which can be highly variable between individuals. This is in part due to the combined influence of differences in activity patterns [208] and the built environment [201, 209]. Even within dwellings, there can be considerable heterogeneity in thermal exposures depending on building characteristics. For example, upper stories, a southern orientation, and an elevated glazing-to-wall ratio are associated with a greater indoor air temperature [210]. Of note, the thermal characteristics and qualities of a home accounts for a greater variation in indoor temperature than the effect of location within the urban environment itself during an extreme heat event [211]. Other factors such as the number of occupants in a home will also have an influence as overcrowding is associated with greater internal heat gains [212]. Because there are differences in how groups of people may respond behaviorally to the same living environment a person's level of exposure to heat can vary. While the use of protective measures (e.g., use of operable windows to enhance air exchange, mechanical ventilation, use of air conditioning, etc.) can mitigate potentially dangerous increases in thermal strain, the appropriate behavioral strategies to implement these measures must occur (e.g., turn on air conditioner, open window, close window blinds, etc.). In the case of vulnerable population such as the elderly, the sick, and others, in the absence of assistance, the activation of protective measures may not be possible.

Occupational Heat Stress in a Changing Climate

Impact of Climate Change and Heat on Occupational Health

At present, nearly 30% of the world's population is frequently exposed to climate conditions that exceed human thermoregulatory capacity [50]. Even if aggressive mitigation measures are adopted by countries across the globe, half of the planet's population will still be exposed to such conditions by 2100 [50], leading to ever-increasing levels of occupational heat stress [30]. Occupational heat stress typically originates in industries from harsh environmental conditions (e.g., increased air temperature and humidity, radiant heat sources, limited air flow), the requirement to wear insulated and/or impermeable protective clothing, and the high metabolic heat load from performing physically demanding tasks, especially when wearing heavy equipment [85, 213]. While the definition/threshold of occupational heat stress can vary based on these factors, in a recent systematic review and meta-analysis of the relevant literature, we found that occupational heat stress is defined in the vast majority of studies as air temperature beyond 27 °C or 33 °C for moderate-/high- or low-intensity work, respectively, or WBGT beyond 22.0 °C or 25 °C for moderate-/high- or low-intensity work, respectively [30]. Working under occupational heat stress conditions leads to progressive rises in core temperature, cardiovascular strain, and fluid depletion [214], which can lead to heat stroke or death [215]. In fact, the core temperature of individuals working under occupational heat stress is increased by 0.7 °C beyond normal, and their urine-specific gravity (a marker of hydration status) is increased by 14.5% compared to the start of the work shift 30. Moreover, 15% of individuals who typically work under occupational heat stress experience kidney disease or acute kidney injury [30]. It is not surprising, therefore, that recent large-scale epidemiological studies on heat-related illness and mortality show that occupational heat stress is responsible for 13–36 deaths per year in the United States alone [216, 217].

Physiological Strain During Work in the Heat

The term occupational heat strain is used to describe the abovementioned physiological and psychophysical effects of occupational heat stress on the worker and his/her performance. In this sense, the occupational heat strain refers to the physiological consequences of occupational heat stress, and a number of studies report that these consequences directly threaten workers' health, with associated negative impacts on productivity, poverty, and socioeconomic inequality [10, 23, 30]. Indeed, nearly one million "work-life years" (similar notion as DALYs) will be lost by 2030 due to occupational heat stroke fatalities, and 70 million "work-life years" will be lost due to reduced labor productivity [218, 219].

While the definition/threshold of occupational heat strain can vary based on environmental conditions, the requirement to wear insulated and/or impermeable protective clothing, and the high metabolic heat load from performing physically demanding tasks, in a recent systematic review and meta-analysis of the relevant literature, we defined occupational heat strain as present if one or more of the following criteria were met:

- Core body temperature higher than 38 °C, according to international occupational health and safety standards [220–222]
- At least one occupational heat strain symptom, as defined by international health and safety guidelines [220, 222–225]

    (a) Serum creatinine concentration of >1·2 mg/dL (indicating acute kidney injury) [226, 227]
    (b) Diagnosed urinary lithiasis (indicating acute kidney injury) [226, 227]
    (c) Urine-specific gravity ≥1·020 (indicating dehydration) [224]
    (d) Heat-associated self-reported nausea or vomiting (indicating heat stroke) [223]
    (e) Painful muscular spasms (indicating heat cramps) [223]
    (f) Confusion, dizziness, or fainting (indicating heat syncope, heat exhaustion, or heat stroke) [223]
    (g) Hot dry skin (indicating heat stroke) [223]
    (h) Self-reported heat strain (indicating heat exhaustion) [223]

- Cholesterol concentration higher than 6·7 mmol/L or low-density lipoprotein concentration higher than 3·4 mmol/L (indicating heat-induced dyslipidemia) [228, 229]

Indices of Occupational Heat Stress and Strain

In the past century, more than 160 environmental heat stress indices have been developed [230] and, as outlined earlier, the most widely used are WBGT and UTCI. The vast majority of these indices consider meteorological factors (e.g., temperature, humidity, wind, solar radiation) and elements of the physical environment that can be measured with instruments to estimate the psychophysical impact on the human body (i.e., the heat strain). Despite their wide usage, the efficacy of these indices for the management of heat strain imposed upon individuals during work or leisure activities is limited and has received some criticism [231–236]. This is illustrated by the fact that heat injuries have been documented in a wide range of air temperatures (26–49 °C) and water-vapor pressures (0.8–3.5 kPa, corresponding to 10–100% relative humidity) [52, 237, 238].

Studies attempting to develop heat stress indices have shown that heat injuries are more prevalent in unfit, obese, and unacclimatized individuals [231]. However, the vast majority of existing heat stress indices do not consider these attributes. While some indices do consider human factors (e.g., activity level, clothing, posture) [230], this aspect has received much less attention. More importantly, as discussed above, additional intrinsic factors for heat injury prevention that are known to increase an individual's susceptibility to heat stress – such as sex [41], age [39], body composition [239], and fitness [44] – have not been considered. To address this gap, we recently identified and validated sex-specific simple and practical screening criteria for susceptibility to heat stress during work and leisure activities in hot environments in a recent large-scale calorimetric study of 167 individuals aged 31–70 years [140]. A total of five screening criteria were developed from simple information derived from age, anthropometry, and cardiorespiratory fitness. In total, men and women aged 31–70 years who test positive in two or more of the following screening criteria have a higher risk for being unable to dissipate a sufficient amount of heat to avert marked increases in thermal strain and, therefore, are more likely to succumb to heat-related injuries (males/females) [140]:

 (i) Age $\geq 53.0/55.8$ years
 (ii) Body mass index $\geq 29.5/25.7$ kg·m^{-2}
(iii) Body fat $\geq 28.8/34.9\%$
(iv) Body surface area $\leq 2.0/1.7$ m^2
 (v) Peak oxygen uptake $\leq 48.3/41.4$ mlO2·fat free kg^{-1}·min^{-1}

Worker Productivity Under Occupational Heat Strain

In parallel to physiological changes, occupational heat stress generates discomfort and fatigue [214], which can lead to labor losses by compromising worker productivity [23, 240]. Indeed, recent meta-analytic data shows that 30% of individuals who work under heat stress report productivity losses [30]. The same systematic review and meta-analysis reports an average 2.6% productivity decline for every degree increase beyond 24 °C WBGT [30]. In occupational settings, problems are already felt by millions of workers [30], especially those above 53/56 years old (males/females) who are especially susceptible to heat illness [140]. The available data suggest that in future decades, individuals working even in temperate climates may be at risk for heat illness on nearly 40 days/year [241]. In line with this, the extent of the damaging potential of heat on human productivity is evident in estimations for 2030, according to which the heat-related labor productivity losses may be 70 times more damaging to healthy, productive, and disability-free life years, than those resulting by occupational heat stroke fatalities [219].

Overview of Occupational Heat-Related Illnesses

Occupational heat-related illnesses – a fully preventable range of conditions – generate deleterious health and productivity outcomes, and it is vital that they are recognized globally as a public health problem [30, 242]. It is necessary to international attention and take action on this problem, particularly in light of climate change and the anticipated rise in environmental heat stress. Developing a surveillance system to monitor prevalence of occupational heat strain throughout the world could be a first step. In parallel, workers and employers should be educated about the health and performance effects of occupational heat strain, while effective screening and mitigation protocols should be incorporated within health and safety legislation.

Heat Health Planning and Protection for General Population

The Current State of Planning and Prevention

A direct relationship between acute mortality and exposure to high temperature has been recorded in almost all populations where it has been studied [243]. As discussed earlier, a well-known analysis of published temperature-mortality relationships in populations living in temperate and cold climates has shown that this association is U- or V-shaped, with exponential mortality risk increase at both high and low temperatures [244]. These results suggest that populations are adapted to their local climates [245] and that mortality risk is increased beyond a location-specific optimum temperature range. Work by the World Health Organization [246] has shown that the factors (economic development, infrastructure, health systems, etc.) that affect the ability of developed countries to prepare for and respond to climate-related hazards such as heat waves vary widely. Additionally, the resilience and adaptive capacity of populations and health systems is different among and within countries. More importantly, the same work [246] highlighted that the interest or capacity of government agencies to collect and circulate information on heat wave response should not be assumed, despite the widely publicized and unanimously agreed health effects of climate-related hazards on health and productivity. The willingness and adaptive capacity reflect each country's specific conditions and priorities, while factors such as location, socioeconomic development, and recorded mortality do not appear to play important roles. Instead, the single most important factor that appears to determine action or inaction across developed countries pertains to the existence (or absence) of a culture for protecting health from climate change [246].

Community Adaptation Programming and Health Advisory Systems for Heat Events

Early warning systems for extreme weather events have been piloted during the past 10 years in some developed countries [247]. Specifically, a recent report by the World Meteorological Association [223] lists a total of 21 countries where

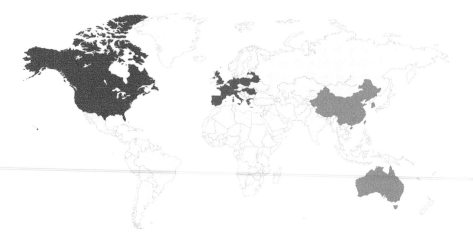

Fig. 12.3 Overview of the geographical representation of the 21 countries where early warning systems for heat waves have been tested according to the World Meteorological Association 224. Color codes representing the different World Health Organization regions: Americas (*red*), Europe (*blue*), and Western Pacific (*green*) (no studies have reported on early warning systems tested in Africa, Eastern Mediterranean, or Southeast Asia)

early warning systems for heat waves have been tested. These are illustrated in Fig. 12.3, showing that the vast majority are in Europe (16 of 21), while none have been reported in Africa, Eastern Mediterranean, or South-East Asia. These early warning systems include forecasting extreme events, predicting potential health impacts, and providing action plans for vulnerable populations. In most cases (e.g., Austria, Belgium, the Czech Republic, France, Germany, Greece, Hungary, Slovenia, Sweden, the Netherlands, the United States), meteorological institutes inform the general public via mass media, and the health professionals are informed directly [247]. Moreover, in a small number of some countries (e.g., the Netherlands), the public health services provide information to the local stakeholders (nursery homes, organizations for the homeless, local communities, etc.).

In light of the above discussion on occupational heat stress and strain, it is crucial to note that the existing early warning systems are designed for the general population whose needs and exposure to heat are vastly different from those of workers. For instance, the typical adaptation strategy in existing systems is to advise individuals to stay indoors throughout the day or to remain in "cooling shelters" at public buildings. However, such strategies are not an option for industrial actors given their need to maintain productivity regardless of the prevailing environmental conditions. Moreover, existing systems have a forecasting capacity limited to a few days which is insufficient for industrial actors who need to plan their activities weeks (or months) in advance to ensure a high level of productivity. Therefore, a different approach is needed to address the health needs of the European workforce.

Heat Protection and Management Strategies for Workers

As noted in the subsection above (*Occupational Heat Stress in a Changing Climate*), heat stress is a deadly, yet common, occupational hazard, reported to be responsible for 37 fatal and 2830 nonfatal occupational injuries and illnesses in the United States in 2015 [248]. Given the increasing frequency and intensity of heat waves due to global warming, heat-related deaths in workers have been estimated to increase by as much as 37% for each ~0.55 °C (1 °F) rise in average daily summer temperature [249], with workers facing a four- to sevenfold greater risk of experiencing a heat-related illness during a heat wave [250]. Excessive heat strain can also cause psychophysical strain (e.g., discomfort, fatigue), which can exacerbate the risk of injury and cause reductions in worker productivity [23, 251–253], costing up to US$6.2 billion in heat-related labor losses [254]. However, while heat stress management guidelines have been recommended by the National Institute for Occupational Safety and Health (NIOSH) [255] and other safety institutions for some time, heat stress continues to compromise worker health and productivity. The following subsections describe the current approach to occupational heat stress management and future directions to better protect and maximize the productivity of individuals working in our warming global climate.

Occupational Heat Stress Management: Common Practices and Methodologies

To reduce the risks associated with heat stress, NIOSH recommends upper heat stress limits defined by the environment (assessed with WBGT) and metabolic rate, expressed as a time-weighted average [255]. Two sliding-scale limits are then specified, the Recommended Alert Limits (RALs) and the Recommended Exposure Limits (RELs), which are analogous to the American Conference of Governmental Industrial Hygienists (ACGIH) Action Limit Values and Threshold Limit Values (TLV®) [256], respectively. The RALs are directed at protecting unacclimatized workers (i.e., individuals who do not possess thermoregulatory adaptations associated with repeated heat exposure), while the less conservative RELs are directed at protecting acclimatized workers. Both upper limits are designed so that healthy workers, who are adequately hydrated, unmedicated, and wearing only a single clothing layer (~1 Clo) should be able to tolerate an 8-hour exposure to such heat stress without incurring adverse health effects for a 5-day workweek. Since additional insulated or impermeable clothing can restrict heat exchange [257], the WBGT associated with the RAL and REL is lowered to consider these effects (e.g., two-layered clothing requires that the WBGT for each limit is lowered by 2 °C). In instances where these thresholds are exceeded, engineering (e.g., ventilation, shade) and administrative controls (e.g., work-to-rest allocations), hygiene practices (e.g., personal cooling devices, fluid consumption schedule), and physiological monitoring are prescribed.

    While current occupational heat exposure limits such as the RALs and RELs may provide a relatively simple means to manage heat stress, recent laboratory-based evaluations of the ACGIH TLV® (analogous to the RELs) indicate that unsafe rises in body core temperature ($\geq$38.0 °C) would occur during work shifts $\geq$4 h in young [234] and especially in older workers [236] when work is performed within these limits. Several instances of peak core temperatures exceeding the ACGIH guidelines for acclimated workers ($\geq$38.5 °C) as well as two instances of more severe heat strain ($\geq$39.5 °C) have also been observed during field-based evaluations of heat strain in electric utilities workers [83]. It has therefore been suggested that current guidelines may provide only moderate protection to worker health [258]. This is because the heat strain one may experience in response to a given level of heat stress can differ markedly among individuals due to various interindividual factors and intraindividual factors both within and beyond a worker's control (see section "Inter- and Intraindividual Determinants of Heat Strain" for additional details). As such, the assessment of heat stress alone can result in the over- or under-protection of workers from heat-related illness, with the former leading to a reduction in productivity in more heat-tolerant workers (false positive) and the latter compromising safety in less heat-tolerant workers who may develop heat-related illness even in mild conditions (false negative).

    To provide more individualized protection, it has been suggested that future emphasis be directed toward the development of guidelines that consider interindividual factors that commonly differ among workers (e.g., sex, age, chronic disease), as well as critical intraindividual factors that can be identified indirectly with basic worker information (e.g., consecutive work days, shift duration) or pre-work assessments (e.g., urine-specific gravity to assess hydration state) [99]. This may involve making adjustments to existing RELs to consider how such factors may impair or improve heat dissipation and the resulting increase in heat strain in response to a given heat stress. These individualized guidelines would therefore serve as a risk stratification tool to identify individuals who may be more susceptible to heat-related illness, even in mild heat stress conditions, while identifying those individuals who are better equipped to continue work in higher heat stress conditions. In instances where these individualized guidelines are exceeded, targeted protective strategies could be employed to alleviate heat strain.

    Although individualized heat stress guidelines may better protect workers health than a generalized exposure limit, it is challenging and perhaps impossible to comprehensively consider all individual factors and their interactive effects on heat strain. For this reason, a more comprehensive solution to managing occupational heat stress may involve monitoring one or more physiological indices of heat strain (e.g., noninvasive or indirect measures of body core temperature and cardiovascular strain, among others), as opposed to the level of heat stress [255, 258]. This approach therefore prevents the over- or under-protection of workers from heat-related illness (i.e., false positives and false negatives) by ensuring that productivity is maximized in more heat-tolerant employees when working in high heat stress conditions and that heat-related illness is prevented in less heat-tolerant workers when working in temperate conditions. These physiological data can also be used to provide alert thresholds to management to ensure that safety limits are not exceeded and to provide physiological feedback to workers to ensure that they control their work rate to optimize productivity while preventing excessive heat strain [259]. Given the added protection offered by physiological monitoring and the recent increases in the development of wearable monitors providing a noninvasive and portable means of quantifying physiological strain, heat strain monitoring may represent the future of occupational heat stress management, especially given our diverse working population.

An occupational heat stress management program that incorporates physiological monitoring may provide a more comprehensive solution to protect worker health, although the implementation of such technology is not without its challenges [258]. Indeed, while some monitoring systems are certified for use in hazardous areas and possess water- and dust-resistance, future research is needed to evaluate the utility of these systems in harsh industrial environments for wearable monitoring to be successful. Further, materials that are nonflammable or flame resistant, noncombustible, hypoallergenic, as well as resistant to arc flash and electromagnetic fields must be used in the construction of a wearable heat strain monitor to satisfy existing safety requirements in many industries. While some of the systems available satisfy such requirements, others would require modification prior to use. Moreover, despite their benefits, the costs associated with purchasing wearable monitors for all employees may be prohibitive for some companies. These costs, however, could be reduced by restricting monitoring to "high-risk" work and/or weather conditions and/or by monitoring employees who, due to their age, health status, or physically demanding occupation, may be more vulnerable to heat-related illness, a process that could be aided by the individualized guidelines noted above [99]. Finally, it is possible that physiological monitoring per se may modify worker behavior (reactivity). This may be characterized by an increase in work intensity and a reluctance to cease work even when experiencing excessive heat strain or a reduction in work effort to avoid displaying greater fatigue than their co-workers. Unfortunately, the former may exacerbate heat strain, while the latter may reduce productivity. Although such behavior modifications may be minimized if physiological monitoring was routine or if management intervened, future research is needed to identify if and to what extent physiological monitoring may modify worker behavior.

Summary

Climate change projections show that there will be continuing increases in the occurrence and severity of some extreme heat events over the next decades placing. As a consequence, there is immediate need to use best scientific practices and other evidence-based methods to protect the public and workers against the potentially harmful effects of exposure to extreme heat. This includes formulating culturally sensitive solutions, policies, and guidelines to protect health, safety, and performance as well as prevent disease exacerbated by heat across different spheres – healthcare, civil protective agencies, military, industry, sports, and others – against the harmful effects of heat.

References

1. Intergovernmental Panel on Climate Change. Global warming of 1.5oC. 2018. https://www.ipcc.ch/sr15/. Accessed 29 Apr 2019.
2. Lindemann U, Stotz A, Beyer N, et al. Effect of indoor temperature on physical performance in older adults during days with normal temperature and heat waves. Int J Environ Res Public Health. 2017;14(2):186. https://doi.org/10.3390/ijerph14020186.
3. Tham KW, Willem HC. Room air temperature affects occupants' physiology, perceptions and mental alertness. Build Environ. 2010;45:40–4.
4. Chartered Institution of Building Services Engineers. Environmental design: CIBSE guide A. 7th ed. London, CIBSE; 2006.
5. van Loenhout JA, le Grand A, Duijm F, Greven F, Vinak NM, Hoek G, Zuurbier M. The effect of high indoor temperatures on self-perceived health of elderly persons. Environ Res. 2016;146:27–34.
6. van Hoof J, Kort HSM, Hensen JLM, Duijnstee MSH, Rutten PGS. Thermal comfort and the integrated design of homes for older people with dementia. Build Environ. 2010;45:358–70.
7. van Hoof J, Schellen L, Soebarto V, Wong JKW, Kazak JK. Ten questions concerning thermal comfort and ageing. Build Environ. 2017;120:123–33.
8. Guo Y, Gasparrini A, Li S, Sera F, Vicedo-Cabrera AM, de Sousa Zanotti Stagliorio Coelho M, et al. Quantifying excess deaths related to heatwaves under climate change scenarios: a multi-country time series modelling study. PLoS Med. 2018;15(7):e1002629.
9. Noe RS, Jin JO, Wolkin AF. Exposure to natural cold and heat: hypothermia and hyperthermia Medicare claims, United States, 2004–2005. Am J Public Health. 2012;102(4):e11–8.
10. Kenny GP, Groeller H, McGinn R, Flouris AD. Age, human performance, and physical employment standards. Appl Physiol Nutr Metab. 2016;41(6 Suppl 2):S92–S107.
11. Canadian Diabetes Association. An economic tsunami: the cost of diabetes in Canada. Toronto; 2009. https://doi.org/10.1175/BAMS-85-8-1067.
12. Luber G, McGeehin M. Climate change and extreme heat events. Am J Prev Med. 2008;35(5):429–35.
13. Borden KA, Cutter SL. Spatial patterns of natural hazards mortality in the United States. Int J Health Geogr. 2008;7:64. https://doi.org/10.1186/1476-072X-7-64.
14. Kenny GP, Yardley J, Brown C, Sigal RJ, Jay O. Heat stress in older individuals and patients with common chronic diseases. CMAJ. 2010;182(10):1053–60.
15. Government of Canada. Canada in a changing climate: sector perspective on impacts and adaptation. Ottawa: Natural Resources Canada; 2014.
16. Kenny GP, Flouris AD. The human thermoregulatory system and its response to thermal stress. In: Wang F, Gao G, editors. Protective clothing: managing thermal stress. Cambridge: Elsevier; 2014. p. 319–65.
17. Kenny GP, Jay O. Thermometry, calorimetry, and mean body temperature during heat stress. Compr Physiol. 2013;3(4):1689–719.
18. Kenny GP, Wilson TE, Flouris AD, Fujii N. Heat exhaustion. Handb Clin Neurol. 2018;157:505–29.
19. De Blois J, Kjellstrom T, Agewall S, Ezekowitz JA, Armstrong PW, Atar D. The effects of climate change on cardiac health. Cardiology. 2015;131(4):209–17.
20. Wang Y, An S, Xing M, Wan Y, Liu Q. Global warming and heart disease prevention. Eur J Prev Cardiol. 2018;25(12):1342.
21. Stearns RL, O'Connor FG, Casa DJ, Kenny GP. Exertional heat stroke. In: Casa DJ, Stearns RL, editors. Emergency management for sport and physical activity. Burlington, MA: Jones and Bartlett Learning; 2015. p. 61–79.
22. Razmjou S. Mental workload in heat: toward a framework for analyses of stress states. Aviat Space Environ Med. 1996;67(6):530–8.
23. Ioannou LG, Tsoutsoubi L, Samoutis G, Bogataj LK, Kenny GP, Nybo L, et al. Time-motion analysis as a novel approach for evaluating the impact of environmental heat exposure on labor loss in agriculture workers. Temperature (Austin). 2017;4(3):330–40.

24. Legault G, Clement A, Kenny GP, Hardcastle S, Keller N. Cognitive consequences of sleep deprivation, shiftwork, and heat exposure for underground miners. Appl Ergon. 2017;58:144–50.

25. Schmitt LH, Graham HM, White PC. Economic evaluations of the health impacts of weather-related extreme events: a scoping review. Int J Environ Res Public Health. 2016;13(11):1105. https://doi.org/10.3390/ijerph13111105.

26. Wondmagegn BY, Xiang J, Williams S, Pisaniello D, Bi P. What do we know about the healthcare costs of extreme heat exposure? A comprehensive literature review. Sci Total Environ. 2019;657:608–18.

27. Knowlton K, Rotkin-Ellman M, Geballe L, Max W, Solomon GM. Six climate change-related events in the United States accounted for about $14 billion in lost lives and health costs. Health Aff (Millwood). 2011;30(11):2167–76.

28. Larrivée C, Sinclair-Desgagné N, Da Silva L, Desjarlais C, Revéret JP. Évaluation des impacts des changements climatiques et de leurs coûts pour le Québec et l'État québécois. Rapport d'étude. Ouranos; 2015. http://www.environnement.gouv.qc.ca/changementSclimatiques/evatuation-impacts-cc-couts-qc-etat.pdf. Accessed 29 Apr 2019.

29. Knowlton K, Rotkin-Ellman M, King G, Margolis HG, Smith D, Solomon G, et al. The 2006 California heat wave: impacts on hospitalizations and emergency department visits. Environ Health Perspect. 2009;117(1):61–7.

30. Flouris AD, Dinas PC, Ioannou LG, Nybo L, Havenith G, Kenny GP, Kjellstrom T. Workers' health and productivity under occupational heat strain: a systematic review and meta-analysis. Lancet Planet Health. 2018;2(12):e521–31.

31. UK Department for International Development. Impacts of higher temperatures on labour productivity and value for money adaptation: lessons from five DFID priority country case studies. London; 2017. https://doi.org/10.1175/BAMS-85-8-1067.

32. Burke M, Hsiang SM, Miguel E. Global non-linear effect of temperature on economic production. Nature. 2015;527(7577):235–9.

33. Saniotis A, Bi P. Global warming and Australian public health: reasons to be concerned. Aust Health Rev. 2009;33(4):611–7.

34. Landis WG, Rohr JR, Moe SJ, Balbus JM, Clements W, Fritz A, et al. Global climate change and contaminants, a call to arms not yet heard? Integr Environ Assess Manag. 2014;10(4):483–4.

35. Fouillet A, Rey G, Wagner V, Laaidi K, Empereur-Bissonnet P, Le Tertre A, et al. Has the impact of heat waves on mortality changed in France since the European heat wave of summer 2003? A study of the 2006 heat wave. Int J Epidemiol. 2008;37(2):309–17.

36. Boyson C, Taylor S, Page L. The national heatwave plan – a brief evaluation of issues for frontline health staff. PLoS Curr. 2014;6. (pii: ecurrents.dis.aa63b5ff4cdaf47f1dc6bf44921afe93).

37. Ebi KL, Teisberg TJ, Kalkstein LS, Robinson L, Weiher RF. Heat watch/warning systems save lives: estimated costs and benefits for Philadelphia 1995–98. Am Meteorol Soc. 2004:1067–73. https://doi.org/10.1175/BAMS-85-8-1067.

38. Larose J, Boulay P, Sigal RJ, Wright HE, Kenny GP. Age-related decrements in heat dissipation during physical activity occur as early as the age of 40. PLoS One. 2013;8(12):e83148.

39. Stapleton JM, Poirier MP, Flouris AD, Boulay P, Sigal RJ, Malcolm J, Kenny GP. At what level of heat load are age-related impairments in the ability to dissipate heat evident in females? PLoS One. 2015;10(3):e0119079.

40. Larose J, Wright HE, Sigal RJ, Boulay P, Hardcastle S, Kenny GP. Do older females store more heat than younger females during exercise in the heat? Med Sci Sports Exerc. 2013;45(12):2265–76.

41. Gagnon D, Kenny GP. Sex modulates whole-body sudomotor thermosensitivity during exercise. J Physiol. 2011;589(Pt 24):6205–17.

42. Gagnon D, Kenny GP. Sex differences in thermoeffector responses during exercise at fixed requirements for heat loss. J Appl Physiol. 2012;113(5):746–57.

43. Gagnon D, Kenny GP. Does sex have an independent effect on thermoeffector responses during exercise in the heat? J Physiol. 2012;590(Pt 23):5963–73.

44. Stapleton JM, Poirier MP, Flouris AD, Boulay P, Sigal RJ, Malcolm J, Kenny GP. Aging impairs heat loss, but when does it matter? J Appl Physiol (1985). 2015;118(3):299–309.

45. Stapleton JM, Larose J, Simpson C, Flouris AD, Sigal RJ, Kenny GP. Do older adults experience greater thermal strain during heat waves? Appl Physiol Nutr Metab. 2014;39(3):292–8.

46. Kenny GP, Flouris AD, Dervis S, Friesen BJ, Sigal RJ. Older adults experience greater levels of thermal and cardiovascular strain during extreme heat exposures. Med Sci Sports Exerc. 2015;46(5):S396.

47. Larose J, Boulay P, Wright-Beatty HE, Sigal RJ, Hardcastle S, Kenny GP. Age-related differences in heat loss capacity occur under both dry and humid heat stress conditions. J Appl Physiol (1985). 2014;117(1):69–79.

48. Kenny GP, Poirier MP, Metsios GS, Boulay P, Dervis S, Friesen BJ, et al. Hyperthermia and cardiovascular strain during an extreme heat exposure in young versus older adults. Temperature (Austin). 2017;4(1):79–88.

49. Kenny GP, Stapleton JM, Yardley JE, Boulay P, Sigal RJ. Older adults with type 2 diabetes store more heat during exercise. Med Sci Sports Exerc. 2013;45(10):1906–14.

50. Mora C, Dousset B, Caldwell IR, Powell FE, Geronimo RC, Bielecki CR, et al. Global risk of deadly heat. Nat Clim Chang. 2017;7:501–6.

51. Epstein Y, Moran DS. Thermal comfort and the heat stress indices. Ind Health. 2006;44(3):388–98.

52. Yaglou CP, Minard D. Control of heat casualties at military training centers. AMA Arch Ind Health. 1957;16(4):302–16.

53. Steadman RG. The assessment of sultriness. Part I: a temperature-humidity index based on human physiology and clothing science. J Appl Meteorol. 1979;18:861–73.

54. Bröde P, Fiala D, Błażejczyk K, Holmér I, Jendritzky G, Kampmann B, Tinz B. Deriving the operational procedure for the Universal Thermal Climate Index (UTCI). Int J Biometeorol. 2012;56(3):481–94.

55. Sherwood SC, Huber M. An adaptability limit to climate change due to heat stress. Proc Natl Acad Sci U S A. 2010;107(21):9552–5.

56. Perkins SE. A review on the scientific understanding of heatwaves – their measurement, driving mechanisms, and changes at the global scale. Atmos Res. 2015;164-165:242–67.

57. Della-Marta PM, Luerbacker J, von Weissenfluh H, Xoplaki E, Brunet M, Wanner H. Summer heat waves over western Europe 1880–2003, their relationship to large-scale forcings and predictability. Clim Dyn. 2007;29(2–3):251–75.

58. Mishra V, Ganguly AR, Nijssen B, Letenmaier DP. Changes in observed climate extremes in global urban areas. Environ Res Lett. 2015;10:024005.

59. Russo S, Sillmann J, Sterl A. Humid heat waves at different warming levels. Sci Rep. 2017;7(1):7477.

60. Matthews T. Humid heat and climate change. Prog Phys Geogr: Earth Environ. 2018;42(3):391–405.

61. Gaffen DJ, Ross RJ. Increased summertime heat stress in the U.S. Nature. 1998;396:529–30.

62. Grundstein A, Dowd J. Trends in extreme apparent temperatures over the United States, 1949–2010. J Appl Meteorol Climatol. 2011;50(8):1650–3.

63. Schoof JT, Ford TW, Pryor SC. Recent changes in U.S. regional heat wave characteristics in observations and reanalysis. J Appl Meteorol Climatol. 2017;56:2621–36.

64. Jacobs SJ, Pezza AB, Barras V. An analysis of the meteorological variables leading to apparent temperature in Australia: present climate, trends, and global warming simulations. Glob Planet Change. 2013;107:145–56.

65. Desai MS, Dhorde AG. Trends in thermal discomfort indices over western coastal cities of India. Theor Appl Climatol. 2018;131(3–4):1305–21.

66. Willet KM, Jones PD, Gillett NP, Thorne PW. Recent changes in surface humidity: development of the HadCRUH Dataset. J Clim. 2008;21:5364–83.

67. Knutson TR, Ploshay JJ. Detection of anthropogenic influence on a summertime heat stress index. Clim Chang. 2016;148:25–39.

68. Lee D, Brenner T. Perceived temperature in the course of climate change: an analysis of global heat index from 1979 to 2013. Earth Syst Sci Data. 2015;7:193–202.

69. Hayhoe K, Edmonds J, Kopp RE, Le Grand A, Sanderson BM, Wehner MF. Climate models, scenarios, and projections. Washington, DC: U.S. Global Change Research Program; 2017.
70. Meehl GA, Tebaldi C. More intense, more frequent, and longer lasting heat waves in the 21st century. Science. 2004;305(5686):994–7.
71. Cowan T, Purich A, Perkins S, Peza A, Boschat G, Sadler K. More frequent, longer, and hotter heat waves for Australia in the twenty-first century. J Clim. 2014;27(15):5851–71.
72. Wenger CB. Heat of evaporation of sweat: thermodynamic considerations. J Appl Physiol. 1972;32(4):456–9.
73. Gagnon D, Jay O, Kenny GP. The evaporative requirement for heat balance determines whole-body sweat rate during exercise under conditions permitting full evaporation. J Physiol. 2013;591(11):2925–35.
74. Sawka MN, Young AJ, Latzka WA, Neufer PD, Quigley MD, Pandolf KB. Human tolerance to heat strain during exercise: influence of hydration. J Appl Physiol (1985). 1992;73(1):368–75.
75. Hensel H. Thermoreceptors. Annu Rev Physiol. 1974;36:233–49.
76. Jessen C. Thermal afferents in the control of body temperature. Pharmacol Ther. 1985;28(1):107–34.
77. Pierau FK, Wurster RD. Primary afferent input from cutaneous thermoreceptors. Fed Proc. 1981;40(14):2819–24.
78. Boulant JA, Dean JB. Temperature receptors in the central nervous system. Annu Rev Physiol. 1986;48:639–54.
79. Flouris AD, Schlader ZJ. Human behavioral thermoregulation during exercise in the heat. Scand J Med Sci Sports. 2015;25(Suppl 1):52–64.
80. Gisolfi CV, Wenger CB. Temperature regulation during exercise: old concepts, new ideas. Exerc Sport Sci Rev. 1984;12:339–72.
81. Belding HS, Kamon E. Evaporative coefficients for prediction of safe limits in prolonged exposures to work under hot conditions. Fed Proc. 1973;32(5):1598–601.
82. Bouchama A, Knochel JP. Heat stroke. N Engl J Med. 2002;346(25):1978–88.
83. Meade RD, Lauzon M, Poirier MP, Flouris AD, Kenny GP. An evaluation of the physiological strain experienced by electrical utility workers in North America. J Occup Environ Hyg. 2015;12(10):708–20.
84. Meade RD, D'Souza AW, Krishen L, Kenny GP. The physiological strain incurred during electrical utilities work over consecutive work shifts in hot environments: a case report. J Occup Environ Hyg. 2017;14(12):986–94.
85. Poulianiti KP, Havenith G, Flouris AD. Metabolic energy cost of workers in agriculture, construction, manufacturing, tourism, and transportation industries. Ind Health. 2018;57(3):283–305.
86. Soule RG, Goldman RF. Energy cost of loads carried on the head, hands, or feet. J Appl Physiol. 1969;27(5):687–90.
87. Dorman LE, Havenith G. The effects of protective clothing on energy consumption during different activities. Eur J Appl Physiol. 2009;105(3):463–70.
88. Taylor NA, Lewis MC, Notley SR, Peoples GE. A fractionation of the physiological burden of the personal protective equipment worn by firefighters. Eur J Appl Physiol. 2012;112(8):2913–21.
89. Montain SJ, Sawka MN, Cadarette BS, Quigley MD, McKay JM. Physiological tolerance to uncompensable heat stress: effects of exercise intensity, protective clothing, and climate. J Appl Physiol (1985). 1994;77(1):216–22.
90. Havenith G. Heat balance when wearing protective clothing. Ann Occup Hyg. 1999;43(5):289–96.
91. Muir IH, Bishop PA, Kozusko J. Micro-environment changes inside impermeable protective clothing during a continuous work exposure. Ergonomics. 2001;44(11):953–61.
92. Nielsen B, Rowell LB, Bonde-Petersen F. Cardiovascular responses to heat stress and blood volume displacements during exercise in man. Eur J Appl Physiol Occup Physiol. 1984;52(4):370–4.
93. Brengelmann GL. Circulatory adjustments to exercise and heat stress. Annu Rev Physiol. 1983;45:191–212.

94. Rowell LB, Brengelmann GL, Blackmon JR, Twiss RD, Kusumi F. Splanchnic blood flow and metabolism in heat-stressed man. J Appl Physiol. 1968;24(4):475–84.

95. Senay LC Jr. Effects of exercise in the heat on body fluid distribution. Med Sci Sports. 1979;11(1):42–8.

96. Sawka MN, Toner MM, Francesconi RP, Pandolf KB. Hypohydration and exercise: effects of heat acclimation, gender, and environment. J Appl Physiol Respir Environ Exerc Physiol. 1983;55(4):1147–53.

97. Gisolfi CV, Copping JR. Thermal effects of prolonged treadmill exercise in the heat. Med Sci Sports. 1974;6(2):108–13.

98. Buono MJ, Wall AJ. Effect of hypohydration on core temperature during exercise in temperate and hot environments. Pflugers Arch. 2000;440(3):476–80.

99. Notley SR, Flouris AD, Kenny GP. Occupational heat stress management: does one size fit all? Am J Ind Med. 2019; https://doi.org/10.1002/ajim.22961.

100. Lamarche DT, Notley SR, Poirier MP, Kenny GP. Fitness-related differences in the rate of whole-body total heat loss in exercising young healthy women are heat-load dependent. Exp Physiol. 2018;103(3):312–7.

101. Lamarche DT, Notley SR, Louie JC, Poirier MP, Kenny GP. Fitness-related differences in the rate of whole-body evaporative heat loss in exercising men are heat-load dependent. Exp Physiol. 2018;103(1):101–10.

102. Notley SR, Poirier MP, Hardcastle SG, Flouris AD, Boulay P, Sigal RJ, Kenny GP. Aging impairs whole-body heat loss in women under both dry and humid heat stress. Med Sci Sports Exerc. 2017;49(11):2324–32.

103. Larose J, Wright HE, Stapleton J, Sigal RJ, Boulay P, Hardcastle S, Kenny GP. Whole body heat loss is reduced in older males during short bouts of intermittent exercise. Am J Physiol Regul Integr Comp Physiol. 2013;305(6):R619–29.

104. Kenny GP, Gagnon D, Dorman LE, Hardcastle SG, Jay O. Heat balance and cumulative heat storage during exercise performed in the heat in physically active younger and middle-aged men. Eur J Appl Physiol. 2010;109(1):81–92.

105. Taylor NA. Human heat adaptation. Compr Physiol. 2014;4(1):325–65.

106. Poirier MP, Gagnon D, Kenny GP. Local versus whole-body sweating adaptations following 14 days of traditional heat acclimation. Appl Physiol Nutr Metab. 2016;41(8):816–24.

107. Poirier MP, Gagnon D, Friesen BJ, Hardcastle SG, Kenny GP. Whole-body heat exchange during heat acclimation and its decay. Med Sci Sports Exerc. 2015;47(2):390–400.

108. Meade RD, Notley SR, D'Souza AW, Dervis S, Boulay P, Sigal RJ, Kenny GP. Interactive effects of age and hydration state on human thermoregulatory function during exercise in hot-dry conditions. Acta Physiol (Oxf). 2019;226(1):e13226.

109. Notley SR, Meade RD, D'Souza AW, Friesen BJ, Kenny GP. Heat loss is impaired in older men on the day after prolonged work in the heat. Med Sci Sports Exerc. 2018;50(9):1859–67.

110. Notley SR, Meade RD, D'Souza AW, McGarr GW, Kenny GP. Cumulative effects of successive workdays in the heat on thermoregulatory function in the aging worker. Temperature (Austin). 2018;5(4):293–5.

111. Dewasmes G, Bothorel B, Hoeft A, Candas V. Regulation of local sweating in sleep-deprived exercising humans. Eur J Appl Physiol Occup Physiol. 1993;66(6):542–6.

112. Yoda T, Crawshaw LI, Nakamura M, Saito K, Konishi A, Nagashima K, et al. Effects of alcohol on thermoregulation during mild heat exposure in humans. Alcohol. 2005;36(3):195–200.

113. Freund BJ, Joyner MJ, Jilka SM, Kalis J, Nittolo JM, Taylor JA, et al. Thermoregulation during prolonged exercise in heat: alterations with beta-adrenergic blockade. J Appl Physiol (1985). 1987;63(3):930–6.

114. Persson PB, Persson AB. Water is life. Acta Physiol (Oxf). 2018;224(2):e13173.

115. Yu W, Mengersen K, Wang X, Ye X, Guo Y, Pan X, Tong S. Daily average temperature and mortality among the elderly: a meta-analysis and systematic review of epidemiological evidence. Int J Biometeorol. 2012;56(4):569–81.

116. Rey G, Jougla E, Fouillet A, Pavillon G, Bessemoulin P, Frayssinet P, et al. The impact of major heat waves on all-cause and cause-specific mortality in France from 1971 to 2003. Int Arch Occup Environ Health. 2007;80(7):615–26.

117. Rey G, Fouillet A, Bessemoulin P, Frayssinet P, Dufour A, Jougla E, Hémon D. Heat exposure and socio-economic vulnerability as synergistic factors in heat-wave-related mortality. Eur J Epidemiol. 2009;24(9):495–502.
118. Fouillet A, Rey G, Laurent F, Pavillon G, Bellec S, Guihenneuc-Jouyaux C, et al. Excess mortality related to the August 2003 heat wave in France. Int Arch Occup Environ Health. 2006;80(1):16–24.
119. Yardley J, Sigal RJ, Kenny GP. Heat health planning: the importance of social and community factors. Glob Environ Chang. 2011;21:670–9.
120. Ishigami A, Hajat S, Kovats RS, Bisanti L, Rognoni M, Russo A, Paldy A. An ecological time-series study of heat-related mortality in three European cities. Environ Health. 2008;7(1):5.
121. Naughton MP, Henderson A, Mirabelli MC, Kaiser R, Wilhelm JL, Kieszak SM, et al. Heat-related mortality during a 1999 heat wave in Chicago. Am J Prev Med. 2002;22(4):221–7.
122. Kilbourne EM, Choi K, Jones TS, Thacker SB. Risk factors for heatstroke. A case-control study. JAMA. 1982;247(24):3332–6.
123. Semenza JC, Rubin CH, Falter KH, Selanikio JD, Flanders WD, Howe HL, Wilhelm JL. Heat-related deaths during the July 1995 heat wave in Chicago. N Engl J Med. 1996;335(2):84–90.
124. Rey G, Jougla E, Fouillet A, Hemon D. Ecological association between a deprivation index and mortality in France over the period 1997–2001: variations with spatial scale, degree of urbanicity, age, gender and cause of death. BMC Public Health. 2009;9:33.
125. Klinenberg E. Heat wave: a social autopsy of disaster in Chicago. Chicago: Chicago University Press; 2002.
126. Robine JM, Cheung SL, Le Roy S, Van Oyen H, Griffiths C, Michel JP, Herrmann FR. Death toll exceeded 70,000 in Europe during the summer of 2003. C R Biol. 2008;331(2):171–8.
127. Barriopedro D, Fischer EM, Luterbacher J, Trigo RM, Garcia-Herrera R. The hot summer of 2010: redrawing the temperature record map of Europe. Science. 2011;332(6026):220–4.
128. Ye X, Wolff R, Yu W, Vaneckova P, Pan X, Tong S. Ambient temperature and morbidity: a review of epidemiological evidence. Environ Health Perspect. 2012;120(1):19–28.
129. Smargiassi A, Goldberg MS, Plante C, Fournier M, Baudouin Y, Kosatsky T. Variation of daily warm season mortality as a function of micro-urban heat islands. J Epidemiol Community Health. 2009;63(8):659–64.
130. Curriero FC, Heiner KS, Samet JM, Zeger SL, Strug L, Patz JA. Temperature and mortality in 11 cities of the eastern United States. Am J Epidemiol. 2002;155(1):80–7.
131. Anderson BG, Bell ML. Weather-related mortality: how heat, cold, and heat waves affect mortality in the United States. Epidemiology. 2009;20(2):205–13.
132. Lin S, Luo M, Walker RJ, Liu X, Hwang SA, Chinery R. Extreme high temperatures and hospital admissions for respiratory and cardiovascular diseases. Epidemiology. 2009;20(5):738–46.
133. Ng CF, Ueda K, Ono M, Nitta H, Takami A. Characterizing the effect of summer temperature on heatstroke-related emergency ambulance dispatches in the Kanto area of Japan. Int J Biometeorol. 2014;58(5):941–8.
134. Guirguis K, Gershunov A, Tardy A, Basu R. The impact of recent heat waves on human health in California. J Appl Meteorol Climatol. 2012;53(1):3–19.
135. Hajat S, Kovats RS, Atkinson RW, Haines A. Impact of hot temperatures on death in London: a time series approach. J Epidemiol Community Health. 2002;56(5):367–72.
136. Sheridan SC, Lin S. Assessing variability in the impacts of heat on health outcomes in New York City over time, season, and heat-wave duration. EcoHealth. 2014;11(4):512–25.
137. Davis RE, Knappenberger PC, Michaels PJ, Novicoff WM. Changing heat-related mortality in the United States. Environ Health Perspect. 2003;111(14):1712–8.
138. Kovats RS, Hajat S, Wilkinson P. Contrasting patterns of mortality and hospital admissions during hot weather and heat waves in Greater London, UK. Occup Environ Med. 2004;61(11):893–8.
139. McGinn R, Poirier MP, Louie JC, Sigal RJ, Boulay P, Flouris AD, Kenny GP. Increasing age is a major risk factor for susceptibility to heat stress during physical activity. Appl Physiol Nutr Metab. 2017;42(11):1232–5.

140. Flouris AD, McGinn R, Poirier MP, Louie JC, Ioannou LG, Tsoutsoubi L, et al. Screening criteria for increased susceptibility to heat stress during work or leisure in hot environments in healthy individuals aged 31–70 years. Temperature (Austin). 2018;5(1):86–99.

141. Ellis FP. Mortality from heat illness and heat-aggravated illness in the United States. Environ Res. 1972;5(1):1–58.

142. Semenza JC, McCullough JE, Flanders WD, McGeehin MA, Lumpkin JR. Excess hospital admissions during the July 1995 heat wave in Chicago. Am J Prev Med. 1999;16(4):269–77.

143. Bar-Or O, Lundegren HM, Buskirk ER. Heat tolerance of exercising obese and lean women. J Appl Physiol. 1969;26(4):403–9.

144. Havenith G, Coenen JM, Kistemaker L, Kenney WL. Relevance of individual characteristics for human heat stress response is dependent on exercise intensity and climate type. Eur J Appl Physiol Occup Physiol. 1998;77(3):231–41.

145. Conti S, Meli P, Minelli G, Solimini R, Toccaceli V, Vichi M, Beltrano C, et al. Epidemiologic study of mortality during the Summer 2003 heat wave in Italy. Environ Res. 2005;98(3):390–9.

146. Vandentorren S, Bretin P, Zeghnoun A, Mandereau-Bruno L, Croisier A, Cochet C, et al. August 2003 heat wave in France: risk factors for death of elderly people living at home. Eur J Pub Health. 2006;16(6):583–91.

147. Henschel A. Obesity as an occupational hazard. Can J Public Health. 1967;58(11):491–3.

148. Yardley JE, Stapleton JM, Sigal RJ, Kenny GP. Do heat events pose a greater health risk for individuals with type 2 diabetes? Diabetes Technol Ther. 2013;15(6):520–9.

149. Hoffmann B, Hertel S, Boes T, Weiland D, Jockel KH. Increased cause-specific mortality associated with 2003 heatwave in Essen, Germany. J Toxicol Environ Health A. 2008;71:759–65.

150. Dematte JE, O'Mara K, Buescher J, Whitney CG, Forsythe S, McNamee T, et al. Near-fatal heat stroke during the 1995 heat wave in Chicago. Ann Intern Med. 1998;129(3):173–81.

151. American Academy of Pediatrics Committee on Environmental Health. American Academy of Pediatrics Committee on Environmental Health. In: Etzel RA, editor. Pediatric environmental health. 2nd ed. Elk Grove Village: American Academy of Pediatrics; 2003.

152. Falk B. Effects of thermal stress during rest and exercise in the paediatric population. Sports Med. 1998;25(4):221–40.

153. Basu R, Ostro BD. A multicounty analysis identifying the populations vulnerable to mortality associated with high ambient temperature in California. Am J Epidemiol. 2008;168(6):632–7.

154. O'Neill MS, Hajat S, Zanobetti A, Ramirez-Aguilar M, Schwartz J. Impact of control for air pollution and respiratory epidemics on the estimated associations of temperature and daily mortality. Int J Biometeorol. 2005;50(2):121–9.

155. Shea KM, American Academy of Pediatrics Committee on Environmental Health. Global climate change and children's health. Pediatrics. 2007;120(5):e1359–67.

156. Diaz J, Linares C, Garcia-Herrera R, Lopez C, Trigo R. Impact of temperature and air pollution on the mortality of children in Madrid. J Occup Environ Med. 2004;46(8):768–74.

157. Hashizume M, Wagatsuma Y, Hayashi T, Saha SK, Streatfield K, Yunus M. The effect of temperature on mortality in rural Bangladesh–a population-based time-series study. Int J Epidemiol. 2009;38(6):1689–97.

158. Bartlett S. Climate change and urban children: impacts and implications for adaptation in low- and middle-income countries. Environ Urbanization. 2008;20(2):501–19.

159. Inbar O, Bar-Or O, Dotan R, Gutin B. Conditioning versus exercise in heat as methods for acclimatizing 8- to 10-yr-old boys to dry heat. J Appl Physiol Respir Environ Exerc Physiol. 1981;50(2):406–11.

160. Drinkwater BL, Kupprat IC, Denton JE, Crist JL, Horvath SM. Response of prepubertal girls and college women to work in the heat. J Appl Physiol Respir Environ Exerc Physiol. 1977;43(6):1046–53.

161. Haymes EM, McCormick RJ, Buskirk ER. Heat tolerance of exercising lean and obese prepubertal boys. J Appl Physiol. 1975;39(3):457–61.

162. Leppaluoto J. Human thermoregulation in sauna. Ann Clin Res. 1988;20(4):2403.

163. Wagner JA, Robinson S, Tzankoff SP, Marino RP. Heat tolerance and acclimatization to work in the heat in relation to age. J Appl Physiol. 1972;33(5):616–22.

164. Falk B, Bar-Or O, Calvert R, MacDougall JD. Sweat gland response to exercise in the heat among pre-, mid-, and late-pubertal boys. Med Sci Sports Exerc. 1992;24(3):313–9.

165. Falk B, Bar-Or O, MacDougall JD. Thermoregulatory responses of pre-, mid-, and late-pubertal boys to exercise in dry heat. Med Sci Sports Exerc. 1992;24(6):688–94.

166. Falk B, Bar-Or O, MacDougall JD, Goldsmith CH, McGillis L. Longitudinal analysis of the sweating response of pre-, mid-, and late-pubertal boys during exercise in the heat. Am J Hum Biol. 1992;4(4):527–35.

167. Bar-Or O. Climate and the exercising child – a review. Int J Sports Med. 1980;1:53–65.

168. O'Neill MS, Zanobetti A, Schwartz J. Modifiers of the temperature and mortality association in seven US cities. Am J Epidemiol. 2003;157(12):1074–82.

169. Schwartz J. Who is sensitive to extremes of temperature?: A case-only analysis. Epidemiology. 2005;16(1):67–72.

170. Schuman SH. Patterns of urban heat-wave deaths and implications for prevention: data from New York and St. Louis during July, 1966. Environ Res. 1972;5(1):59–75.

171. Medina-Ramon M, Zanobetti A, Cavanagh DP, Schwartz J. Extreme temperatures and mortality: assessing effect modification by personal characteristics and specific cause of death in a multi-city case-only analysis. Environ Health Perspect. 2006;114(9):1331–6.

172. Alter DA, Iron K, Austin PC, Naylor CD. Influence of education and income on atherogenic risk factor profiles among patients hospitalized with acute myocardial infarction. Can J Cardiol. 2004;20(12):1219–28.

173. Ward H, Tarasuk V, Mendelson R. Socioeconomic patterns of obesity in Canada: modeling the role of health behaviour. Appl Physiol Nutr Metab. 2007;32(2):206–16.

174. Oliver LN, Hayes MV. Neighbourhood socio-economic status and the prevalence of overweight Canadian children and youth. Can J Public Health. 2005;96(6):415–20.

175. Hall KD, Stephen AM, Reeder BA, Muhajarine N, Lasiuk G. Diet, obesity and education in three age groups of Saskatchewan women. Can J Diet Pract Res. 2003;64(4):181–8.

176. Willms JD, Tremblay MS, Katzmarzyk PT. Geographic and demographic variation in the prevalence of overweight Canadian children. Obes Res. 2003;11(5):668–73.

177. Green C, Hoppa RD, Young TK, Blanchard JF. Geographic analysis of diabetes prevalence in an urban area. Soc Sci Med. 2003;57(3):551–60.

178. Tanuseputro P, Manuel DG, Leung M, Nguyen K, Johansen H. Risk factors for cardiovascular disease in Canada. Can J Cardiol. 2003;19(11):1249–59.

179. Butler GP, Orpana HM, Wiens AJ. By your own two feet: factors associated with active transportation in Canada. Can J Public Health. 2007;98(4):259–64.

180. Mo F, Turner M, Krewski D, Mo FD. Physical inactivity and socioeconomic status in Canadian adolescents. Int J Adolesc Med Health. 2005;17(1):49–56.

181. Choiniere R, Lafontaine P, Edwards AC. Distribution of cardiovascular disease risk factors by socioeconomic status among Canadian adults. CMAJ. 2000;162(9 Suppl):S13–24.

182. Hemingway H, Shipley M, Macfarlane P, Marmot M. Impact of socioeconomic status on coronary mortality in people with symptoms, electrocardiographic abnormalities, both or neither: the original Whitehall study 25 year follow up. J Epidemiol Community Health. 2000;54(7):510–6.

183. Mardby AC, Akerlind I, Jorgensen T. Beliefs about medicines and self-reported adherence among pharmacy clients. Patient Educ Couns. 2007;69(1–3):158–64.

184. Kulkarni SP, Alexander KP, Lytle B, Heiss G, Peterson ED. Long-term adherence with cardiovascular drug regimens. Am Heart J. 2006;151(1):185–91.

185. Klepeis NE, Nelson WC, Ott WR, Robinson JP, Tsang AM, Switzer P, et al. The National Human Activity Pattern Survey (NHAPS): a resource for assessing exposure to environmental pollutants. J Expo Anal Environ Epidemiol. 2001;11(3):231–52.

186. Leech JA, Nelson WC, Burnett RT, Aaron S, Raizenne ME. It's about time: a comparison of Canadian and American time – activity patterns. J Expo Anal Environ Epidemiol. 2002;12:427–32.

187. Bouchama A, Dehbi M, Mohamed G, Matthies F, Shoukri M, Menne B. Prognostic factors in heat wave related deaths: a meta-analysis. Arch Intern Med. 2007;167(20):2170–6.

188. Foroni M, Salvioli G, Rielli R, Goldoni CA, Orlandi G, Zauli Sajani S, et al. A retrospective study on heat-related mortality in an elderly population during the 2003 heat wave in Modena, Italy: the Argento Project. J Gerontol A Biol Sci Med Sci. 2007;62(6):647–51.
189. Hajat S, Kovats RS, Lachowycz K. Heat-related and cold-related deaths in England and Wales: who is at risk? Occup Environ Med. 2007;64(2):93–100.
190. Kramarow EA. The elderly who live alone in the United States: historical perspectives on household change. Demography. 1995;32(3):335–52.
191. Gronlund CJ. Racial and socioeconomic disparities in heat-related health effects and their mechanisms: a review. Curr Epidemiol Rep. 2014;1(3):165–73.
192. Kravchenko J, Abernethy AP, Fawzy M, Lyerly HK. Minimization of heatwave morbidity and mortality. Am J Prev Med. 2013;44(3):274–82.
193. Madrigano J, Mittleman MA, Baccarelli A, Goldberg R, Melly S, von Klot S, Schwartz J. Temperature, myocardial infarction, and mortality: effect modification by individual- and area-level characteristics. Epidemiology. 2013;24(3):439–46.
194. Pillai SK, Noe RS, Murphy MW, Vaidyanathan A, Young R, Kieszak S, et al. Heat illness: predictors of hospital admissions among emergency department visits—Georgia, 2002–2008. J Community Health. 2014;39(1):90–8.
195. McMichael AJ, Wilkinson P, Kovats RS, Pattenden S, Hajat S, Armstrong B, et al. International study of temperature, heat and urban mortality: the "ISOTHURM" project. Int J Epidemiol. 2008;37:1121–31.
196. Gabriel KM, Endlicher WR. Urban and rural mortality rates during heat waves in Berlin and Brandenburg, Germany. Environ Pollut. 2011;159(8–9):204450.
197. Hondula DM, Davis RE, Leisten MJ, Saha MV, Veazey LM, Wegner CR. Fine-scale spatial variability of heat-related mortality in Philadelphia County, USA, from 1983 to 2008: a case-series analysis. Environ Health. 2012;11:16.
198. Laaidi K, Zeghnoun A, Dousset B, Bretin P, Vandentorren S, Giraudet E, Beaudeau P. The impact of heat islands on mortality in Paris during the August 2003 heat wave. Environ Health Perspect. 2012;120(2):254–9.
199. Basu R, Samet JM. Relation between elevated ambient temperature and mortality: a review of the epidemiologic evidence. Epidemiol Rev. 2002;24(2):190–202.
200. Kolokotroni M, Giannitsaris I, Watkins R. The effect of the London urban heat island on building summer cooling demand and night ventilation strategies. Sol Energy. 2006;80(4):383–92.
201. Smargiassi A, Fournier M, Griot C, Baudouin Y, Kosatsky T. Prediction of the indoor temperatures of an urban area with an in-time regression mapping approach. J Expo Sci Environ Epidemiol. 2008;18(3):282–8.
202. Stone B Jr. Urban sprawl and air quality in large US cities. J Environ Manag. 2008;86(4):688–98.
203. Stone B, Hess JJ, Frumkin H. Urban form and extreme heat events: are sprawling cities more vulnerable to climate change than compact cities? Environ Health Perspect. 2010;118(10):1425–8.
204. Harlan SL, Brazel AJ, Prashad L, Stefanov WL, Larsen L. Neighborhood microclimates and vulnerability to heat stress. Soc Sci Med. 2006;63:2847–63.
205. Wolf T, Chuang WC, McGregor G. On the science-policy bridge: do spatial heat vulnerability assessment studies influence policy? Int J Res Public Health. 2015;12:13321–49.
206. Gachon P, Bussières L, Gosselin P, Raphoz M, Bustinza R, Martin P, et al. Guide to identifying alert thresholds for heat waves in Canada based on evidence. Co-edited by Université du Québec à Montréal, Environment and Climate Change Canada, Institut National de Santé Publique du Québec, and Health Canada, Montréal, Québec, Canada; 2016.
207. Bao J, Li X, Yu C. The construction and validation of the heat vulnerability index, a review. Int J Environ Res Public Health. 2015;12(7):7220–34.
208. Kuras ER, Richardson MB, Calkins MM, Ebi KL, Hess JJ, Kintziger KW, et al. Opportunities and challenges for personal heat exposure research. Environ Health Perspect. 2017;125(8):085001.

209. Quinn A, Tamerius JD, Perzanowski M, Jacobson JS, Goldstein I, Acosta L, Shaman J. Predicting indoor heat exposure risk during extreme heat events. Sci Total Environ. 2014;490:686–93.
210. McLoed RS, Hopfe CJ, Kwan A. An investigation into future performance and overheating risks in Passivhaus dwellings. Build Environ. 2013;70:189–209.
211. Oikonomou E, Davies M, Mavrogianni A, Biddulph P, Wilkinson P, Kolokotroni M. Modelling the relative importance of the urban heat island and the thermal quality of dwellings for over-heating in London. Build Environ. 2012;57:223–38.
212. Vellei M, Ramallo-González AP, Coley D, Lee J, Gabe-Thomas E, Lovett T, Natarajan S. Overheating in vulnerable and non-vulnerable households. Build Res Inf. 2017;45(1–2):102–18.
213. Pogacar T, Znidarsic Z, Kajfez Bogataj L, Flouris AD, Poulianiti K, Crepinsek Z. Heat Waves occurrence and outdoor workers' self-assessment of heat stress in Slovenia and Greece. Int J Environ Res Public Health. 2019;16(4) https://doi.org/10.3390/ijerph16040597.
214. Piil JF, Lundbye-Jensen J, Christiansen L, Ioannou L, Tsoutsoubi L, Dallas CN, et al. High prevalence of hypohydration in occupations with heat stress-perspectives for performance in combined cognitive and motor tasks. PLoS One. 2018;13(10):e0205321.
215. Leon LR, Bouchama A. Heat stroke. Compr Physiol. 2015;5(2):611–47.
216. Arbury S, Jacklitsch B, Farquah O, Hodgson M, Lamson G, Martin H, Profitt A, Office of Occupational Health Nursing, Occupational Safety and Health Administration (OSHA). Heat illness and death among workers – United States, 2012–2013. MMWR Morb Mortal Wkly Rep. 2014;63(31):661–5.
217. Gubernot DM, Anderson GB, Hunting KL. Characterizing occupational heat-related mortality in the United States, 2000–2010: an analysis using the Census of Fatal Occupational Injuries database. Am J Ind Med. 2015;58(2):203–11.
218. Kjellstrom T, Lemke B, Otto M, Hyatt O, Briggs D, Freyberg C. Threats to occupational health, labor productivity and the economy from increasing heat during climate change: an emerging global health risk and a challenge to sustainable development and social equity. Mapua: Health and Environment International Trust; 2014.
219. Kjellstrom T, Lemke B, Otto M, Hyatt OKD. Occupational heat stress: contribution to WHO project on "Global assessment of the health impacts of climate change", which started in 2009. Mapua: Health and Environment International Trust; 2014.
220. American Conference of Governmental Industrial Hygienists. Heat stress and strain: TLV physical agents documentation. Cincinnati; 2007. https://doi.org/10.1175/BAMS-85-8-1067.
221. ISO. Ergonomics of the thermal environment – analytical determination and interpretation of heat stress using calculation of the predicted heat strain (ISO 7933:2004). London: The British Standards Institution; 2004.
222. World Health Organisation. Health factors involved in working under conditions of heat stress. Technical report 412. WHO Scientific Group on Health Factors Involved in Working under Conditions of Heat Stress. Geneva, Switzerland; 1969. https://doi.org/10.1175/BAMS-85-8-1067.
223. World Meteorological Organization, World Health Organization. Heatwaves and health: guidance on warning-system development. Geneva, Switzerland; 2015. https://doi.org/10.1175/BAMS-85-8-1067.
224. Sawka MN, Burke LM, Eichner ER, Maughan RJ, Montain SJ, Stachenfeld NS. American College of Sports Medicine position stand. Exercise and fluid replacement. Med Sci Sports Exerc. 2007;39(2):377–90.
225. World Health Organization. International expert consultation on chronic kidney disease of unknown etiology. Colombo, Sri Lanka; 2016. https://doi.org/10.1175/BAMS-85-8-1067.
226. Menon M, Resnick MI. Urinary lithiasis: etiology, diagnosis, and medical management. In: Walsh PC, Retik AB, Vaughan EDJ, Wein AJ, eds. Campbell's urology. 8th ed. Philadelphia: WB Saunders; 2002:3229–3234.

227. Acute Kidney Injury Work Group. Kidney Disease: Improving Global Outcomes (KDIGO). KDIGO Clinical Practice Guideline for Acute Kidney Injury. Kidney Inter. 2012;2(Suppl):1–138.
228. Halonen JI, Zanobetti A, Sparrow D, Vokonas PS, Schwartz J. Outdoor temperature is associated with serum HDL and LDL. Environ Res. 2011;111(2):281–7.
229. Vangelova K, Deyanov C, Ivanova M. Dyslipidemia in industrial workers in hot environments. Cent Eur J Public Health. 2006;14(1):15–7.
230. de Freitas CR, Grigorieva EA. A comprehensive catalogue and classification of human thermal climate indices. Int J Biometeorol. 2015;59(1):109–20.
231. Budd GM. Wet-bulb globe temperature (WBGT)–its history and its limitations. J Sci Med Sport. 2008;11(1):20–32.
232. d'Ambrosio Alfano FR, Palella BI, Riccio G. Thermal environment assessment reliability using temperature-humidity indices. Ind Health. 2011;49(1):95–106.
233. D'Ambrosio Alfano FR, Palella BI, Riccio G. On the problems related to natural wet bulb temperature indirect evaluation for the assessment of hot thermal environments by means of WBGT. Ann Occup Hyg. 2012;56(9):1063–79.
234. Meade RD, Poirier MP, Flouris AD, Hardcastle SG, Kenny GP. Do the threshold limit values for work in hot conditions adequately protect workers? Med Sci Sports Exerc. 2016;48(6):1187–96.
235. Ramsey JD, Chai CP. Inherent variability in heat-stress decision rules. Ergonomics. 1983;26(5):495–504.
236. Lamarche DT, Meade RD, D'Souza AW, Flouris AD, Hardcastle SG, Sigal RJ, et al. The recommended Threshold Limit Values for heat exposure fail to maintain body core temperature within safe limits in older working adults. J Occup Environ Hyg. 2017;14(9):703–11.
237. Cook EL. Epidemiological approach to heat trauma. Mil Med. 1955;116(5):317–22.
238. Schickele E. Environment and fatal heat stroke; an analysis of 157 cases occurring in the Army in the U.S. during World War II. Mil Surg. 1947;100(3):235–56.
239. Dervis S, Coombs GB, Chaseling GK, Filingeri D, Smoljanic J, Jay O. A comparison of thermoregulatory responses to exercise between mass-matched groups with large differences in body fat. J Appl Physiol (1985). 2016;120(6):615–23.
240. Quiller G, Krenz J, Ebi K, Hess JJ, Fenske RA, Sampson PD, et al. Heat exposure and productivity in orchards: implications for climate change research. Arch Environ Occup Health. 2017;72(6):313–6.
241. Maloney SK, Forbes CF. What effect will a few degrees of climate change have on human heat balance? Implications for human activity. Int J Biometeorol. 2011;55(2):147–60.
242. Nybo L, Kjellstrom T, Bogataj LK, Flouris AD. Global heating: attention is not enough; we need acute and appropriate actions. Temperature (Austin). 2017;4(3):199–201.
243. Intergovernmental Panel on Climate Change. Human health: impacts, adaptation, and co-benefits. In: climate change 2014 – impacts, adaptation and vulnerability: Part A: global and sectoral aspects: working group II contribution to the IPCC Fifth Assessment Report. Cambridge: Cambridge University Press; 2014. p. 709–754. doi:https://doi.org/10.1017/CBO9781107415379.016. Accessed 30 Apr 2019.
244. Baccini M, Biggeri A, Accetta G, Kosatsky T, Katsouyanni K, Analitis A, et al. Heat effects on mortality in 15 European cities. Epidemiology. 2008;19(5):711–9.
245. Kovats RS, Hajat S. Heat stress and public health: a critical review. Annu Rev Public Health. 2008;29:41–55.
246. Wolf T, Martinez GS, Cheong HK, Williams E, Menne B. Protecting health from climate change in the WHO European Region. Int J Environ Res Public Health. 2014;11(6):6265–80.
247. Lowe D, Ebi KL, Forsberg B. Heatwave early warning systems and adaptation advice to reduce human health consequences of heatwaves. Int J Environ Res Public Health. 2011;8(12):4623–48.
248. Statistics BoL. The economics daily, work injuries in the heat in 2015. 2015.; https://www.bls.gov/opub/ted/2017/work-injuries-in-the-heat-in-2015.htm.

249. Mirabelli MC, Richardson DB. Heat-related fatalities in North Carolina. Am J Public Health. 2005;95(4):635–7.
250. Xiang J, Hansen A, Pisaniello D, Bi P. Extreme heat and occupational heat illnesses in South Australia, 2001–2010. Occup Environ Med. 2015;72(8):580–6.
251. Axelson O. Influence of heat exposure on productivity. Work Environ Health. 1974;11(2):94–9.
252. Fogleman M, Fakhrzadeh L, Bernard TE. The relationship between outdoor thermal conditions and acute injury in an aluminum smelter. Int J Ind Ergonom. 2005;35(1):47–55.
253. Kjellstrom T, Kovats RS, Lloyd SJ, Holt T, Tol RS. The direct impact of climate change on regional labor productivity. Arch Environ Occup Health. 2009;64(4):217–27.
254. Zander KK, Botzen WJW, Oppermann E, Kjellstrom T, Garnett ST. Heat stress causes substantial labour productivity loss in Australia. Nat Clim Chang. 2015;5(7):647–51.
255. The National Institute for Occupational Safety and Health. Occupational exposure to heat and hot environments: revised criteria 2016. Cincinnati, OH; 2016. https://doi.org/10.1175/BAMS-85-8-1067.
256. American Conference of Governmental Industrial Hygienists. TLVs and BEIs based on the documentation of the threshold limit values for chemical substances and physical agents & biological exposure indices. Cincinnati, OH; 2017. https://doi.org/10.1175/BAMS-85-8-1067.
257. Poirier MP, Meade RD, McGinn R, Friesen BJ, Hardcastle SG, Flouris AD, Kenny GP. The influence of arc-flash and fire-resistant clothing on thermoregulation during exercise in the heat. J Occup Environ Hyg. 2015;12(9):654–67.
258. Notley SR, Flouris AD, Kenny GP. On the use of wearable physiological monitors to assess heat strain during occupational heat stress. Appl Physiol Nutr Metab. 2018;43(9):869–81.
259. Buller MJ, Welles AP, Friedl KE. Wearable physiological monitoring for human thermal-work strain optimization. J Appl Physiol (1985). 2018;124(2):432–41.

Index

© Springer Nature Switzerland AG 2020
W. M. Adams, J. F. Jardine (eds.), *Exertional Heat Illness*,
https://doi.org/10.1007/978-3-030-27805-2